KEY THEMES IN HEALTH AND SOCIAL CARE

Key Themes in Health and Social Care is a learning resource for students in health and social care. It provides an overview of foundational issues and core themes in the field and introduces key areas of debate, moving from an introductory level to in-depth discussion as the book progresses. Divided into three parts:

- Part 1 sets the scene, addressing introductory psychology and sociology, social policy, equality and diversity, skills for practice, and working with people.
- Part 2 considers key themes such as the contribution of philosophy and politics, criminal justice, management of services, the relationship between place and well-being, research in health and social care, theories of counselling and housing and the built environment.
- Part 3 looks at discrete areas of practice such as mental health, substance abuse, protection work, health promotion, disability studies, working with men, child welfare and public responsibility.

Each chapter begins with an outline of the content and learning outcomes and includes reflective exercises to allow students to reflect on what they have read, review their learning and consolidate their understanding. Time-pressed readers wanting to 'dip into' the book for relevant areas can do so but, read from cover to cover, the book provides a comprehensive introduction to the key areas of contemporary health and social care practice. It will be particularly helpful for students undertaking health and social care undergraduate and foundation degrees.

Adam Barnard is a Senior Lecturer at Nottingham Trent University, UK.

We can all expect health and social care to gain greater importance in our lives as the times we live in become less certain and more complex. Those working in these fields can expect greater challenges and demands to be placed on them. They will need many forms of help to enhance their learning and develop their critical capacity to convert that into positive practice. This will come from many sources: fellow learners, teachers, experienced practitioners and service users. But I think there will also be a place for books like this. It will be one of the friends that offers learners more than a little help to get by, supporting them to move from learning to doing, challenging unhelpful boundaries and questionable assumptions, and equipping them to develop their own experiential wisdom.

Professor Peter Beresford, *Brunel University, UK*

This book provides a comprehensive picture of different areas of health and social care policy and intervention. Clear and well researched, with many suggestions for further reading, it will be useful to students and practitioners across a range of health and social care professions. I thoroughly recommend this publication because it provides an up to date exploration of dynamic complexities relevant to fast changing public sector services.

Professor Patricia Higham, *University of Northampton* and *Nottingham Trent University, UK*; and *independent consultant*

KEY THEMES IN HEALTH AND SOCIAL CARE

A COMPANION TO LEARNING

Edited by Adam Barnard

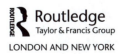

LONDON AND NEW YORK

First published 2011
by Routledge
2 Park Square, Milton Park, Abingdon, Oxon OX14 4RN

Simultaneously published in the USA and Canada
by Routledge
270 Madison Avenue, New York, NY 10016

Routledge is an imprint of the Taylor & Francis Group, an informa business
© 2011 Adam Barnard; individual chapters, the contributors.

The right of Adam Barnard to be identified as editor of this work has been asserted by him in accordance with sections 77 and 78 of the Copyright, Designs and Patents Act 1988.

Typeset in Sabon by GreenGate Publishing Services, Tonbridge, Kent
Printed and bound in Great Britain by TJ International Ltd, Padstow, Cornwall

British Library Cataloguing in Publication Data
A catalogue record for this book is available from the British Library
Library of Congress Cataloging-in-Publication Data
Key themes in health and social care : a companion to learning / [edited by] Adam Barnard.
p. ; cm.
Includes bibliographical references and index.
1. Medical care. 2. Medical policy. 3. Social service. I. Barnard, Adam.
[DNLM: 1. Delivery of Health Care. 2. Social Work. W 84.1 K44 2010]
RA393.K49 2010
362.1--dc22   2010006491

ISBN: 978-0-415-47637-9 (hbk)
ISBN: 978-0-415-47638-6 (pbk)
ISBN: 978-0-203-84585-1 (ebk)

For Ngaio, Edie, Kirsty, Bill and Mairi

CONTENTS

FIGURES AND TABLES

FIGURES

TABLES

NOTES ON CONTRIBUTORS

ADAM BARNARD (Dr) is a senior lecturer in Human Services at Nottingham Trent University. His latest work is on the *Value Base of Social Work and Social Care* published by Open University Press. He has worked in higher education for fifteen years and has published articles from findings from his research, in political and social theory. His research and teaching interests are in the value base of health and social care, social and political theory, moral and political philosophy, ethics and values in health and social care. He is programme leader for Professional Doctorates in Social Practice.

KIRSTY BEART teaches on the areas of philosophy of care and practicalities of practice in health and social care. This involves consideration of philosophical foundations of care and their application into a practice arena. She has specialist knowledge in health care, particularly mental health. This research and practice experience resulted in the publication of a text, *Fundamental aspects of care of a person with dementia* published by Quay Books (2007).

JILL BERRISFORD is a senior lecturer on the BA (Hons) Social Work degree at Nottingham Trent University. She has worked as a social worker for over twenty years. She works at Nottingham Trent University for half of the week and in the other half is employed as a Team Manager in Learning and Development with Nottinghamshire County Council. In this role she commissions and manages postgraduate teaching for social workers and other professionals. Her teaching interests focus primarily on working with children and families, with a particular expertise in fostering and adoption. She is keen to encourage students to critically analyse and reflect on their practice. The concepts of well-being and emotional intelligence are also of interest to her.

HELEN BURROWS is a senior lecturer in Social Work. Her research interests are anti-oppressive practice in service provision and working conditions for lesbian, gay and bisexual (LGB) service users and staff in social care, and service provision for unaccompanied asylum seeking children.

ADRIAN M. CASTELL is principal lecturer in the Division of Information Management and Systems at Nottingham Business School. He is the programme director for the Management Masters Programme in the Business School and has led MBA and MSc Management awards for over a decade. His research, scholarly and professional interests lie in critical management development education, participation in information systems design and methodologies for information systems development.

BARBARA COULSON is programme leader for the BA (Hons) Social Work, full-time route. Barbara teaches sociology, methods and models of social work, and disability. In addition, she supervises dissertations and is Learning Adviser to social work students and coordinates the Learning Adviser group. Her research areas are working with adults including disability and learning disability, domestic violence and adult abuse, and gender and sexuality.

MATTHEW GOUGH is a senior lecturer in Social Work. Matthew is module leader for key themes in social work, statutory interventions in social work, and working with adults, and a contributing teacher on reflective practice. He is a member of the Practice Assurance Committee, a Learning Advisor, a third year tutor and a champion for service user involvement in the programme. He has a MSW which focused upon user involvement in palliative care services. He has worked extensively in the voluntary sector and local authority settings. His study interests include the voluntary sector, service user involvement, Fair Access to Care Services, suicide, mental health and the Mental Capacity Act. He has published work on the need for informed consent in mental health treatments.

BRIDGET HALLAM joined Nottingham Trent University nine years ago, from a professional background in nursing and health visiting, specialising for several years in child protection. She is programme leader for the BA (Hons) Health and Care degree and also acting second year tutor. Bridget teaches a range of subjects across the programme including human growth and development, health and social care policy and practice, child and adult protection, and health promotion. Her research interests include multi-agency working in health and social care, including evaluation of local Sure Start programmes, and work and health.

MARTYN HARLING (Dr) is a senior lecturer in Health and Social Care. He has many years of experience of working within the substance misuse field and is currently undertaking research looking at the attitudes of health and social care students toward illicit substance use. He has previous experience of conducting research within the substance misuse field, completing studies with intravenous and recreational users of illicit drugs. He has a particular interest in projects involving the use of grounded theory in health and social care settings.

PHILIP HODGSON (Dr) is a senior lecturer in Criminology at Nottingham Trent University and Director of the Crime Research Unit. He has over twenty years experience of working within the criminal justice system across a range of agencies and he is currently a member of the Nottinghamshire Police Authority.

KRISTAN HOPKINS-BURKE teaches research methods and study skills across a range of degree programmes within the School of Social Sciences at Nottingham Trent University. Her activities and research interests range widely from running peer observation programmes to developing online survey tools, teaching and learning issues, and mentoring for academics.

ROGER HOPKINS-BURKE is subject leader for the Criminology Group in the Division of Criminology, Public Health and Policy Studies in the School of Social Sciences. Roger's research, scholarly and professional interests include: criminological theory; young people, crime and justice; generic (and state sponsored) policing and social control; and crime prevention, community safety and regeneration. He is widely published and is the author of *Zero Tolerance Policing* (Perpetuity Press, 1998), *An Introduction to Criminological Theory* (Willan Publishing, 2001; third edition, 2009), *Hard Cop/Soft Cop* (Willan Publishing, 2004) and *Young People, Crime and Justice* (Willan Publishing, 2008). Roger is currently researching future books on criminal justice theory and crime and the postmodern condition.

JAMES HUNTER is a senior lecturer in the Division of Criminology, Public Health and Policy Studies. He teaches on a range of courses addressing policy studies, places, neighbourhood and regeneration. His research is focused on policy issues and their spatial elements and he coordinates the Research Excellence Framework activity for the School of Social Sciences.

ANN MCCARTHY is a senior lecturer within the School of Social Sciences, specialising in housing regeneration, public health and professional skill development. She is a Chartered Environmental Health Practitioner and a qualified housing practitioner, working in local authorities within both environmental health and housing, before becoming involved in lecturing in 1988. She led the Environmental Health Course at Nottingham Trent University between 1990 and 2000, which is where her teaching interest in experiential learning and reflective practice began to develop. She currently manages the placement and work experience aspects of the Public Health group and teaches sustainability, community and policy, and practice on a Masters programme in Public Health. She is Vice-Chair on the board of management of a housing association within the East Midlands region and is active within the Greater Nottingham Health and Environment Partnership.

VICKY PALMER worked variously as a Probation Officer, Youth Justice Social Worker and Youth Offending Team Officer, initially in Leicestershire and then in Nottinghamshire. Her experience in the field of criminal justice spans some twenty years, during which time she specialised in working with serious sex offenders, facilitating group work with high-risk offenders and training colleagues in the area of criminal law. In her capacity as accredited Practice Teacher, Vicky supervised a number of final placement Social Work students, many of whom gained subsequent employment in Youth Offending Teams. She joined Nottingham Trent University in October 2005. She is interested in youth and criminal justice, criminal law, criminology and media.

MICHELE RAITHBY is principal lecturer in Social Work at Swansea University and is currently completing her PhD on Strangers in the House: Older persons' experiences of Home Care Services. Her research and teaching interests are in health and care work with older people and evidence based practice.

CHRIS RING is senior lecturer in Social Work at Nottingham Trent University. On qualifying as a mature student in 1994, he worked in research, practice and quality assurance roles, principally in mental health, and has published work in this area.

He holds a MSc in Social Work from London South Bank University, has substantial experience of leading research projects, and has taught research practice in NHS and university settings. He has particular interests in systems approaches, social inclusion, and the impact of large-scale changes on health and social care provision. He currently leads a research project in Yorkshire examining the impact of service reconfiguration upon people with mental health problems.

CHRIS TOWERS (Dr) is a senior lecturer in social policy and is currently involved in teaching social policy within the School of Social Sciences. He has special interests in social policy for health and social care students and practioners.

SIÂN TRAFFORD has a long history of offering student support for academic writing in the School of Social Sciences. Her research interests are on learning styles and academic writing.

JO WARD is the programme leader and teaches on the PG Dip/BA Hons Child Care Practice (Specialist Award in Child Care Practice) which is a post-qualifying professional award for social workers and other professionals in the children's workforce. Her interests are in the areas of children in the care system; fostering and adoption; and therapeutic interventions to improve the lives of looked after children and their carers. She is also interested in all aspects of social policy affecting children.

GRAHAM WHITEHEAD (MSc MBACP Accred.) is a senior lecturer in Counselling and Human Services who joined the team in 2006. His published work to date explores the challenges facing counselling in a multicultural society. His teaching and research interests include transcultural counselling and psychotherapy, counselling in organizations, counselling sexual minorities and practitioner development. His professional background includes management and clinical experience in further and higher education since 1990. He has been a BACP Accredited Counsellor since 1993 and has extensive experience of supervision in both the private and public sector. Graham has research interests in health, social care and counselling, transcultural approaches to counselling and psychotherapy, and the relevance and efficacy of therapeutic intervention in outplacement work.

All members of staff are working at Nottingham Trent University unless indicated.

ACKNOWLEDGEMENTS

Great thanks to all the contributors who have made this work possible. It is testament to their commitment, insight and humanity that this work has been produced. Thanks also to all the students on the BA (Hons) Health and Social Care degree at Nottingham Trent University that have made this a productive and enjoyable journey. Grace McInnes, Khanam Virjee and the staff at Routledge deserve recognition for making this an adventure full of expertise and advice. Thanks also to Nottingham Trent University for all the support and resources offered to complete this work.

Acknowledgement is given to Margaret Whitehead, Triangle Consulting/Mental Health Providers Forum, and Ann Cunliffe for granting permission to reuse their images and figures.

INTRODUCTION TO KEY THEMES IN HEALTH AND SOCIAL CARE

ADAM BARNARD

The aim of this book is to provide the reader with an introduction to the key themes and debates in health and social care. This can never be exhaustive but is intended to provide a flavour of or orientation to areas that are the lifeblood of study and work in health and social care. The themes discussed in this volume will be of interest to a range of students, practitioners and academics in what might be termed the 'helping professions' or perhaps, more broadly, professionals 'working with people'. This volume arose from research and teaching expertise and interest in these areas from undergraduate and postgraduate programmes at Nottingham Trent University. Contributors bring a wealth and depth of knowledge, skills and expertise from across health and social care. It is hoped that the reader finds the material of use in stimulating ideas, introducing key themes in knowledge and practice, and contributing to the varied and fascinating world of working with people in a supportive way.

As the volume serves as an introduction to key themes it is divided into three parts each building, sequentially, on the previous discussion although the reader is invited to delve into those areas of particular relevance to their interests. The book is designed for those studying for a qualification in health and social care particularly on an undergraduate programme. The book adopts a 'thematic' focus by introducing and exploring themes that are relevant to studying and work within health and social care. **Part 1** is concerned with some of the essentials for an introduction to key themes in health and social care. **Part 2** develops in depth and detail by examining contextual, health, philosophical, political and research questions in health and social care. The different arenas of allied disciplines of health and care are also introduced and examined. Criminal justice, counselling, 'place' and housing are the key focus. **Part 3** anticipates the reader has knowledge of the terrain of health and social care, its allied disciplines and the key themes for this area of work and study. As such, this part introduces students to more discrete areas of health and social care and various services, users or client groups that might use health and social care services. Issues of globalization, management and leadership, evidence based practice, mental health, the practice of counselling, substance misuse, children, service users and criminal justice are the themes developed.

Contained within each chapter are varied 'moments of reflection'. These are useful tools to enable you to pause for thought, perform an activity, and reflect upon the material you have just read. The reflective moments encourage you to engage with material, to think it through critically, and to apply your understanding to health and social care situations. They contribute to this text being a companion to learning so you can develop your critical skills in examining ideas in context and exploring how useful they are.

PART 1

The volume opens by introducing students to the necessary skills to be able to study for a qualification in health and social care. *Siân Trafford* in **Skills for study and practice** introduces writing skills to provide guidance on grammar and punctuation, a glossary of confusing words, and exercises on how to write academically. The section on reading effectively explores reading and notetaking while researching and reviewing literature, and includes summarising, paraphrasing, and citation and referencing using (Harvard) the easy way. Writing a successful essay is discussed and includes: using your essay title, learning outcomes and assignment criteria to create an essay plan; essay structure and signposting; constructing a written argument using your evidence; and how to proofread effectively. Finally, learning from your experience – reflection discusses how to use a portfolio to demonstrate ability to reflect and learn from experience.

Chapter 2 introduces the central theme of **Working with people** – interpersonal communication and people skills in a professional context. *Kirsty Beart, Graham Whitehead* and *Adam Barnard* explore the complexities of working with people in health and social care environments. Interpersonal skills are of vital importance for anyone who needs to take a serious interest in dealing effectively with the other people in their professional or personal lives and effective communication is an essential quality for working with people. Theories and concepts of interpersonal behaviour are highlighted and consideration is given of relevance to health and social care professional roles. Emphasis is given to communication theory and practice, listening skills, assertiveness behaviour, teamwork, interviewing skills, the significance of feedback, and assessment, and of how to use these skills in an applied setting. The reader will gain a clear understanding of how people interact and deal with each other in a health and social care context. These skills are seen as transferable and relevant to study, work and social life. At the end of the chapter there are discussion points, individual, group and reflexive exercises.

Having introduced writing and studying skills, and interpersonal skills, Chapter 3 examines an introduction to the developmental psychology and sociology necessary for health and social care. **The individual in society** by *Barbara Coulson* and *Bridget Hallam* provides an understanding of how human beings grow and change over their lives and is fundamental to effective work with users of health and social care services. This chapter aims to provide an introduction to some of the physical, psychological, emotional and social changes that people experience during their lifespan and the factors that affect those changes. The discussion will be underpinned by reference to relevant traditional and more recent developmental theories. It is easy to think of human growth and development as something that only happens internally and on an individual basis but of course this is not the case. External factors, such as the society in which individuals live, the opportunities they have and the difficulties specific groups may encounter, have a massive impact on people's lives. The chapter therefore includes a brief exploration of key sociological themes and perspectives so that individual development may be set in its wider context. Again, relevant theoretical underpinning informs the discussion. The chapter begins by setting our current understanding of human growth and development in its historical, cultural and sociological context before going on to consider the relative impact of nature and nurture on the developing individual. Key aspects of growth and development are discussed with a particular emphasis on life transitions and how individuals' experiences of these are influenced by factors such as gender, ethnicity and disability. Readers are encouraged to reflect on their own lives, the developmental transitions they have made and the factors that have been significant in shaping the person they are.

Chapter 4 extends those aspects of diversity and examines the concepts of equality and key mechanisms in relation to social differences that facilitate or inhibit the promotion of equality. **Concepts of equality and diversity** by *Adam Barnard* aims to provide a theoretical introduction to the concept of equality. An understanding of the nature and defining features of equality is essential to health and social care work. The notions of equality, inequality and equal opportunity are introduced and explored to see what implications they have for health and social care. The chapter then explores mechanisms that can operate to limit the promotion of equality such as prejudice, stereotyping, discrimination and oppression. Having discussed the theoretical foundations to equality, the discussion moves to consider social differences such as class, gender, ethnicity, culture, age, sexuality and disability. The ways the mechanisms and social differences impact on each other is discussed. The legislative framework that exists to address equality and diversity is also considered.

In the final chapter of Part 1 the context of health and social care is explored in **Introduction to social policy** by *Chris Towers*. Social policies have the potential to affect the lives of the users and the providers of health and social care services and this chapter examines the many ways in which policies can touch lives. The chapter starts with an exploration of what social policy actually is and there is reference to how it relates to other disciplines. It is important to locate the subject and to understand its relevance to people through the life course. Students are also invited to consider how people's wants and needs may or may not be met through social policies. The chapter explores the historical context in which welfare organizations have developed – from the Poor Laws to the development of charities and the birth of the modern welfare state. The impact of this history is examined as are the different perspectives on welfare provision and the role of family and other providers. Current social policy issues from immigration to an ageing population and from homelessness to work and welfare are illustrated with extensive use of case studies. The chapter also features a glossary of terms to help students to become acquainted with the subject. There are also discussion points and exercises to be used in the classroom and to aid individual learning.

PART 2

Building on the first part of the book, Part 2 extends and deepens the discussion around key themes in health and social care. It is an appropriate place to have a clear statement of the emerging key themes that have been considered and that will form the basis for the rest of the book.

Siân Trafford's chapter on **Studying at a higher level in health and social care** examines how to construct written arguments at levels two and three of an undergraduate programme. The discussion takes you through the elements of constructing a good argument, how to use chains of reasoning and produce coherent and comprehensive arguments. The different levels of sophistication of arguments are discussed with central processes for producing a good piece of written work. The chapter also addresses the idea that there are competing and multiple perspectives within health and social care and that a good argument is one that can entertain and critique different perspectives on a topic.

Health and health care in Britain by *Bridget Hallam* begins with a discussion of 'health' and a discussion of different groups in society's experiences of health, and different approaches and attitudes to using health services. This chapter provides a brief introduction to ways of thinking about health, and to health services in Britain. It looks broadly at what we mean by the term 'health' before exploring health inequalities in relation to socio-economic status, ethnicity and gender. The second part of the chapter shifts the focus to look at issues relating to health care and covers the organization of the National Health Service (NHS), the issue of 'quality', and patient and public involvement in health, as three key themes shaping health services in Britain.

Key themes in health and social care by *Chris Ring* examines how social policy and practice respond to emerging health and social needs, and the outcomes experienced. The practical challenges associated with three key policy aims – providing individualized care; protecting adults and children from harm; and the promotion of well-being – are illustrated using experience in areas of particular practice, such as older people's mental health and young people with disabilities.

Focusing on the service users' experience and observed outcomes in these settings, we examine how the contributions of the different professions, and their organization and management, contribute to the quality of health and social care services. Consideration of service users and carers' perspectives on this, and other evidence of effectiveness, leads to discussion of current approaches to performance management. Finally, readers are encouraged to engage in a reflective exercise, examining the extent to which features of contemporary welfare are fit to address emerging challenges to public health and well-being.

Philosophical and political debate in health and social care by *Adam Barnard* will allow you to develop analytical skills that will enable an examination of political and philosophical issues which impact upon health and social care by introducing key philosophical, political and ethical theories. The moral concepts of rights, responsibility, freedom, authority and power are introduced. The structure of this chapter starts with a consideration of philosophy and the purpose of philosophical inquiry for health and social care. Some of the central concepts of philosophy and political philosophical schools are examined. This is not intended to be exhaustive but represents key political philosophies that have informed and continue to inform the practice of health and social care. The discussion then considers key political philosophies and ethical theories. The chapter concludes by suggesting health and social care are centrally involved with philosophy, politics and ethics.

Research in health and social care by *Kristan Hopkins-Burke* begins with the broad question of 'what is research?' and distinguishes between producers and consumers of research. In particular, it highlights the need for students and practitioners to be *critical* consumers of research. The reader is introduced to the traditional dichotomy between quantitative and qualitative research methodologies and the more contemporary adoption of mixed methods and triangulation. The most common methods available to health and social care practitioners are then briefly outlined. Experiments, case studies, interviews, observation and surveys are explored along with the distinction between primary and secondary data sources. Statistical techniques and terms are explained in a student-friendly way in order to help the reader to become more research literate and a better consumer of research. The reader is finally introduced to the minefield of research ethics and their implications for research in general terms. Key issues are emphasized in relation to health and social care research, and in particular those related to access, law, informed consent and data protection. An annotated bibliography is provided at the end of the chapter to enable the reader to follow up ideas along with one or two suggestions for class based activities which students and teachers may find helpful.

Introduction to the criminal justice system by *Philip Hodgson* uses the broad definition of health and social care focused on the promotion of well-being of individuals, communities and society. As such, consideration of health and social care includes central areas such as criminal justice. This chapter focuses on the contours of the criminal justice system, and provides the reader with an introduction to definitions of criminal justice and the key areas of the police, prosecution, the courts, probation, prison, multi-agency working and victims. The chapter concludes with a discussion of the future direction and challenges of the criminal justice system.

Theories of counselling by *Martyn Harling and Graham Whitehead* provides a broad introduction to the body of theory that underpins counselling activity in contemporary Britain. It starts by exploring definitions of counselling and how counselling fits in with contemporary society. It identifies the theoretical bases of major counselling paradigms, putting their development into a historical context. It discusses the work of key theorists in the major counselling approaches and examines the explanations and assumptions about psychological development which underpin these. Consideration is given as to how these explanations engender differing models of helping. A case study invites the reader to consider how theoretical perspectives might be applied in practice, and presents points for discussion and reflection.

Place, neighbourhood and health by *James Hunter* draws upon the wide ranging literature on neighbourhood in order to provide the reader with an understanding of place poverty and neighbourhood effects, and how this shapes the prevalence of, and responses to, social problems. The chapter argues for the need to adopt a holistic understanding of place and neighbourhood – one which takes into account the quality of local services and the ability of local agencies to bring about sustainable change – as well as factors such as neighbourhood function, spill-over effects, the physical and built environment, social capital and community engagement, access to services, resource allocation and local politics. The chapter provides a framework for evaluating the impact of place and neighbourhood upon the prevalence of health and social problems within specific localities. The narrative also explores contemporary policy approaches to measuring and mapping social problems – and the extent to which these successfully encapsulate the aspects of place and neighbourhood explored within the chapter. Overall, the aim of the chapter is to enable the reader to understand the factors that shape the quality of life and opportunities within different localities – and an exercise is provided at the end which enables the reader to relate the issues explored within the narrative to a locality where they currently live or work.

Health, housing and regeneration by *Ann McCarthy* argues it will become increasingly relevant to consider housing as a substantial element of public health and social welfare, and to integrate health aspects into strategies of sustainable housing construction and neighbourhood or urban planning. This chapter examines the relationship between health, housing and well-being to enable you to understand how potential health impacts associated with the built environment can be addressed. The chapter explores the link between health and housing, and considers ways in which potential threats to health might be addressed at an individual property level, through a consideration of a range of physical, social and economic stressors within the built environment that have the potential to impact upon the health of the public, and how to manage the risks they might pose. From here the focus is expanded to consider the influence and operation of the housing systems and housing policy in enabling society to meet the basic need for shelter with a decent, affordable home for the maximum number of citizens. It describes the impact of a complex housing system, including the role of key players and begins to analyse their ability to interact to achieve healthful housing. It explores agencies operating within the built environment and includes a consideration of a range of issues or problems, themes and debates that arise. The aim is to enable you to appreciate the nature and effectiveness of current national and local policies, and to be able to debate current issues and challenges in managing the built environment. Finally, the chapter explores the potential to deliver better health and well-being through considering the wider health issues associated with place-making, and delivering sustainable communities. Effectively the focus broadens into an urban policy and neighbourhood renewal context. The intention is to enable you to begin to appreciate the kind of problems faced in practice and to understand the technical issues facing health and social care professionals working in this field when faced with the real world of delivering healthy housing opportunities to communities. The overall objective of the chapter is to promote exploration of the knowledge and skills necessary for effective professional activity in the public health, housing and regeneration fields, as a health and social care professional with an appreciation of housing issues.

PART 3

In **Globalization and health and social care** by *Adam Barnard* the contemporary context of health and social care is discussed. The current process of globalization is defined and examined to explore how it is having an impact on communities and health and social care services. The definition explores globalization's defining features such as flows, barriers, stretched social relations, interpenetration of cultures and the emergence of global infrastructures. The chapter concludes by examining the impact globalization has had and raising questions of possible future directions for ongoing process.

Contemporary approaches to leadership and management by *Adrian M. Castell* introduces the concept of management and sets out some key stages in its historical development and its expression in the field of health and social care. The chapter examines some of the criticisms that have been made of management theory and practice and introduces some potential implications for the field of health and social care which flow from the debates that these critiques have engendered. The notion of discourse, particularly in relation to the concept of managerialism, is considered. It is argued that managerialism provides only an attenuated and restricting view of, and guide to, understanding management in the health and social care arena.

Evidence based practice by *Michele Raithby* and *Chris Ring* suggests informing and improving practice in health and social care with reference to the best current evidence which is seen as a cornerstone of being a competent practitioner in the helping professions. The ability to keep up with and utilize relevant up-to-date knowledge is now an expectation in cross-professional contexts. This chapter discusses the skills, knowledge and understanding involved in this crucial area of practice. The chapter begins with an overview of key debates on the development and use of evidence informed practice in health and social care, including ethical issues. The nature and range of research and practice knowledge that can impact on helping services is explored, and sources of credible information and research including systematic reviews are discussed. The importance of skills for critical thinking and appraisal in order to judge relevance and applicability to service needs is illustrated throughout with examples and exercises that relate to practice and the potential impact on people who use services. The concluding section discusses potential gateways and barriers to implementing evidence informed practice in the workplace, with suggestions and exercises that can be used by both students and current practitioners. At the end of the chapter, there are further discussion points for individual and group use.

Contemporary mental health care by *Kirsty Beart* explores a range of perspectives in contemporary mental health and social care. This includes conceptual models (medical, social and user), assessment, policy and practice frameworks. It aims to enable you to develop a critical awareness of current provision, policy and legislation and provide you with an opportunity to examine the implications of mental health and illness in society. The chapter aims to introduce you to the nature, role and purpose of 'interventions' in current service frameworks. To achieve this, three main areas are considered. The first is defining mental health and ill health in society, which includes types of illness, age effects, concepts and models, history, terminology, classification and all the relevant legislation to these issues. The second area is health and social care assessment and interventions considering the philosophical perspectives of treatment and care. Accompanying this is consideration of the use of mental health law and its effect on this process, and working and learning with other agencies and professionals. Finally, service user empowerment, long-term intervention and service provision, self awareness of communications skills in specific situations, therapeutic interventions, crime and mental health, vulnerable adults and risk are considered.

The practice of counselling by *Graham Whitehead* explores the application of counselling skills in contemporary Britain. The discussion explores the ethics, principles and purpose underpinning counselling practice; practitioner development of counselling skills; the dynamics of the therapeutic relationship; and encourages an active process of self-exploration and enquiry. The relevance of developing the skills of the reflective practitioner is discussed. Practice issues explored include discussion of counselling settings; boundaries and ethics; assessment and referral; supervision and support; and consideration of how to manage the helping relationship. Case studies are offered to give an understanding of the relevance of counselling in studying health and social care. The chapter also includes discussion points, group and reflective exercises.

Substance misuse by *Martyn Harling* argues behaviour linked to the use of both illegal and legal drugs is of growing concern across many areas of health and social care provision. The twentieth and early twenty-first centuries have seen substance misuse develop from a position of limited state control to a global issue requiring international consideration by the World Health Organization and shaping national and foreign policy in many of the developed nations. This chapter starts by considering the historical development of social policy and legislation linked to substance misuse, from a UK perspective. Biological, psychological and sociological concepts of 'addiction' are discussed, fitting these different perspectives into their historical context and effect on legislation. The range of illegal and legal substances used in contemporary society will be discussed in terms of their effects, health risk and patterns of usage both at a cultural and individual level. The chapter concludes by considering substance misuse service provision in the UK along with a brief discussion of the physiological and psychological treatment options available to individuals presenting to such services. The chapter provides regular discussion points and reflective exercises linked to both illicit and licit drug use. It also provides the reader with references and suggestions for further study resources relating to substance misuse.

Working with children by *Helen Burrows, Jill Berrisford* and *Jo Ward* suggests working with children can occur in many different settings: it may involve working with children who are developing normally and have few apparent problems; alternatively children may have atypical development, be somewhere on the continuum of children with mental health difficulties, or living in a situation of stress or distress where their needs are not being met. This chapter outlines contemporary theories of child development, including attachment and resilience. It then examines the key themes of working in partnership with children and young people to safeguard and promote their development and needs, and support them through transitions. Children and young people are increasingly able to take part in developing the services provided to support and help them; a key question to be considered is how the views, wishes and feelings of children who are not able to articulate these verbally can be known.

Historically, children have often been seen as passive recipients of both health and social care; in many cultures, patriarchy saw children as objects, blank sheets to be moulded in the image of their elders. In western cultures, 'seen and not heard' was the rule. From the nineteenth century, however, with growing understanding of the needs of children and young people to be supported and protected, a children's rights perspective developed, and this has grown to encompass the concept of not only children's welfare being paramount but also their views, wishes and feelings needing to be considered. Children now have a right to be heard in matters concerning them and this influences not only how we work directly with children, but also how public policies affecting children are developed and implemented.

User involvement by *Matthew Gough* explores the drivers behind what is commonly understood by user involvement and clarifies its expectations. It distinguishes between the different models of user involvement and evaluates their strengths and flaws. There is a critique of unhelpful but common approaches to involvement ranging from consumerist attempts to ill thought out, but well meaning, approaches. The chapter outlines a model of best practice in user involvement and establishes what the function of authentic user involvement can achieve. It makes a case that, far from being a desirable end goal, user involvement is a vital and integral part of a process that cultivates outcomes of genuine respect, meaningful partnership, real transfers of power and true citizenship. The chapter is written by an author with direct experience of using services and includes contributions from user led organizations. There is also a consideration of the practical, often financial, barriers to satisfactory involvement and examples are provided of creative solutions which take into account current policy and legislation. At the end of the chapter there is a best practice checklist for auditing user involvement.

In **Young people and youth justice**, *Roger Hopkins-Burke* explores the involvement of children and young people in criminality and the ways in which the criminal justice authorities have responded to their activities both in the past and in the present. In contrast to the many academic youth crime texts written from a predominantly critical criminological perspective, and which emphasize the admitted reality that many children and young people become involved in offending behaviour but invariably grow out of it, this chapter recognizes that for a small minority involvement in ongoing criminality is a real and serious problem that requires some form of intervention, not just to protect society from their troublesome activities, but is also in their best interests. This paper thus adopts a left realist perspective that recognizes the need to deal with the problematic actions of individuals *and* the conditions which encourage those behaviours not least for the good of the young person involved. It is a chapter thus compatible but not uncritical of the contemporary youth justice system. It commences with a reflexive consideration of the involvement of young people in crime and considers some recent statistics, and the rest of the chapter is divided into two parts. The first considers the problem of youthful criminality in an historical and theoretical context with societal attempts to discipline and educate children and young people in the interest of a myriad of groups not least ourselves. The second considers the development of a specific juvenile/youth justice system charged with intervention in the lives of young people from the justice/punishment model to the welfare/treatment model and beyond into the more ambiguous recent territory of 'excluded tutelage' and 'reintegrative tutelage'.

In **The professionalization of the youth justice workforce**, *Vicky Palmer* discusses the evolution of the modern youth justice system and the elusive nature of the professionalization of youth justice by considering the teaching of knowledge, and the status of semi-professions. The 'modernization' of this profession by government administrations is discussed before contextualising youth justice training as justice versus welfare. The tensions of the modernization process with the rise of bureaucracy are contrasted with the feelings and assessment of service users and practitioners. The chapter continues by reflecting on the nature of youth justice and the lack of focus on the historical emergence of this area of health and social care. The development of youth justice training is located within the rise of New Labour's administration and the chapter considers the impact this has had on training and practice within youth justice.

The conclusion summarizes the key themes in health and social care that have been discussed to provide a trajectory of the themes considered. Again this is not exhaustive but intended to open dialogue and give air to debates that are central to health and social care.

Before the reader embarks on the journey through *Key Themes in Health and Social Care*, there are some caveats that should be added. Although this text provides an introduction to pertinent and relevant themes in the field there are some omissions or gaps in coverage. For example, race and ethnicity, service users' voices and practitioner views are not foregrounded or brought centre stage. A planned second volume in this series will address these omissions. This volume also includes broader discussion of discipline and practice areas beyond health and social care. This transdisciplinary approach has the strengths of considering individuals, groups and communities in their widest sense and of considering the social and well-being aspects of health and social care rather than any narrow definition or focus to the term. Finally, this text represents a plurality of voices and a range of perspectives from within (and from outside) health and social care. The different styles, visions and voices represent the contested field of activity, in theory and practice, in health and social care. It is hoped that this book represents an attempt to problematize or open for debate key areas and key themes in health and social care.

QUICK NAVIGATION AND HOW TO USE THIS BOOK

There are four ways of reading this book. The first is to read it from cover to cover, line by line, chapter by chapter. The authors would be delighted if readers felt they were able and wanted to navigate through the book in this way from front to back but the reality of most people's lives is that this is a luxury they can seldom afford. For the more time pressed, 'gutting the literature' or 'ram-raiding' what is required is the second option for reading the book. Using the index to find specific topics, 'topping and tailing' chapters by reading the introduction and conclusion, and skimming, scanning and reading in depth allow a quicker and more focused reading of the book. The third way is to read the book by chapters. Each chapter contains a discrete discussion on a specific area within health and social care and the reader is invited to dip into (and out of) chapters as required or desired. The fourth way to read the book is thematically. The text is woven together from key themes that inform and underpin theory and practice in health and social care. For reading, writing and research skills, *Skills for study and practice, Studying at a higher level in health and social care, Research in health and social care,* and *Evidence based practice in health and social care* would be appropriate. For theoretical, conceptual, philosophical and political understanding and knowledge, *The individual and society, Concepts of equality and diversity, Working with people, Key themes in health and social care, Philosophical and political debate in health and social care, Place, neighbourhood and health, Globalization and health and social care,* and *Contemporary approaches to leadership and management* would be helpful. For readers wanting an introduction to policy and legislation, *Introduction to social policy* and *Key themes in health and social care* address these issues.

Health is directly addressed in *Key themes in health and social care, Health and health care in Britain, Health, housing and regeneration,* and *Contemporary mental health care.* Criminal justice is considered in *Introduction to the criminal justice system, Young people and youth justice,* and *The professionalization of the youth justice workforce.* Counselling is discussed in *Theories of counselling* and *The practice of counselling.*

Similarly there are key themes that emerge through each of the chapters but also across the book as a whole. Four examples should be illustrative. First, the idea of well-being is a central theme that runs throughout the book. This is conceived as a social form of flourishing rather than just the absence of illness in a medical sense. The critique of purely medical or biological approaches to health and social care is one of the central themes to emerge. The challenge to 'common sense' or taken-for-granted ideas, concepts, and essentialist understanding and beliefs also figures prominently. The relationship of theory to practice is a fundamental theme that is found in many chapters, or by extension the relationship of the abstract to the concrete. Finally, the commitment, focus, desire and professionalism of health and social care workers and students in an attempt to provide high quality services on a personal basis that is respectful of diversity is a further unifying theme that runs throughout the book.

The book is constructed to aid students and readers in exploring knowledge and understanding in health and social care and theory's application to practice.

Key Themes in Health and Social Care: Mapping the field

	Key themes	Key terms
Part 1		
Skills for study and practice	Writing skills, reading, essay plans, essay structure, written arguments	Grammar, punctuation, summarising, paraphrasing, citation, referencing, proofreading
Working with people	Interpersonal skills, communication theory, listening skills, skills development, interviewing, person-centred approach, health care models	Attitudes, values, health care planning and self-awareness feedback, non-verbal communication, para-verbal communication, anti-oppressive practice, anti-discriminatory practice, team work
The individual in society	Psychology and sociology theories	Life transitions, gender, ethnicity, disability, prenatal, early years, teenagers, adolescence, adulthood
Concepts of equality and diversity	Equality, barriers, diversity and legislation	Inequality, equal opportunity, prejudice, stereotyping, discrimination, oppression, class, gender, ethnicity, culture, age, sexuality, disability
Introduction to social policy	Social policy, wants and needs, welfare provision	Social security, health, education, employment and housing. New right, socialism, social democracy, New Labour
Part 2		
Studying at a higher level in health and social care	Level 1 to Level 3, supporting arguments, critical reading, reflective practice	Argument, critical reading, critical literature review, reflective practice
Health and health care in Britain	Health, health inequalities, models of health	Socio-economic status, ethnicity, gender, National Health Service, comprehensive services, 'quality', patient centred
Key themes in health and social care	Health, social care, outcomes, lived experience, protection from harm	Personalization, safeguarding, partnership, quality of life, 'abuse', 'care', failures
Philosophical and political debate in health and social care	Philosophy, politics, ethics	Freedom, authority, rights, justice, liberalism, socialism, social democracy, conservatism, new right, New Labour, utilitarianism, deontology, virtue
Research in health and social care	Research, epistemology and theories of knowledge, quantitative and qualitative research, questionnaires, research methodologies, and ethics	Quantitative, qualitative, methodology, method, evidence based practice, research design, experiments, natural experiments, surveys, questionnaires, observation, case studies, action research, grounded theory, narrative and content analysis
Introduction to criminal justice	Criminal justice, the police, the national offender management service – the prison and probation services	The police, prosecution, courts, probation, prison, multi-agency working, victims
Theories of counselling	Counselling, history and theory of counselling	Psychodynamic, cognitive behavioural, humanistic, multicultural

Continued

Key Themes in Health and Social Care: Mapping the field (continued)

	Key themes	Key terms
Part 2 (continued)		
Place, neighbourhood and health	Place poverty, neighbourhood effects, mapping social problems	Neighbourhood function, spill-over effects, the physical and built environment, social capital and community engagement, access to services, resource allocation and local politics
Health, housing and regeneration	Public health, housing and regeneration	Healthy housing, poor housing, housing hazards, sustainable development, neighbourhood
Part 3		
Globalization and health and social care	Globalization	Flows, barriers, stretched social relations, interpenetration of cultures, infrastructure, heterogeneity, homogeneity, McDonaldization
Contemporary approaches to leadership and management	Management, leadership	Managerialism, values, leadership, scientific management, discourse, human relations, critical management studies
Evidence based practice in health and social care	Evidence based practice	Critical thinking, evidence base, knowledge
Contemporary mental health care	Mental health	Deinstitutionalization, community care, needs, positive practice, mental illness, humanistic theory, medical model, integrative model
The practice of counselling	Practice issues, counselling skills, self awareness	Therapeutic relationship, ethics, confidentiality, assessment, referral, supervision
Substance misuse	History of substance misuse, concepts of 'addiction', substance misuse service provision	Ecstasy, LSD, cocaine, heroin, amphetamine, cannabis, anabolic steroids, alcohol, tobacco
Working with children	Historical context, child development, and values	'Rights', 'paternalism', attachment, resilience, transition, communication, participation
User involvement	Personalization, service user involvement, best practice	Consumerist approaches, citizenship, empowerment, partnership
Young people and youth justice	Young people, criminology, youth justice system	Justice/punishment, welfare/treatment, excluded tutelage, reintegrated tutelage
Professionalization of the youth justice workforce	Youth justice system, 'professionalization'	Modernization, case managers, agency, structure, managerialism, rights, responsibilities, Third Way, McDonaldization, effective practice, rehabilitation, crime prevention

PART 1

CHAPTER 1

SKILLS FOR STUDY AND PRACTICE

SIÂN TRAFFORD

O B J E C T I V E S

After reading this chapter you should be able to:

- Have an awareness of writing academically.

- Understand the process of writing and preparing to write.

- Understand how to structure and review your written work.

After reading this chapter you will know the meaning of the following terms: Grammar, punctuation, summarising, paraphrasing, citation, referencing, proofreading.

There is a Moment of Reflection at the end of the chapter.

INTRODUCTION

This chapter opens by introducing the necessary skills to be able to study for a qualification in health and social care. It begins with a stepped approach to getting started. Writing skills are introduced to provide guidance on sentences and grammar, subject–verb agreement and punctuation of full stops, commas, colons and semicolons. Using reading effectively explores reading, managing reading lists and using the internet, skimming, scanning and reviewing, before paraphrasing and citation and referencing are discussed. Essay writing skills examine planning, structure, sign posting and cohesion, conclusions and proofreading. Examples in the conclusion, at the end of chapter, allow you to apply the skills to real situations.

GETTING STARTED

Writing at university involves skills in reading critically and writing in a manner which is understandable and credible. This chapter will assist you in developing these skills so that your experience of learning will be enjoyable: you will learn how to learn.

Step 1

Identify available time and space for study – a separate room or a corner of a room to accommodate the necessary equipment (paper, pens, PC and printer, books and learning resources, and so on). Work out how much time has to be spent on commitments such as lectures, seminars, tutorials, family, paid or voluntary work, and so on, and then plan how to use the remaining time effectively by setting targets to achieve specific goals. (See SMART targets under essay writing skills.)

Step 2

Become familiar with the library and read – reading is vital, not just to gather the information needed to complete assignments, but because it introduces the academic writing style necessary at university. Pay attention to the words and expressions used, sentence and paragraph structure and referencing conventions, and consider how they can be used in your own writing.

Step 3

Identify any problems with your skills in studying – such as not being clear about computers or writing well. Get help from tutors or sources of student support as early as possible before problems become overwhelming.

WRITING SKILLS

The object of good academic writing is to communicate ideas and evidence clearly and effectively. Academic writing therefore needs to be well structured and analytical, with a strong argument that takes the reader logically step by step to a persuasive conclusion. Correct grammar and punctuation are two of the tools which help writers to achieve clarity so this chapter will explain how to write clear, well-formed sentences and avoid the pitfalls of ungrammatical or incomplete sentences.

Punctuation is important because it helps the reader to make sense of what has been written. When speaking, facial expression, hand gestures, tone and pitch of the voice are used to convey meaning, but with written material, the reader has to rely on punctuation. This chapter will, therefore, also consider the use of punctuation, particularly commas, full stops, semicolons and colons.

This chapter will cover some of these fundamental writing skills because although many students are confident about how to study, some are less sure of their writing abilities.

Sentences

Children learn in primary school that sentences begin with a capital letter, end with a full stop and make complete sense on their own, but problems can arise with the more sophisticated constructions required for academic writing. Common problems include beginning sentences with conjunctions (words such as although, because, while, whereas, and so on) or with a continuous version of a verb (words such as judging, listening, working, and so on) because this can result in incomplete sentences.

For example:

- Suggesting that removing children from families is not always effective.
- Whereas the Youth Justice Board wants to ensure that custody is only used as a last resort.

These phrases do not make sense on their own because they only provide limited information so they are called sentence fragments. In the first example, there is no indication of *what* demonstrates that removing children from families is not always effective. In the second example, *whereas* indicates that the information is providing a contrasting point yet there is no other information to contrast it with. These fragments could be converted into complete sentences with a simple adjustment.

For example:

- Looked-after children frequently underachieve educationally, suggesting that removing children from families is not always effective.
- Public opinion regularly demands that all criminals should be jailed whereas the Youth Justice Board wants to ensure that custody is only used as a last resort.

OR

- Whereas the Youth Justice Board wants to ensure that custody is only used as a last resort, public opinion regularly demands that all criminals should be jailed.

Subject–verb agreement

Another issue which causes problems for students is subject–verb agreement. The subject of a sentence (the person or thing doing the action) has to match the form of the verb (the action word). This is because the subject of a sentence can be singular (there is only one of them) or plural (there are lots of them) and the verbs change accordingly.

For instance, if the above sentence read *Looked-after children frequently underachieves educationally* it would sound incorrect because the subject is plural (children) while the verb (underachieves) is in the singular form.

This adjustment is usually made automatically when speaking, and when writing too. The problem arises when writing becomes more sophisticated and sentences become longer, such as in academic writing, so extra care needs to be taken to clarify the subject of a sentence.

- The group of social workers (agree, agrees) to meet the following week.
- A wide range of sentences (is, are) available to the youth justice system.

- In the gym, only three treadmills (was, were) unoccupied.
- All of the assignments, including the one submitted electronically, (was, were) marked before the end of the week.

- The group of social workers **agrees** to meet the following week. *Because 'the group' is the subject of the sentence and is singular.*
- A wide range of sentences **is** available to the youth justice system. *Because 'a wide range' is the subject of the sentence and is singular.*
- In the gym, only three treadmills **were** unoccupied. *Because 'treadmills' are the subject of the sentence and are plural.*
- All of the assignments, including the one submitted electronically, **were** marked before the end of the week. *Because 'all of the assignments' are the subject, not just 'the one submitted electronically'.*

PUNCTUATION

Correct punctuation makes meaning clear to the reader. Incorrect punctuation can make written work confusing or even incomprehensible so it is vital to get it right.

Full stops

Full stops separate one statement from another and indicate to the reader that a sentence is complete. As has been stated, a sentence must express a complete idea and make sense on its own.

Commas

Commas are used to separate items in a list and to separate parts of a sentence. They are also used to link simple sentences, but care needs to be taken not to use a comma when a full stop is required.

- The student dropped her pens, books and lecture notes.
- The pathways included working with children, caring for the elderly and supporting offenders.
- The social work profession, which is frequently criticised by the press, provides a vital service for vulnerable people.

The first two examples show commas being used to separate listed items. In the second sentence, the listed items are more complex but they all have the same grammatical structure.

In the third example, the commas are separating parts of the sentence. Indeed the section contained between the commas could be omitted and there would still be a complete grammatical sentence. This allows the writer to place the emphasis on the vital service provided by social workers rather than on the press criticism (Rose 2001).

Colons

Colons provide a pause before introducing items in a list.

- There are many assessment formats at university: essays, spoken presentations, reports, poster presentations and exams.

They can also indicate further information about or amplification of a preceding point.

- Social work is gruelling: it can be highly rewarding or very distressing.

Semicolons

Semicolons can separate items in a list when a comma is already in use.

- The speakers at the conference were: Dr Sally Jones, Sheffield; Dr Martin Long, Leeds; Prof. Jane Davies, Swansea; and Dr Phil White, Nottingham.

OR

- The new system has been introduced to reduce paperwork, especially form filling; to reduce staff time, including administrative staff; to improve clarity and transparency; and to utilise IT more effectively.

Each phrase after the first semicolon has to follow the same grammatical pattern. Semicolons can also link closely related sentences but each side of the semicolon **must** be a complete sentence.

- I read the textbook in one sitting; it was not very inspiring.

READING SKILLS

University reading lists can be intimidating but some simple tips can make reading more manageable and enable the student to take notes effectively.

Managing the reading lists

Students are not expected to read every single book from cover to cover – an important part of study at university is learning to identify and select relevant information to use as evidence in their work. Ways can be found to prioritise the books on the list: tutors or fellow students can make recommendations, an author's name might be familiar from a previous course, some texts might be more up to date than others, or the title might suggest the level of the book (for example, 'introduction' or 'advanced') (Habeshaw, Habeshaw and Gibbs 1989).

USING THE INTERNET FOR RESEARCH

Caution needs to be exercised when using the internet for research. There are undoubtedly many excellent websites with academic and peer-reviewed material. Unfortunately, because of the nature of the internet, there is also a lot of material that is inaccurate, false, out of date, fraudulent or even malicious. Readers need to be aware of bias, credibility and reliability (*see* Critical reading, thinking and writing section in Chapter 6 and Place *et al.* 2006).

SKIMMING AND SCANNING

SQ3R (Survey, Question, Read, Recall, Review)

When reading it is useful to have some questions in mind that might be answered by the text because this will help to focus attention. Habeshaw, Habeshaw and Gibbs (1989) suggest that adopting the SQ3R technique (Survey, Question, Read, Recall, Review) can help concentration and reading will therefore be more effective. Begin by skimming (surveying) the chapter or journal article, using the title and sub-headings, to get an idea of what will be covered. Abstracts, contents and index lists are also useful sources of information.

Next, write down the questions to be answered by the text. The above survey will help in compiling the questions as will the assignment title or exam questions (*see* Essay writing skills, page 10). Burns and Sinfield (2008: 159) suggest questions such as 'What am I looking for?'; 'Where and how will I use the information?'; 'Which bit of the assignment will it help me with?'; and 'Which of the learning outcomes will it help me with?'.

Now read the text while looking for answers to the questions. Aim to understand the information before making notes, although Burns and Sinfield (2008: 159) advocate 'getting physical' with texts by highlighting, underlining or annotating text. They point out, however, that other people's books must not be defaced in this way – students need to buy their own books or photocopy relevant pages from library books.

Put the book to one side and attempt to recall the answers to your questions from memory. Notes should be made in the student's own words, paraphrasing accurately. This will help to avoid plagiarism later on. This method highlights what has been learned and what still needs to be worked on.

Finally, review by checking that the answers are correct and that the meaning of the original has not been lost by being paraphrased. Any errors need to be amended. Special attention should be paid to anything that could not be recalled (Habeshaw, Habeshaw and Gibbs 1989).

Paraphrasing

Paraphrasing is your own version of the key points you have read. To paraphrase effectively, aim to understand the text and then 'translate' it into your own words (University of Wisconsin 2009). Successful paraphrasing involves more than just using synonyms: sentence structure and grammar needs to be significantly altered. Break up long sentences or combine short sentences, swap verbs for nouns or nouns for verbs, change verbs from active to passive and vice versa. By using their own words students demonstrate their understanding of the text and avoid the trap of using too many quotes. Too many direct quotes can make tutors question whether students have really understood the issues and can also lead to accusations of plagiarism if material has not been properly referenced. Paraphrases also have to be correctly referenced of course, and this is dealt with in the next section.

CITATION AND REFERENCING

Citation and referencing are the ways a writer identifies his/her sources. Accurate referencing is an integral part of academic writing. As well as being courteous to the originator, it demonstrates effective reading and research skills, it allows the student and the tutor to find the material again easily and it dispels any suspicion that students are trying to pass someone else's ideas off as their own.

Harvard referencing is the preferred method at many universities, but check with tutors to find out what is expected. Citations must be included in assignments for quotes or paraphrases, and a complete reference in the reference list at the end of the work must also be provided. The Harvard style requires a name and a date for any material used within an assignment such as a text book or journal article. If a direct quote has been used (the words have been taken from the text and not altered at all) then a page number will also have to be included and the quote will have to be enclosed in quotation marks. This is the convention for including a quote:

> According to Rose (2001, p131) 'a reference is a note that you make of where you found a particular idea or a sentence or two that you have quoted'.

The quotation marks indicate that these are the actual words as they were published in the book.

These are conventions for including a paraphrase:

> Rose (2001) defines a reference as a personal record of the location of any specific thoughts or words used in an assignment.

> A reference can be defined as a personal record of the location of any specific thoughts or words used in an assignment (Rose 2001).

When paraphrasing, there are two methods of indicating the author. The originator is either included as part of the sentence (as in example (a)), in which case only the date needs to be included in brackets. In example (b) the statement has been made and then attributed to the originating author. This technique requires the author's name and the date to be included in the brackets, and the brackets need to be included in the appropriate sentence, so the full stop has to come after the brackets otherwise it will be unclear which sentence the citation refers to.

References in the reference list follow clearly defined patterns and, as long as these patterns are followed, all will be well. There are five basic elements for books – author(s)'(s) name(s), year, title, place of publication, publisher. There are, obviously, variations for different sources such as websites or journals, but if you learn the basic patterns you should not go wrong. The title of the book, the journal or the website page should always be highlighted because that is the information that will be used to search for it.

> Author(s)'(s) name or names (Year) *Title,* Place of publication: Publisher.

> Rose, J. (2001) *The Mature Student's Guide to Writing,* Basingstoke: Palgrave.

If the book is a second or subsequent edition, this needs to be included with the title because editions can vary substantially in content.

Cottrell, S. (2003) *The Study Skills Handbook* (2nd edition), Basingstoke: Palgrave McMillan.

Journal references are slightly different in that there are technically two titles, the title of the article and of the journal. However, it is the journal title which needs to be highlighted as it is the journal title you would search for if you wished to source the material.

Author(s)'(s) name or names (Year) Article title, *Journal title,* Volume (issue/part number), page numbers.

Jack, G. (2005) Assessing the impact of community programmes working with children and families in disadvantaged areas, *Child and Family Social Work,* 10, pp. 293–304.

Website references also differ slightly from book references but again they have a set pattern. If no author can be found, it is acceptable to use the 'editor' or 'owner' of the website. In this example we have used NSPCC. The term '[online]' can be said to be the place of publication.

Author(s) or Editor(s) (Year) *Title* [online] Place of publication, publisher. Available at … (Accessed date).

NSPCC (2008) *What is Child Abuse?* [online] NSPCC. Available at http://www. nspcc.org.uk/helpandadvice/whatchildabuse/whatischildabuse_wda36500.html (Accessed on 20 November 2008).

ESSAY WRITING SKILLS

Realistic planning is key to writing a good essay, not only planning the structure of the essay but also planning and setting targets for completing the different stages of the essay. It is advisable to work backwards from the submission date, allowing enough time to plan, research, draft, edit and proofread the work.

Anxiety about assignments can be reduced by breaking each task down into smaller and smaller tasks and setting SMART targets. SMART targets are **S**pecific, **M**easurable, **A**chievable, **R**elevant and **T**ime related, meaning that the targets need to be realistic, attainable and quantifiable. For example, 'I will do some reading' would become 'From 7–9pm (time related) I will read Chapters 1–3 of XXX (specific and achievable) after which I will be able to describe the range of under-18 custody options (measurable)'. This goal setting allows the student to exercise control over their workload which reduces stress and can increase motivation because something tangible has been achieved.

Planning

First of all, the essay title needs to be analysed as this will help with formulating an essay plan. Planning the essay is important as it provides the opportunity to sort and order the information, and to ensure that all the important issues are included. What is the question really asking? What are the key words or issues mentioned in the title? What exactly is the key instruction? (for example, compare, contrast, assess, discuss or evaluate). How can the question be answered? What knowledge or information is required to produce this answer and how much of this knowledge or information is already known, and how much still needs to be researched?

In addition to the title, the assignment criteria and learning outcomes can all be used to construct an essay plan. These sources will provide information about what needs to be included: points that must be covered, issues that need to be discussed and skills that will need to be demonstrated in order to obtain a good mark.

There are many essay planning techniques, including spider diagrams, mind maps (Buzan 2006), linear plans (lists, headings and sub-headings), and horizontal plans (columns headed by key terms from the essay title and containing important points to be analysed, explained or explored). Colour coding using coloured pens and/or paper is also a useful planning aid, and not just for essays. Different colours can be used for different modules or themes and issues within those modules, making organisation and retrieval of information easier and faster to accomplish as well as easier to remember.

Below is an example of how to plan an essay by breaking down the title into key terms, using the horizontal plan method. This enables the writer to identify the main issues that need to be addressed within the essay and to list the themes, concepts and so on that must be discussed in order to answer the question. It also allows the student to see whether the information is arranged in a logical order, and to make adjustments if necessary.

Discuss the view that an understanding of cultural diversity is important in health and social care.

Introduction	Cultural diversity	Health and social care	Importance	Conclusion
What will the essay talk about? Will the essay show that the writer agrees or disagrees with the statement?	Aspects of cultural diversity, for example race or gender	How and when do cultural diversity and health and social care impact on each other?	Respect Appreciation of others' values/beliefs Power relations – use of language	Summarise the main points. Is the writer's view clear? Is there an obvious conclusion?

Structure

Essays need to be well structured to make them easy to read. The most basic structure is introduction, main body (where the argument is developed (Cottrell 2003)), and conclusion, not forgetting the title and references.

It is important to include the title for several reasons. It can provide a useful reminder of what needs to be covered in the essay so that the writer can check that they are not straying from the subject and introducing irrelevant material. Similarly, it allows the person reading, and perhaps marking, the essay to ascertain whether the writer has answered the question set. Students may assume that the tutor is aware of the title but assignments are frequently read and marked by individuals other than the tutor, such as external examiners. If the title is not included the reader is unsure of the writer's task and, therefore, whether they have succeeded in achieving it.

Composing the introduction can be problematical, but questions such as: What am I writing about? Why am I doing this? How will I do it? (Dissc live 2008) can help to get ideas flowing. The introduction can show that the implications of the title question have been understood by stating how it will be interpreted. For example, the introduction can explain why the subject is important and how it will be dealt with. This in turn will demonstrate an understanding of the subject and of the issues behind the title. This kind of introduction can also act as a broad essay plan, again allowing the student to check back that they are adhering to the subject matter and to their own structure.

Of course, the introduction need not be the first part of the essay to be written. Some writers prefer to start with the main body and compose the introduction later in the process once they are more confident of the direction of the essay.

A major part of the essay will be the formulation and development of the argument, that is, the writer's point of view and the reasons and evidence that support it. In order to influence or persuade the reader to a particular way of thinking, the writer needs to 'state a point of view or opinion, and a clear line of reasoning to support it' (Cottrell 2003: 186). Supporting evidence for these reasons could include examples, proven facts, reliable statistics, causes or effects. In effect, the reader is being persuaded to believe in or accept a certain standpoint because of the evidence being presented by the writer.

Similarly, the presentation of counter arguments will demonstrate that the writer has not discounted contradictory viewpoints but has examined and evaluated them and found them unconvincing. This displays balanced and informed opinion while establishing the superiority of the main argument.

Signposting and cohesion

The parts of an essay need to be smoothly connected to each other (known as cohesion). The reader needs to have an indication of what will be said next and how it links to what has already been said. These 'signposts' perform various tasks such as imposing sequence (recently, primarily), introducing additional points (in addition, moreover), introducing a contrasting or opposing idea (however, conversely) or presenting a consequence (thus, as a result) and so on.

Cohesion can also be achieved by using words and phrases to refer backwards and forwards in your work, within and between sentences and paragraphs. Pronouns such as 'he', 'she', 'it', 'they', 'this', 'that', 'these' or 'those' can be used as this avoids repetition and provides cohesion. For example, 'Vulnerable adults need to be protected by legislation as **they** can be subject to abuse', or 'Many people are faced with violence in their daily lives – teachers, health professionals, bus and train staff. **This** problem discourages people from entering **these** professions.'

Conclusions

The function of the conclusion is to sum up the key issues in the essay and show how the evidence has lent support to the writer's point of view. It can be useful to refer back to key words and phrases in the title, thus linking the ending to the beginning. It is vital not to introduce any new material at this stage and it is advisable not to finish with a quotation. Above all, ensure conclusions are clear and that a sense of ending is provided.

PROOFREADING

Once the essay is finished it can be tempting to submit it without further checking, but proofreading is vital. Proofreading can detect grammatical, spelling and typographical errors and is best done after a break away from the work to become 'unfamiliar' with it (Burns and Sinfield 2008). Reading it straight away on screen increases the likelihood of the eyes 'seeing what should be there rather than what is there' (Burns and Sinfield 2008: 199). Leaving a break, printing the work out and reading it aloud will produce the best results because this will force a slower pace so that more attention is paid to the actual words as written. Punctuation should also be taken into account and if there are too many pauses, or not enough, then it needs to be adjusted (*see* Writing skills, page 4).

CONCLUSION

The key to a successful university career is planning. Be prepared by having all the necessary equipment (pens, paper, PC, books, and so on) and by allowing adequate time to complete the work. Breaking the work down into a series of manageable targets gives the student control and makes it easier to succeed. This is where self awareness is useful. Learn to recognise your learning style and be realistic about how much time is needed for tasks. Be honest about your strengths and problem areas and seek help early if you need it.

Feedback from students demonstrates that attending lectures and seminars is also crucial because lecturers do a lot of the necessary groundwork for their students. They introduce the main theories and thinkers and then summarise the main aspects: their strengths and weaknesses and how they relate to other theories. This in turn directs students to the important texts where selection and reading skills can be used to sort the relevant from the irrelevant. In addition, reading widely helps to make the conventions of academic writing more familiar (the language and terms used, the structure of academic writing, referencing styles, and so on) and this can help boost confidence.

Another benefit of attending taught sessions regularly is getting to know other students. This has two advantages. First, it allows students to discuss the course content and work and to share ideas and recommend resources such as useful books or websites. It also makes it more enjoyable, and therefore more likely that students will attend if they feel they are going to meet with familiar, friendly faces.

Asking questions is an important part of being a student. Ask tutors if you are unclear about an assignment or a point made in a lecture or if there are other problems affecting your study. If they cannot sort it out they can refer you to someone who can.

Use assignment guidelines, marking criteria and learning outcomes to find out what is expected in written assignments and use them to plan your writing. Then, when reading and writing, ask yourself questions – who, what, when, where, why, what for? – to focus your thoughts and to stimulate ideas.

Finally, make sure you are getting your meaning across by using words and sentences you are confident with, rather than using long words and even longer sentences because you think it is more academic.

Above all, value the skills and experience you already possess. Rather than concentrate on what you cannot do (yet), think about what you can do and put steps in place to achieve your goals. Health and social care requires clear but elegant, simple and accessible written work.

Now that you have read this chapter, read the following two paragraphs. Which of the two is the more academic? Why is it more academic?

MOMENT OF REFLECTION

Example A

Substance misuse can also be a factor which plays a major role in homelessness, being addicted to a substance is more often than not a downward spiral, often resulting in homelessness, and can also possibly lead to criminal behaviour. I think this can be seen as a personal responsibility in many respects, because you could prevent this happening by not becoming mixed up in it in the first place. In my opinion it becomes a public responsibility when a person is addicted to a substance, and all they can think about is where their next 'hit' will come from, and will stop at nothing to get it, even if it means losing their home and committing crime.

Example B

Another factor which may contribute to homelessness is substance misuse. Addiction can cause a downward spiral, resulting not only in homelessness but also in criminal behaviour. An individual could prevent this situation arising by taking personal responsibility and avoiding becoming involved in substance misuse. However, there is also an element of public responsibility in such a situation because the addict will become fixated on acquiring their next 'hit' regardless of the cost to themselves or the impact on society.

Example B is the more academic because Example A has some stylistic errors, as detailed below	
Punctuation	'Being addicted…' is the beginning of a new sentence
Use of 1st instead of 3rd person	I think, in my opinion
Colloquialisms (language used in conversations)	More often than not; in many respects; mixed up in; all they can think about; in the first place; stop at nothing. The word 'hit' has been used in both and it is in inverted commas which indicates that the writer is aware that it is colloquial but that it fits the context

SUMMARY OF MAIN POINTS

You should be able to:

*   Understand writing academically.
*   Understand the process of writing and preparing to write.
*   Understand how to structure and review your written work.

REFERENCES

Burns, T. and Sinfield, S. (2008) *Essential Study Skills. The Complete Guide to Success at University* (2nd edition), London: Sage.

Buzan, Tony (2006) *Mind Mapping: Kick-start your creativity and transform your life*, Harlow: BBC Active.

Cottrell, S. (2003) *The Study Skills Handbook* (2nd edition), Basingstoke: Palgrave McMillan.

Dissc live (2008) *What should an introductory paragraph do?* [online] University of Teesside. Available at http://dissc.tees.ac.uk/Writing/paragraphs/page9.htm (Accessed 23 December 2008).

Habeshaw, T., Habeshaw, S. and Gibbs, G. (1989) *53 Interesting Ways of Helping your Students to Study* (2nd edition), Bristol: Technical and Educational Services.

Place, E., Kendall, M., Hiom, D., Booth, H., Ayres, P., Manuel, A. and Smith, P. (2006) *Internet Detective: Wise up to the Web* (3rd edition) [online] Intute Virtual Training Suite. Available at http://www.vts.intute.ac.uk/detective/ (Accessed 16 December 2009).

Rose, J. (2001) *The Mature Student's Guide to Writing*, Basingstoke: Palgrave.

University of Wisconsin (2009) *Quoting and Paraphrasing Sources* [online] University of Wisconsin. Available at http://writing.wisc.edu/Handbook/QPA_paraphrase2.html (Accessed 6 March 2009).

CHAPTER 2

WORKING WITH PEOPLE

*KIRSTY BEART, GRAHAM WHITEHEAD
AND ADAM BARNARD*

OBJECTIVES

After reading this chapter you should be able to:

- Have an awareness of working with people in a health and social care environment.

- Understand interpersonal skills in an applied setting.

- Understand models and philosophical models of health and social care.

After reading this chapter you will know the meaning of the following terms: Interpersonal skills, communication theory and practice; listening skills; assertiveness behaviour; group and teamwork; interviewing skills; giving and receiving feedback.

There are five Moments of Reflection to work on throughout the chapter.

INTRODUCTION

The significance of the development of interpersonal skills for students and workers in health and social care cannot be underestimated. The awareness and skills development necessary will be of central importance to your learning and work and this chapter explores your attitudes, values, self-awareness and skills development in a health and social care setting.

This chapter covers the relevant theoretical understanding necessary to inform this process and will encompass communication theory, health care planning and the significance of self-awareness in working with people in health and social care settings.

ESSENTIAL QUALITIES IN HEALTH AND SOCIAL CARE

Working in health and social care settings requires significant consideration of interpersonal skills so that service users are offered a professional and responsive service. There is a need for students and workers to develop and reflect upon their interpersonal skills and learn about how they interact with other people. This exploration can be both rewarding and challenging but the outcome is an increased awareness of how communication can be used effectively in a professional setting to respond effectively to service user needs. The starting point is for students to understand the dynamics of communication and consider some of the challenges that may be faced. Working with people not only demands patience and the ability to listen closely to identified needs, but also the ability to operate within the context of organisational constraints which at times can result in the need to reach a compromise with service users on what can be provided within the given resource limitations.

MOMENT OF REFLECTION

Activity One

What qualities are needed in health and social care?

Make a list of the qualities you think a health and social care professional needs to demonstrate to a service user. Choose a specific role, for example health adviser and make a list of desired qualities.

The qualities you have identified will hopefully have highlighted the need to listen closely to what the service user is asking for. Using the example of the health adviser, the service user may be asking for very specific information about a health condition, requiring the adviser to listen closely to the particular aspects that s/he will be required to respond to. Listening is an essential skill at this point in the professional relationship. There are many factors that may get in the way of hearing exactly what is being requested of you. Developing your understanding of what might get in the way of hearing exactly what is required in a health and social care setting will assist you in responding effectively. Activity Two is designed to make you think about your own listening skills and to reflect on what you might do differently to develop a professional and proactive approach.

MOMENT OF REFLECTION

Activity Two

What kind of a listener are you?

Reflect upon whether you think you are a good listener:

- What do you do that is effective?
- What do you do that could be improved?

Make a list of professional roles in health and social care where listening skills are particularly important.

Think of a scenario in which you have been personally involved in which active listening skills were important.

The above activities are aimed to develop your thinking around the necessary skills required in health and social care roles. These activities will have ideally identified the significance of communication in the process of developing your range of skills. Moss (2008: 5) discusses the significance of skill development for 'people-workers' and identifies the importance of skill levels. He cites Trevithick (2005: 65) in the discussion of the journey from basic, intermediate to advanced skills for health and social care workers. This development is a process and will include the development of basic skills in communication to the more advanced skills of developing professional confidence and competence to work closely with patients and service users. Feedback from role-play and group activities is an essential component of this process. Useful guidelines are offered by Pendleton and Hasler (1983) to develop feedback processes. These are cited by Moss (2008: 113) as:

1   When the interview is finished, the interviewer is asked to comment on what went well, followed by the role player giving their feedback.
2   The observer/trainer gives feedback with examples of what went well.
3   Next, the interviewer has the opportunity to suggest what might have been done differently.
4   The role player makes suggestions about what might have been more helpful responses to the scenario.
5   The observer/trainer then can add comments about how things might have been handled differently.
6   Finally, with the role player coming out of role, the concluding discussion can highlight learning points that have been identified. These points need to be specific and detailed so that the interviewer can use the feedback to improve on specific aspects of their performance.

It is the ability to reflect closely on performance in such activities that allows the participants to develop their learning and progress their skills through the skill levels discussed above. Close attention to interpersonal skills is an essential requirement for students of health and social care as is a direct, honest and supportive level of feedback.

CENTRAL TENETS OF COMMUNICATION

At its most simple, communication is a transmission between sender and recipient which was the focus of early work by Cherry (1961). Within the context of health and social care, the aim of the interaction is to provide a safe environment for the patient or service user to explore issues they bring to the meeting and to provide appropriate information and emotional support. Service delivery hence aims to maximise patient or service user health and well-being.

MOMENT OF REFLECTION

Activity Three: Communication

Think about the last time you visited a health professional, maybe your GP or practice nurse. What do you remember about the visit? What aspects of communication were important? Was the meeting useful? What was missing from the interaction? Did you come away satisfied with the outcome?

The central tenets of communication include non-verbal communication, para-verbal communication, verbal communication and listening skills. Try applying these aspects of communication to understand the activity you considered in Activity Three (above):

- *Non-verbal (body language).* Think about appearance, eye contact, facial expressions, proximity posture, personal space, and touch.
- *Para-verbal (accompaniments to speech which give emphasis).* Think about hand gestures, facial expressions, tone of voice, speed of conversation, volume and clarity of speech.
- *Verbal (the spoken word).* Think about the language that was used, was it technical or delivered to clarify your understanding?
- *The ability to offer active and empathic listening.* Did the health and social care professional pay close attention to your concerns? Did s/he understand your concerns? Did you feel listened to? Did you leave the meeting with a clear understanding of future options?

Kadushin and Kadushin (1997) offer a further definition of communication as 'the sharing of thoughts, feelings, attitudes and ideas through the exchange of verbal and non-verbal symbols. We share our private thoughts and feelings with others through communication'.

This definition offers an insight into the intricate mix of thoughts and feelings that are conveyed in communication both verbally and non-verbally. Trevithick (2005: 8) goes further by highlighting the relationship between communication and professional practice:

As human beings we are, in fact, always communicating something, although this may not be intelligible to ourselves or to others. It may require some deciphering, which can be likened to learning a different language or, more precisely, a new dialect. As practitioners, to achieve an understanding about what is being communicated means using everything at our disposal in order to come alongside the experiences of the people with whom we work. From this perspective, I do not believe that it is possible to be an effective practitioner without being an effective communicator.

BARRIERS TO COMMUNICATION

When there is a disparity between a verbal and non-verbal message, the non-verbal message is more likely to be believed in a health and social care interaction. If a service user misinterprets the meaning of a verbal communication, miscommunication occurs with the result that s/he can be left unsure of the outcome of the interaction. As a result, especially within the field of health and social care, miscommunication can be more damaging than no communication.

MOMENT OF REFLECTION

Activity Four: Barriers to communication

Think back to the meeting you reflected on in Activity Three above. Do you recall any barriers to communication between the health and social care professional and yourself? Thinking more widely, what other barriers do you see to communication in health and social care settings?

Table 2.1 offers some examples of barriers to communication. When reviewing Activity Four check against these barriers to clarify your understanding of how miscommunication can occur in a health and social care setting.

Table 2.1 Barriers to communication in health and social care interactions

PRACTITIONER	COMMUNICATION	SERVICE USER
	PHYSICAL (hearing, sight, comprehension)	
	PSYCHOLOGICAL (state of mind, status differential)	
	CULTURAL (class, gender, race, ethnicity, age, sexuality, identity, beliefs and values)	
	LANGUAGE (difference to meaning, interpretation, values)	
	ENVIRONMENT (noise, setting, seating arrangements)	

Within a multicultural context, health and social care practitioners need to pay very close attention to intercultural communication. Language and the use of language can be problematic between people of different ethnic backgrounds. This can lead to significant misunderstandings around terminology and the meaning to phrases that are used in the health and social care interaction. Where service delivery is in English and the service user does not speak or has minimal English ability, the use of a translator is invariably necessary. There is, however, a strong case for the provision of health and social care services in the mother-tongue for non-English speaking service users, which inevitably requires the recruitment of non-English speaking practitioners where necessary.

ETHICS AND VALUES AND ANTI-OPPRESSIVE PRACTICE

Ethics and values are central to health and social care theory, practice and communication. A person's value base can facilitate effective communication or act as a barrier to communication. Ethics are coherent bodies of ideas that deal with morals (distinguishing between right and wrong) and are often seen as moral philosophy. This is the systematic study of ethical principles that can form 'schools' or traditions, such as Marxist or feminist ethics. Values are more personal in nature and include what individuals or groups see as having moral worth and value and what we choose to see as ethically relevant or worthy. For example, religion, spirituality and culture are all social areas of people's lives that are significant and inform their moral, ethical and value perspective. Values are 'a set of fundamental moral/ethical principles' to which workers 'are/should be committed' (Banks 1995: 4). These fundamental moral principles form the basis of professional codes of conduct or practice.

DEVELOPING ANTI-OPPRESSIVE PRACTICE

'In order for the oppressed to be able to wage the struggle for their liberation they must perceive the reality of oppression, not as a closed world from which there is no exit, but as a limited situation which they can transform' (Freire 1972: 14).

For the student or professional working and studying in health and social care there is a need for individuals, groups and organisations to work in ways that are anti-discriminatory. Anti-discriminatory practice is an approach to practice which recognises the pervasiveness of discrimination and oppression. As such, it is practice that needs to ensure discrimination and oppressions are, first, taken into consideration, and second, countered and challenged. Commentators such as Thompson and Mullender (2004) have suggested that anti-discriminatory practice is work that is designed to address specific, legally defined injustice and inequalities. The difficulty of this type of practice is that it is narrow and legal in its focus. Therefore, the preferred term, in theory and practice is anti-oppressive practice. This type of practice is health and social care work that involves a wider social analysis. It attempts to challenge structures and aids people in challenging oppression. Communication is a central process in developing this type of practice, to allow individuals and groups to express and say what difficulties they are having and to have effective communication between people to address these forms of oppression.

Anti-discriminatory and anti-oppressive practice are aimed at challenging inequalities and injustices but also at combating prejudice, stereotypes, discrimination and oppression. These processes have real consequences and effects on oppressed groups. For example, Dominelli (2002) suggests privileges, socio-economic discrimination, isolation and intimidation, verbal threats and emotional abuse, sexual abuse and physical assaults, attacks on children, political marginalisation, and cultural betterment are all consequences for groups and individuals on the receiving end of inequalities, discrimination and oppression. Health and social care planning are a fundamental way to challenge oppressive practices and conditions and being able to communicate in effective and accessible ways is a central element to this process. Clear communication is a central element to health and social care planning.

HEALTH AND SOCIAL CARE PLANNING – APPROACHES TO CARE

Working with people who are vulnerable because of health or social circumstances can be a very time consuming and emotionally draining experience. Professionals who work with service users and carers often find they have less time than they need to develop an effective and positive professional relationship.

Despite this problem there are ways of becoming more efficient when planning care with people. The basis of this chapter is all about the need to recognise your skills and use them effectively. Part of the process of planning care involves interviewing the person or people involved in any given situation. To be able to get the most from this arrangement a professional needs to understand the process and the skills they may need for each individual involved.

The goals of any interview are to be:

- objective
- relevant
- prepared.

However, any professional should be critical and ask questions of the techniques they use, such as should we be objective? The person's life is subjective. Decisions need to be made about when it is appropriate to be either objective or subjective (if this is even possible). Alternatively, both can be used interchangeably. The professional evidence based knowledge applied to a subjective situation is the most appropriate approach to planning.

The interview needs to be planned by setting goals of achievement, asking the right questions to gain the information needed. Prevention of repetition by many different professionals is important to avoid too much pressure on the service user. Therefore clear guidance within the team should outline what each professional is dealing with.

During the process Thompson (2003: 120) discusses planning, engaging, responding and ending as a useful structure to plan any interaction with service users. This offers a clear aim to the discussion, an accommodating, empathic and clarifying interview which has clear boundaries and structures.

Moss (2008) discusses active listening as key to any relationship development and the method by which everything that each person has said is received and understood. Other areas identified as useful here are summarising, paraphrasing and clarifying. 'Summarising' helps check the pace of the interview and demonstrates you are listening. 'Paraphrasing' can be used to provide a narrower focus on a particular issue which means that the relationship can be developed with particular priorities, etc. 'Clarifying' helps people to establish what they are trying to say by positively reinforcing their comments and asking them to clarify certain points.

Lishman (2009) offers some useful evaluation of research which identifies helpful and effective communication. SCIE (2004) cited in Lishman (2009: 19) identified a summary of skills that service users want from social workers as follows:

- physically and emotionally available
- supportive, encouraging and reassuring
- respectful
- patient and attentive

- committed to the independence of the individual
- punctual
- trustworthy
- reliable
- friendly but not frightened to tell people how they see things
- empathic and warm.

Therapeutic interviewing skills are key communication skills which are used in many different ways with individuals and can be seen as relative to each situation. However, there are certain common skills which help verbal and non-verbal communication. When using these skills the professional needs to be aware of issues which may impact on the usefulness of the technique used. For example cultural issues, language, age, physical and mental ability, values and attitudes often influence the interview and will have an effect on the outcomes. Allen and Langford (2008) identify accessible language, anti-discriminatory language and special needs communication skills. This combination of skills ensures that these issues are actively acknowledged and dealt with.

The need to be prepared for adaptability within the moment is a key skill.

Therapeutic skills involve:

- *Using silence* which allows time to collect thoughts.
- *Accepting what the person says* indicates understanding.
- *Making observations* encourages examination of behaviour as a means of exploring feelings.
- *Encouraging descriptions of perceptions* increases understanding.
- *Focusing* concentrates on a key issue.
- *Exploring* examines that issue more closely.
- *Reflecting* empowers the service user to make their own choices.
- *Active listening* provides a confirming and definite basis for a relationship.
- *Validation* acknowledges loss or distress whilst continuing to explore.

Non-therapeutic skills involve:

- *reassuring*
- *giving approval*
- *disagreeing*
- *disapproving*.

All of these non-therapeutic actions can take control of emotions and conversation away from the service user. This means that the discussion is guided by the professional's value base only, which can result in demoralising and demeaning behaviour.

Watkins (2001) identifies the need to use a person centred approach in gathering information to ensure understanding about a client's inner and outer worlds, from their own reference. This humanistic philosophical approach allows an ongoing process of understanding a person's despair on their terms. Helping them to explore this encourages a focus on strengths rather than just problems. It also highlights the benefits of learning to live with the problems and encourages clients to consider the connections between feelings and actions.

The interview is the basis of any communications between service user, client, carer and professional. This offers a beginning for an assessment and a plan which will only be useful if the interview is effective.

MODELS OF ASSESSMENT

In the world of health and social care there are many forms of assessment. Areas of practice will usually have developed these to the needs of the service users they work with. The standard format of models ranges from very generalised to very specific and tends to be used as a basis for the interview rather than a formal structure. Downs and Bowers (2008) identify best practice in assessment as finding clarity of its purpose. They go on to describe key questions that should be asked and situations to be prepared for when assessing someone with a dementia type illness. The priorities of what information is needed will vary depending on whether the person is in a social or hospital situation. The plan and interview will also be different from someone who has heart disease or is homeless for example.

The most useful models are those which are integrative and therefore result in the least distortion of the facts. So, how do professionals decide which model of care to follow? Usually, this is about traditional approaches and perspectives of the profession you are in. For example, the medical model is dominant in health care and the social care model is dominant in social care. Specialities are developed along specific routes in line with this and practice frameworks developed accordingly.

Effectively a model of care is whatever it needs to be, based on evidence, theoretical backgrounds and client needs. However, this is also influenced by organisational structures, finances, traditions, professional priorities and accountability and legislation.

Using a model can organise our thinking in a way which can then be translated into measurable, accountable practice (Payne *et al.* 2007). The author goes on to say that not using a model can lead to unfocused, biased and prejudiced non-accountable practice.

The professional must have a philosophical approach which is then translated into a model of care. This is based on evidence of needs rather than anecdotal approaches. An evidence base offers an educated approach which has a wealth of theory and research and can in turn be tailored and adapted to meet individual needs. This is in contrast to an individual approach with no idea of potential benefits of treatments and side effects, care strategies or services. However, using a strict philosophical and model based approach can lead to a lack of adaptability or flexibility when working with individuals or other professionals.

Working with models involves collaboration with all parties, service users, carer(s) and fellow professionals. This is a necessary aspect of care generally and it has ethical implications as well as legal obligations in duty of care. Organisations such as Connexions, community health and social care teams, specialist housing, combined education, specialist roles, health and social care professionals in prisons, schools and offender rehabilitation schemes are all examples of newly formed structures which combine disciplines and service users in their practice.

PHILOSOPHICAL MODELS OF HEALTH AND SOCIAL CARE

There are three main models of health and social care: biomedical, humanistic and social/environmental. In the biomedical model science underpins research based treatments. All problems of behaviour and ultimately society can be explained by the biological functioning of an individual. For example, illness can be explained by changes in physical functioning. The humanistic model builds on existential sociology and the acceptance that there is much more to people than biology. The view is that there are many explanations for behaviour and that science cannot be seen as the only relevant knowledge. Person centred care is borne of this philosophy as it concentrates on the person's own interpretation of the problems they have. The social/environmental model also assumes that there is more than biology to account for behaviours/illness and well-being. The effects of personal environments and socio-economic factors are the key issues.

These models offer professionals a basis for their approach. They are a philosophical standpoint which encourages the person to be responsible for their actions and decisions made with and about service users. Ethically and legally it is essential to have in-depth understanding and comprehension of why and what you believe. Otherwise service users are vulnerable to the values of anyone, right or wrong. They also mean the professional can see the bigger picture and the wider context of the infinitely complex combination of relationships, needs and desires. This opens up flexibility of the service to accommodate people more openly. The development of a value base is an inevitable part of human function and thought. Without the philosophical evidence based approach identified here there is a risk of being limited to internal and parochial perspectives and limiting effective communication when working with people. The use of the models varies between disciplines and therefore it is essential to be aware of the people and skills involved in the situation. Collaboration and teamwork are the next step in learning to use these skills effectively.

TEAMWORK

Working as part of a team is an essential requirement in health and social care settings. Although you may find yourself working in a one-to-one capacity with patients or service users, you will undoubtedly be part of a wider team, very usually a multidisciplinary team, that is, involving professionals from different occupational backgrounds. Students in health and social care will find ample opportunity to develop these skills, but to learn from the process requires careful evaluation and reflection. These activities contribute to greater self-awareness of how you respond in a professional setting.

A team is essentially a group of members who work together on a defined task(s), with a defined goal(s) in mind. This may sound straightforward, when in fact the opposite can hold true when working with people. Levin (2005) distinguishes between groups and teams and suggests that teams are not developed until relationships have developed enough to operate on a professional level. Common obstacles include personality clashes, a battle for leadership, and historical tensions which have a habit of reappearing when a task is faced. Such is the challenge of working in teams.

As discussed above, a central tenet in health and social care interactions is that of communication and this is no less significant in teamwork. Without effective communication, working relationships will fail to develop and teamwork is likely to be unproductive. An understanding of the way in which a team (or group) develops, and of the way in which things can go wrong, is essential for students of health and social care.

Tuckman (1965) described the four distinct stages that a group experiences as it comes together and starts to operate. His focus was primarily aimed at educational groups but his model can be usefully applied to health and social care settings. This process can be subconscious, although an understanding of the stages can help a team to operate more effectively.

Stage 1: Forming

Individual behaviour is driven by a desire to be accepted by the others, and avoid controversy or conflict. Serious issues and feelings are avoided, and people focus on being busy with routines, such as team organisation, who does what, when to meet, etc. But individuals are also gathering information and impressions – about each other, and about the scope of the task and how to approach it. This is a comfortable stage to be in, but the avoidance of conflict and threat means that not much is achieved at this stage.

Stage 2: Storming

Individuals in the group can only remain nice to each other for so long, as important issues start to be addressed. Some people's patience will break early, and minor confrontations will arise that are quickly dealt with or glossed over. These may relate to the work of the group itself, or to roles and responsibilities within the group. Some will observe that it's good to be getting into the real issues, whilst others will wish to remain in the comfort and security of Stage 1. Depending on the culture of the organisation and individuals, the conflict will be more or less suppressed, but it will be there, under the surface. To deal with the conflict, individuals may feel they are winning or losing battles, and will look for structural clarity and rules to prevent the conflict persisting.

Stage 3: Norming

As Stage 2 evolves, the 'rules of engagement' for the group become established, and the scope of the group's tasks or responsibilities is clear and agreed. Having had their arguments, they now understand each other better, and can appreciate each other's skills and experience. Individuals listen to each other, appreciate and support each other, and are prepared to change preconceived views – they feel they are part of a cohesive, effective group. However, individuals have had to work hard to attain this stage, and may resist any pressure to change – especially from the outside – for fear that the group will break up, or revert to a storm.

Stage 4: Performing

Not all groups reach this stage, characterised by a state of interdependence and flexibility. Everyone knows each other well enough to be able to work together, and trusts each other enough to allow independent activity. Roles and responsibilities change according to need in an almost seamless way. Group identity, loyalty and morale are all high, and everyone is equally task orientated and people orientated. This high degree of comfort means that all the energy of the group can be directed towards the task(s) in hand.

Tuckman revisited this developmental model in 1975 and added a further stage to the process. This he called 'adjourning'.

Stage 5: Adjourning

This is about completion and disengagement, both from the tasks and the group members. Individuals will be proud of having achieved much and glad to have been part of the group experience. They need to recognise what they have achieved, and consciously move on. Stage 5 has also been described as 'Deforming and mourning', recognising the sense of loss felt by group members.

Tuckman's original work simply described the way he had observed groups evolve, whether they were conscious of it or not. The significance of this model for health and social care professionals is in recognising where a team is in the process, and helping it to move to the Perform stage. In organisational settings, groups are often forming and changing, and each time that happens, they can move to a different Tuckman stage. A group might be happily 'Norming' or 'Performing' but a new team member might force them back into Storming. Seasoned leaders will be ready for this, and will help the group get back to Performing as quickly as possible. Many work groups live in the comfort of 'Norming' and are fearful of moving back into 'Storming', or forward into 'Performing'. This will govern their behaviour towards each other, and especially their reaction to change.

MOMENT OF REFLECTION

Activity Five: Observing team processes

You can apply this activity to either a workplace experience, or perhaps a seminar group or teamwork exercise in which you have been involved. Choose an experience which is clear in your mind and try to recognise whether the team or group has touched upon the stages identified by Tuckman.

What insight does this give you about performing effectively in teams within a health and social care setting? What insights have you gained about how you work as part of a team?

Individuals will take on different roles within a team activity, and it is worth being mindful and observant about the role which you and others may take. In the 1970s, Belbin and his research team focused on team observation, with a view to finding out where and how these differences come about. They wanted to control the dynamics of teams to discover if and how problems could be pre-empted and avoided. Using psychometric tests, the behaviour and personality of individuals were studied closely. Team success was found to depend more on behaviour than intellect or personality. Belbin (1993) offered nine specific roles which he cites as contributing to effective team work.

Table 2.2 Belbin's team roles

PLANT an individual who generates ideas
SHAPER an individual who motivates others
MONITOR EVALUATOR an individual who can make decisions
COORDINATOR an individual who is able to coordinate the group
IMPLEMENTER an individual who implements decisions
COMPLETER-FINISHER an individual who has the ability to bring a decision-making process to a close
SPECIALIST an individual who offers specialist knowledge
TEAMWORKER an individual who is committed to the team endeavour
RESOURCE INVESTIGATOR an individual who carries out background research

Adapted from Belbin (1993)

Although Belbin's team roles are useful in assisting you to understand the dynamics of teamwork, it is possible that not all roles may be present in any teamwork that you do. It is also worth noting that these roles may not be mutually exclusive and that in fact you may find yourself carrying out more than one role in team activities you are asked to participate in.

THE SIGNIFICANCE OF SELF-AWARENESS

The exercises throughout this chapter have been designed to help you to focus on your self-awareness as a student of health and social care. As health and social care interactions require activities such as assessment, professional judgement and communication, for example assisting to explain medical terminology, at the centre of the interaction between service user and health and social care professional is the need to be acutely aware of the impact you are making in any given scenario.

Practitioner self-awareness is hence central to this process. Dryden (2007: 114) highlights the significance of practitioner self-awareness. Here he is talking about the qualities of effective therapists but the same is true for any health and social care professional: 'self-awareness combined with empathy are the key to effective [therapeutic] intervention'. On a similar theme, Johns (2004) introduces the significance of knowing and managing the self in professional relationships. It is this ability to reflect and develop a sense of self in health and social care scenarios that will contribute towards effective professional practice. If the practitioner responds without a sense of awareness there is the potential to distort the outcome of the health and social care interaction. This is particularly the case where the professional is not fully aware of how personal material might distort the outcome of the interaction. For example, in a scenario where a helper is supporting a victim of domestic abuse but has personal unresolved issues in relation to a personal relationship, it is possible that the outcome of the intervention may be distorted for the service user should the helper fail to bring self-awareness to the interaction.

As a student of health and social care, you will face many challenging scenarios and situations, many of which may resonate with your personal material. The argument for developing self-awareness is central to developing professional competence which will offer the service user an ethical and effective response.

TECHNIQUES FOR WORKING WITH PEOPLE

There are a range of key skills when working with people. These require knowledge, understanding, and practice to allow students or workers to act professionally with each other and service users.

Egan (1994) in the 'The Microskills of Attending' suggests SOLER is a useful, practical way of being able to demonstrate an engaged internal attitude towards a service user reflected in non-verbal communication.

S   *Face the service user squarely*. Posture is an important part of engaging with people and can give a clear message that we are interested by focusing on the individual interaction (Thompson 2006: 137).

O   *Adopt an open posture*. This gives a clear message that we are not defensive or 'closed', not crossing legs and arms and adopting an open physical position.

L   *Lean forwards*. Leaning forward is a way of showing interest and engagement although ensuring we do not invade someone's personal space.

E   *Maintain eye contact*. Engaged and balanced eye contact rather than constant or staring eye contact establishes interest and concentration.

R   *Try to be relaxed*. Thompson (2006: 138) suggests this is to give the message that you are here to help and can be relied upon so that you are not fidgeting or nervous.

These are simple techniques that need practice and sophistication when working with people. They also need a degree of cultural sensitivity to be used in multicultural and transcultural settings. Working with a diverse range of people also demands a degree of sensitivity to issues of diversity such as class, gender, age, and sexuality.

SARAH (like SOLER) is a tool designed to help people cope with raised levels of emotion. It should help deal with emotional intensity and is presented in a useful, structured way to try and make sure that you respond in a positive and helpful manner. Lambert (1996: 36) suggests 'when things start to go off the rails and signs of roused emotion appear, think SARAH'.

S   *Stop talking*. This emphasises the importance of *listening*. Thompson (2006: 131) suggests if someone is becoming agitated, carrying on talking can make a situation worse, whereas if we show we are listening it can calm someone down by taking seriously the concerns being expressed.

A   *Active listening*. We need to show we are listening actively by nodding our head, giving positive non-verbal feedback and 'attending' to the person (Thompson 2006: 131).

R   *Reflect content or feeling.* Do this by feeding back understanding of the situation, for example by paraphrasing key points and making clear you have understood the issues raised. Thompson (2006: 132) suggests using neutral comments such as 'I can understand why you might be annoyed by this situation but …' is helpful by not adding any judgment to the situation of saying something is good or bad, but showing you are reflecting how the person feels.

A   *Act with empathy.* Empathy is recognising and acknowledging someone's feelings without necessarily feeling them yourself. It is not about sympathy or sharing feelings with someone (Thompson 2006: 132). Sympathy can lead to burn-out, being overloaded, and intensifying feelings. Empathy allows a certain distance to understand feelings but not colluding.

H   *Handle objections.* Lambert (1996: 132) suggests we should listen, reason and deal with any objections raised and allow the service user to do this same process. Trying to second guess what a service user is thinking is often very difficult and can remove the idea that you were listening to them in the first place.

This form of SARAH intervention is useful in a wider range of contexts when working with people. Practice and planning this technique provides a platform for skills development leading to greater levels of confidence for students and those working with people. Thompson (2006: 133) suggests the person that can 'weather the storm of high emotions' can win respect, trust and professional confidence.

Thompson (2006: 65, 114) adds two more useful dimensions to working with people where the situation might become heated. These are the RED approach and the idea of 'elegant challenging'.

The RED approach involves three dimensions:

R   *Recognise conflict.* This addresses avoiding conflict, ignoring it or brushing it under the carpet. It also brings conflict and disagreement into the open as part of working with people so you can address difficult situations.

E   *Evaluate conflict.* This allows us to weigh up difficulties to address the ones that could get worse or that need tackling. This involves a degree of judgment that develops over time with practice.

D   *Deal with conflict.* This allows us to decide how best to deal with conflict and hopefully resolve it with open and clear communication. Thompson (2006: 115) suggests this avoids the 'ostrich' approach of ignoring conflict and the 'sledge-hammer to crack a nut' approach of inappropriate action to tackle minor issues.

Finally, Thompson (2006: 65) provides a helpful and useful way of addressing conflict and difficulties that can arise when working with people. He suggests being constructive in challenging unacceptable behaviour or language can be achieved through 'elegant challenging'. There are two poles to this process, on the one hand collusion or not challenging conflict, on the other 'aggressive challenging'. What we should try and achieve is a balance of a sophisticated, well thought out, and helpful challenge. This allows us to challenge difficult subjects or issues in a constructive and supportive way.

Thompson (2006: 139) suggests there are three stages to developing our interpersonal skills when working with people. The first is when we feel nervous and unconfident and show it in various ways. The second stage is when we still feel nervous but are able to manage it or not show it so readily. The third stage is when we are sufficiently experienced and confident that we no longer feel nervous but are able to engage in working with people. Being reflective on these techniques allows professional and confident interpersonal skills.

CONCLUSION

This chapter has discussed the significance of the development of interpersonal skills for students and workers of health and social care. The awareness and skills development necessary are of central importance to your learning, work and attitudes, values, self-awareness and skills development in a health and social care setting. The chapter considered the relevant theoretical understanding necessary to inform this process, communication theory, health care planning, models of assessment and health and social care, teamwork and techniques of communication and the significance of self-awareness in working with people in health and social care settings.

CASE STUDIES

Case study One

A research study group intends to interview and assess glaucoma patients with a view to determining appropriate community support needs.

Which assessment model would adequately determine patient needs?

Case study Two

The number of people who consult their GP with flu-like illness during the winter varies considerably from year to year (usually the figure is between 50 and 200 for every 100,000 of the population). What measures might a Primary Care Trust consider in assessing patient needs to control the incidence of influenza? How might any recommendations be implemented?

Case study Three

Clifton takes his son Alex to the local GP surgery as he has been complaining of 'tummy ache' and has been off his food.

Alex is given an appointment with Dr Ahmed.

What kind of assessment would most usefully assist to offer Clifton some peace of mind and help Alex to feel better?

SUMMARY OF MAIN POINTS

You should be able to:

- Have an awareness of working with people in a health and social care environment.
- Understand interpersonal skills in an applied setting.
- Understand models and philosophical models of health and social care.
- Describe the issues that affect communication and explain why those issues should be addressed.

REFERENCES

Allen, G. and Langford, D. (2008) *Effective Interviewing in Social Work and Social Care: A practical guide*, Hampshire: Palgrave Macmillan.

Banks, S. (1995) *Ethics and Values in Social Work*, Basingstoke: Macmillan.

Belbin, R.M. (1993) *Team Roles at Work*, London: Butterworth Heinemann.

Burnard, P. (1997) *Effective Communication Skills for Health Professionals*, London: Nelson Thornes.

Cherry, C. (1961) *On Human Communication*, New York: Science Editions.

Dominelli, L. (2002) *Anti-Oppressive Social Work Theory and Practice*, Basingstoke: Macmillan.

Downs, M. and Bowers, B. (2008) *Excellence in Dementia Care; Research into Practice*, Berkshire: Open University Press.

Dryden, W. (2007) (5th edition) *Dryden's Handbook of Individual Therapy*, London: Sage.

Egan, G. (1994) (5th edition) *The Skilled Helper: A Problem-Management Approach to Helping*, Pacific Grove, CA: Brooks/Cole.

Fisher, S.G., Hunter, T.A. and Macrosson, W.D.K. (1998), The structure of Belbin's team roles, *Journal of Occupational and Organizational Psychology*, 71, 283–8.

Freire, P. (1972) *Pedagogy of the Oppressed*, Harmondsworth: Penguin.

Johns, C. (2004) (2nd edition) *Becoming a Reflective Practitioner*, Oxford: Blackwell.

Kadushin, A. and Kadushin, G. (1997) (4th edition) *The Social Work Interview*, New York: Columbia University Press.

Lambert, T. (1996) *Key Management Solutions*, London: Pitman.

Levin, P. (2005) *Successful Teamwork*, Maidenhead: Open University Press.

Lishman, J. (2009) (2nd edition) *Communication in Social Work*, Basingstoke: Palgrave Macmillan.

Moss, B. (2008) *Communication Skills for Health and Social Care*, London: Sage.

Payne, M., Moss, B., Adams, R., Oko, J. and Jackson, M. (2007) Part Two 'Contexts for practice' in Adams, R. (2007) *Foundations of Health and Social Care*, Hampshire: Palgrave Macmillan.

Pendleton, D. and Hasler, J. (1983) *Doctor–patient Communication*, London: Academic Press.

Thompson, N. (2003) *Communication and Language: A handbook of theory and practice*, Basingstoke: Palgrave Macmillan.

Thompson, N. (2006) *People Problems*, Basingstoke: Macmillan.

Thompson, N. and Mullender, A. (2004) *Promoting Equality: Challenging Discrimination and Oppression*, Basingstoke: Palgrave.

Trevithick, P. (2005) (2nd edition) *Social Work Skills: A Practice Handbook*, Maidenhead: Open University Press.

Tuckman, B.W. (1965) Developmental sequence in small groups, *Psychological Bulletin*, 63, 384–99.

Tuckman, B.W. (1975) *Measuring Educational Outcomes*, New York: Harcourt Brace Jovanovitch.

Watkins (2001) *Mental Health Nursing: The art of compassionate care*, Oxford: Butterworth-Heinemann.

FURTHER READING

Argyle, M. (1994) *The Psychology of Interpersonal Behaviour*, London: Penguin.

Guirdham, M. (1990) *Interpersonal Skills at Work*, London: Prentice Hall.

Hargie, O. (Ed.) (2003) *Skilled Interpersonal Communication: Research, Theory & Practice*, London: Routledge.

Hartley, P. (1999) *Interpersonal Communication*, London: Routledge.

Hayes, J. (2002) *Interpersonal Skills at Work*, London: Routledge.

Keats, D. (2000) *Interviewing: a practical guide for students and professionals*, Buckingham: Open University Press.

Thompson, N. (2002) (2nd edition) *People Skills*, Basingstoke: Palgrave Macmillan.

CHAPTER 3

THE INDIVIDUAL IN SOCIETY

BARBARA COULSON AND BRIDGET HALLAM

OBJECTIVES

After reading this chapter you should be able to:

- Explain a number of key sociological and developmental theories and concepts.

- Identify some of the changes that take place in the sequence of growth, development and ageing through the life course.

- Recognize environmental, social and psychological factors that may affect service users' lives and their need for specific health and social care services.

- Understand the impact of life events on growth, development and socialization.

After reading this chapter you will know the meaning of the following terms: Life transitions, gender, ethnicity, disability, prenatal, early years, teenagers, adolescence, adulthood.

There are three Moments of Reflection to work on throughout the chapter.

INTRODUCTION

An understanding of how human beings grow and change over their lives is fundamental to effective work with users of health and social care services. This chapter aims to provide you with an introduction to some of the physical, psychological, emotional and social changes that people experience during their lifespan and the factors that affect those changes. Aspects of biology, psychology, education and sociology will all help to inform our discussion. It is easy to think of human growth and development as something that only happens internally and on an individual basis but of course this is not the case. External factors, such as the society in which individuals live, the opportunities they have and the difficulties specific groups may encounter, have a massive impact on people's lives. Taking this into account we also explore some key sociological themes and perspectives that help to set individual development in its wider context – hence the title of this chapter – 'The individual in society'.

Any exploration of human growth and development has to take into account the historical, cultural and sociological context. The experience of childhood in 2010 would be unrecognizable to children working in domestic service, factories or farms at the beginning of the twentieth century. Similarly, the transition to adulthood of a young person from a traditional Muslim family may be very different from that of a young person who has been brought up in a family without religious beliefs. Old age living on benefits in the United Kingdom will not have the same impact on the individual as old age cushioned by savings and a good pension. It is important to remember that these contexts will shape the way in which changes take place and are experienced throughout people's lives. Further discussion of sociological themes such as gender, race and ethnicity, sexuality and age can be found in Chapter 4, Concepts of equality and diversity. Here we will focus more on perspectives relating to the life course.

A sociological approach can not only help us to understand the context within which individuals develop; it can also help to explain some of the problems encountered in health and social care work, such as domestic violence, youth crime and eating disorders. Seeing incidents as part of a bigger picture informs practice and stops us from blaming individuals, instead encouraging us to help people to find ways to challenge their situations (Cree 2000).

As you read you are encouraged to reflect on your own life, transitions you have made and the individual and wider social factors that have been significant in moulding you into the person you are.

TRANSITIONS

The term 'transition' has been mentioned twice in the previous section but what does it mean and why are transitions important when thinking about how individuals develop? All lives contain periods of rapid growth, change and disruption or imbalance. These are often known as transitions and can be related to physiological changes, role changes or specific rites of passage dependent on the society and culture in which the individual lives. Transitions tend to be followed by periods of relative calm – consolidation where the individual has a chance to adapt to the changes they have experienced. If mapped out on paper an individual's life might look like a range of mountains with peaks and troughs interspersed with rolling foothills of calm.

MOMENT OF REFLECTION

Activity One

Reflect on the transitions that have occurred in your life so far. Draw a map or picture to trace the changes (highs, lows and periods of calm). What does your individual map suggest to you about the factors that influence the way individuals experience the transitions they go through?

COMMENTARY

Your transition map will be unique to you. It might include a number of transitions experienced by many other people but none of those people will have experienced their transitions in exactly the same way that you have. For some individuals a biological and psychological transition such as adolescence might have been a period of turmoil and anxiety whereas others might have found it an exciting period offering new opportunities. This will be the same for any significant changes in life whether this is starting school, becoming a parent or experiencing a significant loss. The way you manage those transitions will be dependent on a whole range of factors including your physical health, personality, family and cultural background as well as your personal and social circumstances at the time of the transition.

This suggests then that individual development, and in effect who we become, is dependent on a mixture of innate characteristics (nature) and environmental influences (nurture). The nature/nurture debate is not new; for centuries philosophers, scientists and sociologists have been debating the relative contributions made by our genetic makeup and our environments (*see* Anastasi and Foley 1948).

THE ROLE OF THEORIES TO INFORM PRACTICE

Theories connect facts and observations and provide a framework to support our understanding. They are important in health and social care because they can provide a rationale for the actions we take, inform contacts with service users, help our understanding of behaviour and support the development of effective practice. Single theories are unlikely to provide the whole explanation in any given situation because they are to some extent based on generalizations and it is always possible to find exceptions to the rule – those situations where the theory does not seem to fit.

It is important that you question and critique different theories in order to get the full picture. Think of them as a toolkit from which you can pick and choose those that seem most effective to help you get the job done effectively. Equally, theories do not come without bias. Remember they are developed by people whose thinking will inevitably be influenced by factors such as the society and time in which they live, their age, gender, race and culture.

Sociological theories

Traditional sociology uses a distinction between what are called 'consensus' and 'conflict' theories. The difference between these two approaches is a bit like belonging to a political group. If you see society through one perspective or the other, your interpretation of what you see and the solutions you think will help are geared towards your favoured approach. Thus consensus sociologists see society with a rosy glow in terms of united endeavours towards a benevolent system. Solutions tend to focus on individuals changing their behaviour to 'fit' better into existing social structures.

Conflict theorists however see society as a competitive forum where different groups vie for scarce resources and the underdog suffers. Solutions demand radical social change to equalize power relations. Consensus theories are generally conflated into analyses of functionalism and conflict theories are most often demonstrated by Marxist and feminist perspectives. You will find descriptions and analyses of consensus and conflict theories in all the major sociology textbooks, particularly Giddens (2009), Haralambos et al. (2008) or Marsh et al. (2009).

Although consensus and conflict theorists see society in vastly different ways, they share what is called a structural or 'macro' view of society. That means their analysis is based on the way that society is structured. On the other hand there is another set of sociological theorists who have a smaller scale focus and believe that society is made up of individual actions and behaviour. Some of those who favour this 'micro' approach include G. H. Mead, Erving Goffman and Harold Garfinkle. Again, any of the major sociological texts provide in-depth analyses of their writings (see Giddens 2009). Some texts refer to this group of theorists by different names, for example social-action, interpretive or interactionist approaches. In this chapter the term interpretive sociology is preferred. The shared ground of interpretive approaches is that they emphasize individual behaviour, the influence of others on the individual, micro-level interactions and the purpose of actions.

So, it becomes clear that there are disputes between sociologists about the nature of society, the impact of social structures and of individual behaviours. This debate will continue to run but how do these competing perspectives help health and social care workers? Professionals are usually confronted with individuals in some kind of distress about some particular aspect of their lives. What sociology can do is to enable the situation to be seen within a social context: thus the service user experiencing stress in the workplace might be seen by Marxism as being subject to exploitation; the woman abused by her husband can be seen by feminism as a victim of patriarchy/male dominance; the anorexic teenager might be asked to examine their perception of society's ideal body type.

However, although essential to our understanding, these theories alone cannot explain how an individual develops the complex range of emotions, abilities and relationships that go together to make that unique human being. For that we have to turn to the discipline of developmental psychology.

Theories of human development

Many theories of human development focus on specific aspects of development and pay less attention to the wider contexts in which development occurs. Beckett (2002) and Smith et al. (2003) provide excellent, accessible explorations of key developmental theories, their strengths and criticisms of them. These include the work of key researchers in the field such as Freud and Erikson, who focused on the development of personality and identity, and Piaget whose research informs our understanding of cognitive development. Whereas these theories tend to emphasize the impact of nature on human (and particularly child) development, theorists such as Watson, Skinner and Bandura were more concerned with the role of environmental forces in shaping behaviour – the nurture argument. Again, you will find a good overview of their ideas in Beckett (2002) and Smith *et al.* (2003).

However, there is one theory that focuses specifically on the interaction between individual and their environment: Bronfenbrenner's Ecological Systems Theory. Uri Bronfenbrenner was one of the founders of Head Start in the United States of America, the scheme upon which Sure Start is based (*see* Department for Children, Schools and Families (DCSF) 2009a). According to Bronfenbrenner the child's world is organized 'as a set of nested structures, each inside the next, like a set of Russian dolls' (1979: 22). These structures or subsystems make up the system:

- **The microsystem** incorporates the most immediate aspects of the child's life including the child itself and the family, peer group and school.
- Surrounding this, **the mesosystem** represents the relationships between the components of the microsystem. So, for example, parents interact with teachers and the school system and health care services interact both with a child's family and her school.
- Next is **the exosystem** which includes settings that impact on a child's development but with which the child has little direct contact. For example, a parent's work may affect the child's life if it requires that he or she travels a great deal or suddenly moves to shift work. If a local planning department decides to run a new road near to the local park, this could impact on the child's safety.
- **The macrosystem** consists of more remote contexts in which the child is not directly involved, such as society's culture and political and legal systems.

As with any systems theory, the argument is that these subsystems are interlinked and change in any one can lead to change in the others. The four subsystems change over time and this can alter the overall system at all levels, from microsystem to macrosystem. Over time both the child and his environment undergo change, which can originate within the individual through, for example, puberty, severe illness or in the external world. Examples of these changes could include events as disparate as the birth of a sibling, divorce of parents, winning the lottery or war.

This theory is particularly useful because it helps us to understand the complexities of the interactions between the individual and their environment which impact on development. The assessment framework, used by social workers in child care and mentioned later in this chapter, is another example of an ecological systems approach to understanding an individual child's development.

So far, the discussion has looked in general at ideas relating to sociology and human growth and development. The next sections focus on specific periods during the lifespan to highlight briefly some important aspects of development and some of the issues within sociology that can inform our understanding of individuals in society. Remember though we have already made the point that each individual is unique so there will inevitably be generalizations that do not apply to all.

THE PRENATAL PERIOD

A normal pregnancy last forty weeks and is split into three stages or trimesters:

Table 3.1 Trimesters of pregnancy

Trimester	Timespan	Details of development
1st trimester	0–12 weeks	The basic structure of the main organs, systems and body parts is completed apart from the central nervous system (CNS) which is still developing.
2nd trimester	13–24 weeks	The foetus becomes discernibly active in the womb and finer features such as fingernails, eyelashes and eyebrows develop.
3rd trimester	25–40 weeks	The baby can often survive outside the womb. Its main systems mature and there is rapid weight gain. The brain and CNS continue to develop after birth.

The majority of babies develop normally but where there are problems these may be caused by genetic errors or by external factors such as drugs, viruses or pollution that interfere with the environment in which the foetus is developing. Most developmental abnormalities arising from these causes occur in the first trimester. The mother's age, physical health and emotional state may also impact on the development of the foetus. It is important therefore that health and social care professionals encourage prospective parents to access antenatal care at an early stage and ensure that effective support systems are in place to address difficulties that could impact on the well-being of the baby and its mother. One such threat is poverty, the negative effects of which can continue to exert an influence throughout the child's life and into adulthood.

The sociological perspective – Poverty

It is not surprising that the impact of poverty is reported by a number of organizations including Save the Children, Barnado's, the Joseph Rowntree Foundation and the Child Poverty Action Group. Statistics on poverty are regularly reported in the quality press but a particularly valuable resource is the Office for National Statistics (ONS) database which can be probed at neighbourhood (post code) level for indices of deprivation. The Labour Government's ambitious *Children's Plan* (2007) aimed, amongst other things, to eradicate child poverty by 2020. The *Children's Plan* aims stem from the five outcomes of the *Every Child Matters* programme, affirmed in the Children Act 2004 in England. The five outcomes are: be healthy; stay safe; enjoy and achieve; make a positive contribution and achieve economic well-being (DCSF 2009b).

Many families are in need of services to ensure that the children are healthy and developing as they should be – this could be in connection with neglect or abuse or because the child is disabled as defined by the Children Act 1989 (Office of Public Sector Information 2009a). *Messages from Research* (Department of Health 2001), reporting on the operation of the Children Act soon after its introduction, found that poverty was a dominant feature in families in need. However, it is not true to say that all families living in poverty will need intervention. O'Loughlin and O'Loughlin (2008) discuss family support and assessment principles for children and families in need.

MOMENT OF REFLECTION

Activity Two

Find out more about levels of deprivation in your neighbourhood by typing your postcode into the Neighbourhood Statistics website and follow it up by searching your local authority website for services for children and families in the area.

THE EARLY YEARS

The first three years are probably the most rapid period of change that an individual will experience in their life. It is during this time that most of the basic elements are set in place for their future development and they develop from being a helpless infant to become a walking, talking individual capable of expressing many emotions (*see* Keenan and Evans 2009 for a clear overview of the key changes). However, babies are not 'blank slates' in terms of their development. They are born with a range of innate reflexes and perceptual skills which are refined through experience with their environment (Piaget 1952).

Central to this change are the brain and nervous system. The growth of nerve connections is very rapid indeed and by the age of two nearly all the connections are in place for any processing that may be necessary through the rest of life. Those that are used and exercised develop and those that are not die away (Shore 1997). It is therefore essential that young children are exposed to a wide range of experiences in whatever setting they are cared for and that any problems with perception or motor skills are picked up at as early a stage as possible (Dawson *et al.* 2000).

Vital to these early experiences is the presence of an attachment figure that the child can use as a safe base from which to explore their world, knowing that they are safe and that their needs will be met (Bowlby 1997). Attachment theory is explored in a later chapter but important to note here is that the formation of strong attachments in this period is crucial for future healthy development. Primary carers such as mother and father as well as other family members are key attachment figures in a young child's life but what do we mean by family? It is hard to define.

The sociological perspective – Family

Giddens (2009: 331) suggests a family is 'a group of persons directly linked by kin connections, the adult members of whom assume responsibility for caring for children'. The forms families take in the twenty-first century are now complex. Less likely to be linked by kinship ties, it might be more useful to refer to households as 'a residential group whose members usually share some basic tasks (like cooking)' (VanEvery in Marsh *et al.* 2009: 448). Dramatic changes in household composition between the early 1970s and the census in 2001 show a decrease in married couple households (from 68 per cent to 45 per cent); a threefold rise in lone parents (from 6 per cent to 19 per cent) and the beginnings of the rising trend in one person households (from 6 per cent to 16 per cent) (Marsh *et al.* 2009: 453).

A functionalist view of the family, popular in the 1950s and 1960s claimed the conventional family as the best structure to work in the modern industrial world. The family provided 'primary socialization' for children – the first place they would learn right from wrong – the rules of behaviour in that particular social culture and the expectations on girls and boys to act in certain ways. The family also provided a structure in which women and men could stabilize their identity in relationship to each other and to undertake roles to support each other and their children. According to functionalists the ideal structure involved the father being the breadwinner and the mother being available to care for the child/ren (Talcott Parsons in Giddens 2009: 834). Early attachment theories supported this view, placing women as the primary carer with little mention of the father's role in physical or emotional aspects of child rearing.

The role of women in this model was questioned by feminists who argued that the mother's role in the private sphere (the home) was assumed in society to be inferior to the father's public persona. Similarly feminists suggested that culturally accepted power relations meant women experienced lower status in the workplace and that the higher power and prestige held by men led to a social acceptance of domestic violence towards women. Although the twenty-first century household might reject both of these sociological approaches, it is easy to identify persistent inequalities in the position of men and women in society both in the home and in the workplace.

MOMENT OF REFLECTION

Activity Three

Think about how families and society are structured and ask how men and women share the breadwinning and the child care. If we lived in a society that was equal we would expect fathers to do 50 per cent of the child care and mothers to bring home 50 per cent of the salary. What are the barriers to this happening?

COMMENTARY

You might have identified full-time work; the relatively short school day; expensive housing and social stereotypes as some of the barriers. With desire for change, these could be overcome.

TODDLERS TO TEENAGERS

Between three and eleven years of age children continue to consolidate and refine the key physical and intellectual skills and the personal attributes developed in the early years. This is a gross oversimplification but theorists such as Freud (*see* Storr 2001) and Erikson (1968) saw this time, particularly the school years, as a period of relative calm between the explosion of growth in all areas of development associated with the early years and the potential crisis of adolescence.

It is during this period that children begin to develop a greater sense of who they are outside the confines of their own family, and to build wider relationships with their peers. This includes beginning to develop a clearer understanding of their gender and racial identity (Daniel *et al.* 1999). Important at this stage is to build the child's sense of self esteem and resilience so that they are more able to cope with the challenges that life may pose them (Newman and Blackburn 2002).

These challenges can include coping with a physical or learning disability. Additionally, many children have some form of psychological or behavioural problem, the causes of which differ but include poor physical health and disability (Green *et al.* 2004). However, many of these difficulties either result from or are worsened by inappropriate parenting styles (*see* Baumrind 1971) and poor attachments. They can be severe enough to cause significant problems to the child and those around him. Health and social care workers have an important support role to play in helping to address these issues.

The sociological perspective – Education

We have already mentioned in this section the importance of school. By law, children in the UK between the ages of five and sixteen must receive full-time education. Parents who do not ensure their children attend school regularly may be ordered to do so and possibly be fined or sentenced to prison (Directgov 2009a). The age of compulsory education in England is due to rise by 2013 to eighteen (BBC News 2007) to address the issue of young people having comparatively low levels of qualifications and workplace skills.

Functionalists maintain education has a vital role to play in the smooth running of a society. School is the source of secondary socialization where children learn the common values in society and are expected to develop a sense of self-discipline. Education teaches skills that are needed in specialist occupations. Finally, children are able to achieve according to merit rather than their ascribed characteristics such as class, sex and race (Giddens 2009: 687). The idea of achieved merit can then be further explored in relation to aspects of equality. If it is true that children achieve according to their merit we would expect to see little difference in the achievement across the boundaries of socio-economic status (class), gender or ethnicity. However, national statistics show some interesting patterns.

In relation to social class, children from lower socio-economic groups achieve fewer GCSEs, at lower grades, and are less likely to go to university than children with professional parents (Marsh *et al.* 2009). Females achieve more GCSEs and A Levels than males and are more likely to go to university (Haralambos *et al.* 2008). Better GCSE results are obtained by Chinese children than any others, but Black Caribbean and African boys have the lowest attainment. There is a growth in the number of Asian females attending university, which is a new feature as this group traditionally has not been seen in higher education (Marsh *et al.* 2009). Statistics in text books easily become outdated – go directly to sources such as the Office for National Statistics and Social Trends for the latest figures.

ADOLESCENCE – A SEARCH FOR IDENTITY

A significant period of transition takes place between eleven and eighteen years of age. It encompasses increased growth and strength with the physical changes associated with becoming sexually mature (puberty) and adaptation to the new roles and responsibilities involved in becoming an adult (adolescence). In some societies the transition from child to adult status is abrupt and marked by a rite of passage but in the Western world it takes place over a number of years (Jaffe 1998).

One of the key psychological features of adolescence is a search for identity, including gender and ethnic identity (Erikson 1968). Early adolescence is often characterized by confusion in young people followed by active experimentation with ideas and behaviours before they find a role and identity for themselves (Marcia 1980). This confusion and searching can lead to risk taking behaviour which, rather than being abnormal, may be part of natural adolescent development associated with gaining peer acceptance, establishing autonomy and coping with anxiety. Though peers become increasingly important in adolescence, family remains an important source of love and support for most young people (Gillies *et al.* 2001).

As in the early years, major changes take place in the adolescent brain. Activity increases in areas at the front of the brain which are responsible for powers of reasoning and more sophisticated language skills. These changes enable the young person to develop over time the ability to balance complex ideas, control impulses and take a more reasoned approach to life (Weinberger *et al.* 2005). Brain remodelling in adolescence may provide another explanation for risk taking, for a sense of confusion in young people and for why adolescents do not see the world in the same way as adults. For some young people a search for identity and risk taking can lead to behaviour which has serious implications.

The sociological perspective – Crime and deviance

Crime or offending is when an activity breaks the law; deviance is behaviour that does not conform to the norms and expectations of a particular society (Haralambos *et al.* 2008). Both are relative and culturally determined because what constitutes crime and deviance changes over time and according to place. Gay men's sexual acts were a criminal offence until 1967. Fixing the age of consent at sixteen for homosexual sex was only made equal to heterosexual consent in the Sexual Offences Amendment Act 2000 in the UK (except in Northern Ireland where it is seventeen) (OPSI 2009b). Some people still consider homosexuality deviant but as the gay rights campaigning group Stonewall say 'Some people are gay – get over it' (Stonewall 2007).

Functionalists, Marxists and feminists all have something to say about crime but interpretive sociology offers an opinion applicable to work in the health and social care sector. 'The deviant is one to whom that label has been successfully applied: deviant behaviour is behaviour that people so label' (Becker 1963 quoted in Haralambos *et al.* 2008: 335). Howard Becker's classic study 'Outsiders: studies in the sociology of deviance' asserts that society creates deviants who break rules and sanctions which are made in order to extract conformity. Once labelled as deviant or delinquent as a young person it becomes an identity by which others see them and they come to see themselves as that label.

What identifies criminals from the general population is that they are labelled as criminal. We cannot identify those who commit crimes but do not get caught (for example, people who drive faster than the speed limit or drink alcohol in pubs before they are legally allowed) nor can we always know whether those who are convicted are actually guilty. Individuals who acquire criminal convictions will find they will always keep the label. This is especially relevant in health and social care work where pre-employment checks are made and convictions are never considered 'spent' right through into adulthood.

BEING AN ADULT

Many theories that explore development in adulthood are stage theories (Erikson 1995, Levinson 1978) and were formulated at a time when the lifespan tended to follow a more predictable course than it does today. Patterns of employment, education and relationships in Western society have undergone huge changes, meaning there is no longer a 'traditional life course'. Having said this, transitions which may cause major shifts in lifestyle such as forming intimate relationships, becoming parents and experiences of loss are not uncommon for many adults (Crawford and Walker 2007).

The way individuals maintain some continuity and consistency through these transitions is dependent on their physical, social and psychological characteristics and the wider social support available to them. Unlike stage theorists, Neugarten (1996) believed men and women tend to measure their lives and achievements against those of their peers to decide if they are 'on schedule'. Stress is experienced when individuals believe their life is not following the expected pattern.

From what has been said it may be clear that relationships between sexual partners, parents and offspring (young or adult), and between friends, are a key feature of the adult years. Researchers Hazan and Shaver (1987 *see* Fraley 2004) explored Bowlby's ideas regarding infant attachment (Bowlby 1997) in the context of romantic relationships and argue that these adult relationships, like infant–caregiver relationships, are attachments. They found attachment patterns in adults appear to mirror those seen in children and that the relationships function in much the same way, in secure attachments providing a secure base and source of support for the adult partners (Fraley 2004).

The sociological perspective – Work and disability in adulthood

Work is a key feature of many adult lives. *Employment* is usually seen as 'paid work' whereby *labour* is exchanged for a wage. There are a range of other activities that are part of what Giddens (2009) refers to as the 'informal' economy; for example cash payments, DIY, housework and voluntary work. All these activities provide goods and services that would otherwise be paid for. Giddens (2009: 886) uses the following explanation:

> We can define WORK, whether paid or unpaid, as being the carrying out of tasks requiring the expenditure of mental and physical effort, which has as its objective the production of goods and services that cater for human needs.

The UK census lists 20,000 jobs which were arranged into eight distinct categories by The National Statistics Socio-Economic Classification 2000 (Office for National Statistics 2009b). As mentioned earlier, the pattern of working lives has changed. For example, 'knowledge economy' is a phrase which describes the way that the economy is based on ideas and information rather than production and manufacture. This applies to Western Germany, the United States, Japan, Britain, Sweden and France where, according to an OECD study, half of all business was knowledge-based as early as the mid-1990s (cited in Giddens 2009: 916).

Employers value workers who are quick to learn, can use their initiative and work alone or in teams. These sorts of personal abilities mean workers can adapt to new technologies and ways of working which is more useful to an organization than someone who is an expert in a specific skill (Meadows 1996 in Giddens 2009: 917). It is rare in the twenty-first century that adults will enter a job for life as was the case for many older retired people when they were of working age. Some may change job roles many times or have periods of unemployment whilst others are excluded from the work environment as a result of mental health illness or disability. Peter Birkett's 1981 cartoon (Figure 3.1) in *Punch* showed three Daleks (like wheelchairs, Daleks move around on wheels) thwarted from conquering the universe because they could not get up a flight of stairs. The cartoon perfectly illustrates the social model of disability. People who use wheelchairs are excluded from society because of the way it is built. Their problem is not their impairment (lack of functioning part of the body) but the lack of access to be able to participate in society. The term 'disabled people' is preferred by the disability movement because it makes clear the 'fault' is with society which dis-ables people who have impairments (Oliver and Sapey 2006).

Disabled people experience discrimination through the environment, the economy and culture (Priestley 2003). Disabled adults want to work but still experience

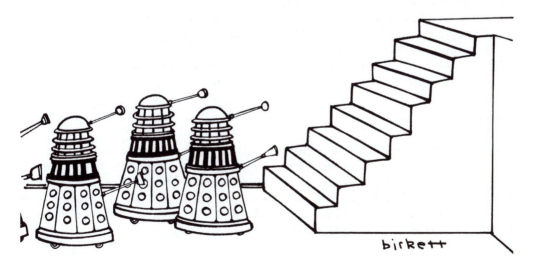

"Well, this certainly buggers our plan to conquer the Universe."

Figure 3.1 Birkett's Daleks (1981, *Punch* Library)

barriers in physical access and unhelpful attitudes. This often results in them living in poverty on state benefits or low incomes. Only 50 per cent of disabled people of working age are in work (Shaw Trust 2009). The Government wants disabled people to join the workforce and has put incentives into place as a result of the Disability Discrimination Acts 1995 and 2005 (Directgov 2009b).

OLDER PEOPLE

Disabled people are only one of the groups facing discrimination in society. Despite the fact that people are living longer and older people make up an increasingly large proportion of the population (Office for National Statistics 2009c), attitudes to ageing in Western culture tend to be negative and ageism, even in health and social care services, is not uncommon (Askham 2008). The way one ages is a mixture of inheritance and environmental factors and an individual's gender and race as well as their experiences in earlier life will have a huge impact on the ageing process. Though it is fair to say that illness and disability become more common in old age, these are not inevitable and many older people describe their health as good (Beckett 2002).

Some theories of ageing explore the older person's interaction with society, either suggesting there is a gradual withdrawal from wider social activity or conversely that ageing is most successful when activities are maintained as far as possible (*see* Hunt 2005). Erikson (1995) focused more on the individual's need to reflect on their life and to integrate past experiences, positive and negative, in order to approach the end of their life with some sense of acceptance. He suggested failure to do this could ultimately lead to fear of death.

Experiences of loss occur throughout the lifespan but particularly in old age where the older person is likely to experience losses through the death of partners and friends and/or their own increasing infirmity. The response to such losses depends on the individual's personality, their circumstances and the coping mechanisms they have built up through life (Sidell 1993). Stage theories to explain the process of coming to terms with bereavement (Parkes 1986) and with one's own imminent death (Kubler-Ross 1970), whilst useful do not tell the whole story. Like everything else in an individual's life, grieving is unique to that person.

CONCLUSION

This chapter has identified developmental and sociological theories which impact on individuals' inherent and environmental situations. It has also considered different periods in the lifespan and explored some of the themes we feel are of particular relevance. We hope that, in your future careers as health and social care workers, you will use your understanding of people and the environment in which they develop to promote effective practice when working with individuals in society.

SUMMARY OF MAIN POINTS

You should be able to:

- Understand a number of key sociological and developmental theories and concepts.
- Understand some of the changes that take place in the sequence of growth, development and ageing through the life-course.
- Understand environmental, social and psychological factors that may affect service users' lives and their need for specific health and social care services.
- Understand the impact of life events on growth, development and socialization.

REFERENCES

Anastasi, A. and Foley, J. (1948) A Proposed Reorientation in the Heredity Environment Controversy, *The Psychological Review,* 5 (55), 239–49.

Askham, J. (2008) *Health and Care Services for Older People: Overview report on research to support the National Service Framework for Older People* [online]. Available at http://www.dh.gov.uk/prod_consum_dh/groups/dh_digitalassets/@dh/@en/documents/digitalasset/dh_088849.pdf (Accessed 13 December 2009).

Baumrind, D. (1971) Current Patterns of Parental Authority, *Developmental Psychology,* 4 (1), Pt. 2, 1–103.

BBC News (12 January 2007) *School Leaving Age set to be 18* [online]. Available at http://news.bbc.co.uk/1/hi/education/6254833.stm (Accessed 19 December 2009).

Beckett, C. (2002) *Human Growth and Development,* London: Sage.

Bowlby, J. (1997/1969) *Attachment,* London: Pimlico.

Bronfenbrenner, U. (1979) *The Ecology of Human Development: Experiments by Nature and Design,* Cambridge, MA: Harvard University Press.

Crawford, K. and Walker, J. (2007) *Social Work and Human Development* (2nd edition), Exeter: Learning Matters.

Cree, V. (2000) *Sociology for Social Workers and Probation Officers,* London: Routledge.

Daniel, B., Wassell, S. and Gilligan, R. (1999) *Child Development for Child Care and Protection Workers,* London: Jessica Kingsley.

Dawson, G., Ashman, S. and Carver, L. (2000) The role of early experience in shaping behavioral and brain development and its implications for social policy, *Development and Psychopathology,* 12 (4), 695–712.

DCSF (2009a) *Every Child Matters: Sure Start Children's Centres* [online]. Available at http://www.dcsf.gov.uk/everychildmatters/earlyyears/surestart/whatsurestartdoes/ (Accessed 11 December 2009).

DCSF (2009b) *Every Child Matters* [online]. Available at http://www.dcsf.gov.uk/everychildmatters/about/aims/aims (Accessed 22 October 2009).

Department of Health (2001) *Messages from Research* [online]. Available at http://www.dh.gov.uk/en/Publicationsandstatistics/Publications/PublicationsPolicyAnd Guidance/ DH_4006258 (Accessed 19 December 2009).

Directgov (2009a) *School Attendance and Absence: The Law* [online] Available at http://www.direct.gov.uk/en/Parents/Schoolslearninganddevelopment/YourChildsWelfareAt School/DG_066966 (Accessed 28 December 2009).

Directgov (2009b) *The Disability Discrimination Act* [online] Available at http://www.direct.gov.uk/en/DisabledPeople/RightsAndObligations/DisabilityRights/DG_4001068 (Accessed 19 December 2009).

Erikson, E. (1995/1968) *Childhood and Society,* London: Vintage.

Fraley, C. (2004) *A Brief Overview of Adult Attachment Theory and Research* [online] Available at http://www.psych.uiuc.edu/~rcfraley/attachment.htm (Accessed 13 December 2009).

Giddens, A. (2009) (6th edition) *Sociology*, Cambridge: Polity.

Gillies, V., Ribbens McCarthy, J. and Holland, J. (2001) *The Family Lives of Young People*, York: Joseph Rowntree Foundation.

Green, H., McGinnity, A., Meltzer, H., Ford, T. and Goodman, R. (2004) *Mental health of children and young people in Great Britain 2004, summary report* [online]. Available at http://www.statistics.gov.uk/downloads/theme_health/summaryreport.pdf (Accessed 11 December 2009).

Haralambos, M., Holborn, M. and Heald, R. (2008) (7th edition) *Sociology: Themes and Perspectives*, London: Collins Education.

Hunt, S. (2005) *The Life Course: A Sociological Introduction*, Basingstoke: Palgrave Macmillan.

Jaffe, M. (1998) *Adolescence*, New York: Wiley.

Keenan, T. and Evans, S. (2009) *An Introduction to Child Development*, London: Sage.

Kubler-Ross, E. (1970) *On Death and Dying*, London: Tavistock.

Levinson, D. (1991/1978) *The Seasons of a Man's Life*, New York: Ballentine.

Marcia, J. (1980) Identity in Adolescence in J. Adleston (Ed.) *Handbook of Adolescent Psychology*, New York: Wiley.

Marsh, I., Keating, M., Punch, S. and Harden, J. (Eds) (2009) *Sociology: Making Sense of Society* (4th edition), Essex: Pearson.

Neugarten, D. (Ed.) (1996) *The Meanings of Age: Selected Papers of Beatrice L. Neugarten*, Chicago: University of Chicago Press.

Newman, T. and Blackburn, S. (2002) *Transitions in the Lives of Children and Young People: Resilience Factors*, Edinburgh: Scottish Education Executive Department.

Office for National Statistics (ONS) (2009a) *Neighbourhood Statistics* [online]. Available at http://www.neighbourhood.statistics.gov.uk/dissemination/LeadHome.do?bhcp=1 (Accessed 19 December 2009).

Office for National Statistics (2009b) *NS-SEC Classes and Collapses* [online]. Available at http://www.ons.gov.uk/about-statistics/classifications/current/ns-sec/cats-and-classes/ns-sec-classes-and-collapses/index.html (Accessed 19 December 2009).

Office for National Statistics (2009c) *Statistical Bulletin: Older People's Day 2009* [online]. Available at http://www.statistics.gov.uk/pdfdir/age0909.pdf (Accessed 13 December 2009).

Office of Public Sector Information (OPSI) (2009a) *Children Act 1989* [online]. Available at http://www.opsi.gov.uk/acts/acts1989/Ukpga_19890041_en_1.htm (Accessed 19 December 2009).

Office of Public Sector Information (2009b) *Sexual Offences Amendment Act (2000)* [online]. Available at http://www.opsi.gov.uk/acts/acts2000/ukpga_20000044_en_1.htm (Accessed 19 December 2009).

Oliver, M. and Sapey, B. (2006) (3rd edition) *Social Work with Disabled People*, Basingstoke: Palgrave Macmillan.

O'Loughlin, M. and O'Loughlin, S. (Eds) (2008) (2nd edition) *Social Work with Children and Families*, Exeter: Learning Matters.

Parkes, C. (1986) (2nd edition) *Bereavement: Studies of Grief in Adult Life*, London: Tavistock.

Piaget, J. (1952) *The Origins of Intelligence in Children* (translated by Margaret Cox), New York: International Universities Press [online]. Available at http://www.archive.org/stream/originsofintelli017921mbp#page/n5/mode/2up (Accessed 11 December 2009).

Priestley, M. (2003) *Disability: A Life Course Approach*, Cambridge: Polity.

Shore, R. (1997) *Rethinking the Brain: New Insights into Early Development*, New York: Families and Work Institute.

Siddell, M. (1993) Death, Dying and Bereavement in Bond, J., Coleman, P. and Peace, S. (Eds) *Ageing in Society: an introduction to social gerontology* (2nd edition), London: Sage.

Smith, P., Cowie, H. and Blades, M. (2003) *Understanding Children's Development* (4th edition), Oxford: Blackwell.

Stonewall (2007) *Education for All Campaign* [online]. Available at http://www.stonewall.org.uk/education_for_all/news/current_news/2043.asp (Accessed 19 December 2009).

Storr, A. (2001) *Freud: A Very Short Introduction*, Oxford: Oxford University Press.

Weinberger, D., Elvevåg, B. and Giedd, J. (2005) *The Adolescent Brain: A Work in Progress* [online] Available at http://www.thenationalcampaign.org/resources/pdf/BRAIN.pdf (Accessed 12 December 2009).

FURTHER READING

Beckett, C. and Taylor, H. (2010) *Human Growth and Development* (2nd edition), London: Sage.

Crawford, K. and Walker, J. (2007) *Social Work and Human Development* (2nd edition), Exeter: Learning Matters.

Giddens, A. (2009) *Sociology* (6th edition), Cambridge: Polity.

Shaw Trust (2009) *Disability and Employment Statistics* [online] Available at http://www.shaw-trust.org.uk/disability_and_employment_statistics (Accessed 19 December 2009).

Thompson, N. (2003) (2nd edition) *Promoting Equality*, Basingstoke: Palgrave.

USEFUL WEBSITES

Directgov – the official UK government website for citizens:
http://www.direct.gov.uk

Office for National Statistics:
http://www.statistics.gov.uk

A link to a whole range of resources on developmental psychology that have been evaluated positively by academics in Higher Education:
http://www.intute.ac.uk/cgi-bin/search.pl?term1=developmental+psychology&limit=0

CHAPTER 4

CONCEPTS OF EQUALITY AND DIVERSITY

ADAM BARNARD

O B J E C T I V E S

After reading this chapter you should be able to:

- Recognize and discuss the theoretical foundations of social difference and begin to apply this theoretical discussion to issues of class, gender, race and ethnicity, age, disability and sexual identity

- Debate the notions of equality, inequality and equal opportunity

- Discuss the consequences of prejudice, stereotyping, discrimination and oppression

- Describe and discuss the human rights framework and identify relevant legislation and the European dimension.

After reading this chapter you will know the meaning of the following terms: Equality, inequality, equal opportunity, prejudice, stereotyping, discrimination, oppression, class, gender, race and ethnicity, age, disability, sexual identity.

There are two Moments of Reflection to work on at the end of the chapter.

AIMS

This chapter provides you with an introduction to the study of concepts of equality and diversity within health and social care. It explores the processes people experience as a consequence of social difference, and considers the relevant legislation surrounding these social differences. The notions of equality, inequality and equal opportunity, prejudice, stereotyping, discrimination and oppression are discussed. Theoretical foundations of social differences are considered to take into account class, gender, race and ethnicity, age, disability and sexual identity. The chapter ends by considering the human rights framework and relevant UK and European legislation on equality and diversity issues.

There exist a range of social differences that characterize contemporary society. Payne (2006: 3) suggests we automatically perceive and pigeonhole different people, individuals and groups and behave towards them in terms of the slots we have put them into. These divisions or differences are often along the divisions of class, gender, 'race', ethnicity, age and sexuality, although this is not exclusively so and there is a degree of 'fuzziness' in these differences. The distinction between division and difference has been widely discussed (Carling 1991; Anthias 1998, 2001; Braham and Janes 2002; Best 2005). Not all differences are homogenous (or the same) and there are many differences and heterogeneity of experience between people in different social divisions. These divisions are socially, culturally, politically and economically constructed and maintained. The taken for granted idea of any biological or natural origin to these differences has been widely discounted and has been part of the difficulty of understanding social difference. However, these differences and divisions often embody or involve inequality, discrimination and oppression.

All individuals have differences and there exist different groups with similarities and differences. Differences often have two sides, for example man/woman, ill health/ good health, or black/white. This ignores many points in between, is often a simplistic representation and usually involves unequal relations between the two sides. These differences are often used in negative ways such as discrimination and oppression (Parekh 1992; Pitt 1992). Discrimination can be a good thing when used to identify difference, for example discrimination between red and green in traffic lights. However, it becomes more difficult when discrimination is used negatively and negative attributes are attached to differences and people or individuals are discriminated against. For example, the Apartheid regime in South Africa discriminated against black people on the basis of their race and ethnicity.

Oppression is the process where discrimination is used to treat people unequally and one group dominates or oppresses another group. Oppression is where discrimination is used to disadvantage groups such as left-handed people. Oppression is a wider concept that takes into account the many structural inequalities and discriminatory thoughts, feelings and actions that individuals or groups may experience. Discrimination and oppression are closely linked and can be experienced as inequalities. At its simplest, inequality is where people have more or less of something such as money, health care, life chances or opportunities. Discrimination and oppression are linked to inequality in a variety of ways. Thompson (2003: 11–12) suggests inequalities can take many forms.

- Economic – different distributions of financial resources (for example, money) and services are a key factor in underpinning poverty, social deprivation, inequality and discrimination and oppression.
- Social – a person's integration into society determines how far they can participate and enjoy the rewards and status distributed in society.
- Political – some groups have more power and can prevent participation according to social divisions.

- Ethical – inequality involves making judgments about behaviour and action, and questions the morality of actions.
- Ideological – controlling ideas, information and representation can maintain inequality.
- Psychological – can be split into three parts:
  - cognitive – thoughts about social division
  - affective – feelings about social division
  - conative – the behavioural norms of a social division.

To understanding inequalities Thompson (2003) suggests a P-C-S or Personal–Cultural–Structural analysis can be useful. This gives three analytically distinct but intersecting levels on which to explore inequality, discrimination and oppression.

The personal level involves the thoughts, feelings and actions of individuals at a personal and psychological level that have a direct impact on discrimination and oppression. For example, on the personal level it could be not liking certain groups or believing 'common sense' ideas such as ideas about 'old age'. The cultural level involves complex questions of ways of life. Culture is an important sociological concept that describes patterns of behaviour shared across particular groups and societies. For example, sexism and derogatory humour operate at a cultural level. The personal is embedded in culture and often personal discriminatory ideas cannot operate without cultural support. For example, discriminatory personal attitudes towards women require an oppressive culture towards women. Culture is embedded in structure where the social, political and economic structures constrain (and enable) people and groups. For example, structures include institutions such as education, housing, schools, family, the police, the health service, and social work. To give an example, the Stephen Lawrence inquiry (Macpherson 1999) into the death of a black teenager found levels of institutional racism within the police force. The suggestion was that it was not necessarily individual racist police officers dealing with the case but the structure and procedures of the police that could be seen as racist.

The personal, cultural and structural levels are a useful way to understand equality and the barriers to promoting equality. Equality is a political term that is contested and used by different people for different reasons. As such it is an ideological term that has been used to justify many situations. For example, it has been used to suggest all men are equal when considering political rights such as voting but ignoring women. Equality does not mean being the same. It is something desirable and not a natural but a social and political thing, it can be promoted and realized and inequality can be removed and decreased. Health and social care, it is often suggested, is the attempt to try and promote equality and reduce inequalities by addressing and challenging discrimination and oppression.

People who experience inequality share a 'common position of marginalization and disadvantage' (Bagilhole 1997: 6) in key areas of health and social care, social policy, service provision, participation and access to opportunities. Inequalities are sustained and reproduced by the processes of discrimination and oppression; and inequality has an impact on life chances, participation, access to power and resources where dominant groups benefit and excluded groups suffer disadvantage. Inequalities are the result of discrimination and/or oppression. Discrimination is a set of processes by which an individual 'receives' unfair or 'less advantageous treatment' (Thompson

2003: 147) and oppression is 'inhuman or degrading treatment of individuals or groups; hardship and injustice brought about by the dominance of one group over another; the negative and demeaning exercise of power' (Thompson 2003: 147) that often involves disregarding rights and citizenship. For example, in Nazi Germany Jewish people were discriminated against until they were oppressed. Discrimination and oppression usually occur along the lines of class, 'race' and ethnicity, gender, age, culture, religion, sexuality or disability and are manifest or brought into being through prejudice and stereotypes.

Prejudice refers to opinions and attitudes held by one group towards another, most often a set of negative assumptions. They are based on incomplete information and are resistant to change. Prejudice is often based on stereotypes which are the attribution of fixed and inflexible characterizations of individuals and groups. Stereotypes are a form of mental shorthand that make a host of assumptions from limited information and experience. For example, Stonewall (2003) found (wrongly) that half of all people who felt hard done by believed that immigrants and ethnic minorities were getting priority over them. Much health and social care work and training is directed towards exploring and challenging prejudicial and stereotypical thoughts, feelings and beliefs.

Within health and social care, discrimination and oppression are the things to be challenged and stereotypes and prejudice are to be countered. These processes are often experienced along the lines of social differences. For example, the United Nations Declaration on Human Rights (1948) Article Two states 'without distinction of any kind, such as race, colour, sex, language, religion, political or other opinion, national or social origin, property, birth or other status'. For our purposes, the social differences that will be examined are class, gender, 'race' and ethnicity, religion, age, sexuality and disability.

CLASS

A person or group's class is their **socio-economic position** that allows a large group of people to share common economic interests, experiences and lifestyles. Scott (2006: 26) suggests class describes economic divisions and inequalities often rooted in property and employment relations. Class cuts across and intersects with other dimensions of difference, for example, women's experience of work. The 'common sense' idea of class falls into upper, middle and working class. This has changed recently to a distinctive occupations-based account to three main groups – the subordinate (manual, wage-paid) classes, the intermediate (salaried or self-employed) classes and the 'advantaged classes' (capital and property owners, and employers). Occupational change, culture, identity, consumption and life-style may blur the picture of class but class situations still have determining effects on inequalities and people's life chances (Payne 2006: 17). For example, the Black Report (DHSS 1980) made a clear case for people's health being closely related to their class position.

Two main theorists have examined class, Karl Marx and Max Weber. For Marx (1978 [1875]), class is central to the exploitative system of relations in capitalism that leads to the oppression of the majority of working people. There are two classes or two warring hostile camps: the property owning and controlling bourgeoisie (or ruling class) and the labouring proletariat (or working class) that sell their labour to make a living. The bourgeoisie exploit the proletariat by exploiting profit from their labour. This has been seen by some as a simplistic model, an unrealistic assessment on the future of capitalism, and ignoring the fluidity of class membership and consciousness (Giddens 2009: 441). However, Marx still provides value in the emphasis on the exploitative and unjust nature of capitalist relations and how these can effect inequality, discrimination and oppression.

Weber's theory of social class sees a number of distinct classes competing for positions. It is similar to but different from Marx. These positions are based on people's places in the occupational hierarchy and success in the labour market. There are many divisions between classes in status and power. For Weber (1979 [1925]), class refers to identifiable groups of individuals who have certain interests in common. These interests are 'market position' – the opportunity to earn income through work or trade. Inequalities in 'life chances' and opportunities in health, education, housing, employment and levels of income are experienced by people of different classes. Weber extends Marx's analysis by introducing party and status. 'Party' refers to any organization or voluntary association that brings together people with common backgrounds, aims or interests in pursuit of particular policies or control of a particular organization, that is power. For example, trades unions, political parties, voluntary associations, community projects are sources of party membership and benefits. Status is the different amount of prestige, honour or social standing that society attaches to different social groups. This has been suggested as similar to 'styles of life'. Whatever the merits of these two approaches, they both make important contributions to understanding how income, wealth, status, and power are centrally involved in reproducing inequalities and the possibilities of challenging discrimination and oppression in relation to socio-economic position.

GENDER

Gender is the psychological, social and cultural differences between males and females. It is different from 'sex' which relates to the physical characteristics of men and women. Gender is closely concerned with the political, cultural and social construction of masculinity and femininity.

Feminism has demonstrated how cultural and media products marketed to children reinforce 'taken for granted' ideas about gender roles and expectations (Weitzman 1972; Oakley 1974; Shaver and Hendrick 1987; Davies 1991). Smith (1979) has argued there is a distinct female life experience that is a reflection of the essentialist, taken for granted and ideological understanding of what it is to be a woman. As De Beauvoir (1972 [1949]) argues 'one is not born a woman but one is made a woman'. Judith Butler (1990) has argued that we 'perform' different genders. Masculinities are an important part of gender relations (Connell 2001, 2009a, 2009b). These perspectives on gender challenge any neutral or uncritical acceptance of common sense ideas and the cultural construction of potentially discriminatory and oppressive practices and beliefs about gender.

Abbot (2006: 99) argues that the characteristic of gender differences, particularly in the UK, is the 'persistence of inequalities between men and women'. Pay, employment and patriarchal power (that work in men's interests) are still, arguably, the dominant experience for most women.

RACE AND ETHNICITY

'Race' is one of the most contested terms and has been used to oppress and discriminate against individuals and groups. It has a long and troubled history of racialization where people have been classified, usually for exclusion and denial of human, civil and political rights. 'Race' often wrongly implies fixed biological characteristics so ethnicity is often the preferred term. Ethnicity refers to the cultural practices, language, history, traditions and outlook of a particular community. For example, some deaf people see themselves as belonging to a particular ethnic community. Bagilhole (2009: xiv) refers to ethnicity as 'the recognition of a group's shared identity based on country of origin, culture, language or religion'. Black and minority ethnic groups (BME) is the preferred term as it emphasizes the diverse experience of different ethnic groups and prevents imposing a false homogeneity (or sameness) of experience. 'Black' is a preferred term for its association with the political position that people find themselves in. 'Race' and ethnicity have a difficult relationship to inequality, discrimination and oppression.

RELIGION

Religion and spirituality are important elements of individuals' personal, cultural and structural beliefs, understandings and action. Berger (1967) suggests there are three key elements to religion. First, it is a form of culture that involves a shared set of beliefs, ideas, world views, values and norms for a particular community. Second, religion involves ritualized practices and particular behaviours for a group of individuals. Third, religion provides a sense of purpose and meaning for a community. As such it is a very significant part of people's identity, beliefs, activity and spirituality. Health and social care work needs to recognize and respect this spiritual dimension.

AGE

Ageism is discrimination against people on the basis of their age. Young people and older people are the most vulnerable groups for ageism. McEwan (1990) has argued that age is the 'unrecognized discrimination' and Age Concern (2006) suggests one third of people surveyed had experienced age discrimination and the over 55s were twice as likely to have experienced age prejudice than any other form of discrimination. Health and social care services need to be aware of age and how this relates to inequality, oppression and discrimination.

SEXUALITY

Everyone moves through the 'life course' or the process of aging. If gender is the social and political shaping of femininity and masculinity to challenge the idea that relations between men and women are determined by nature, 'sexuality' is generally broader in meaning, encompassing erotic desires and identities, as well as practices (Scott and Jackson 2000: 171). Heterosexuality has historically and socially been presented as a 'norm' and 'natural' order to sexual preference and identity, as a dominant social institution and as an example of essentialist thinking. Foucault (1978) has shown that homosexuality is a socially, politically and culturally constructed term that barely existed before the eighteenth century, with diverse sexual behaviour, orientations and identity being normal and natural at different times and in different cultures. Most explanations of sexuality would suggest a complex interplay between biological and social/cultural factors. Plummer (1975) distinguishes 'types' of homosexuality, Siedman (1997) has argued for different ideas of sexuality to challenge established, 'common sense' cultural heterosexuality, and sees sexuality as part of a wider project of political, social and personal solidarity.

Sexuality is historically, culturally and socially constructed to operate as a gender-based form of control promoting a 'normative heterosexuality' at the expense of homosexuality as a valued and equal orientation and identity. Oppressive and discriminatory thoughts and practices around sexuality have led to discrimination and oppression of individuals and groups.

DISABILITY

Disabled people is the preferred term for people who are disabled as it promotes their humanity and highlights the fact that they are disabled by society (Bagilhole 2009: xiii). The Disabled People's International definition is 'the loss or limitation of opportunities to take part in the life of the community on an equal level with others due to physical and social barriers' (Bagilhole 2009: xiii). Hunt (1966) argues 'the problem with disability lies not only in the impairment of function and its effects on us individually, but also, more importantly, in the area of our relationship with "normal" people'. Furthermore, disability has been traditionally viewed from a medical model focusing on impairment or what has become known as the individual model of disability that focuses on an individual's limitations as the main cause of people's difficulties with disability. Finklestein (1980), Barnes (1991) and Oliver (1990, 1996) have put forward a social model of disability that challenges the individual and medical model in favour of an understanding of the social, cultural and political barriers of disability. This sees disability as the way society 'dis-ables' and creates 'invalidity' rather than anything to do with the individual. Shakespeare and Watson (2002: 11) have argued that although identifying the social barriers of disability, the social model also denies a major part of people's biographies if it ignores the everyday experience of impairment.

These social differences or major social differentiation often provide the lines of disadvantage, oppression and discrimination experienced by individuals, groups and societies. Linking this to how people are thought about and treated, Bagilhole (2009: xvii) suggests prejudice may take the following forms:

- **Sexism** – the belief or attitude that women are inferior to men, including practices or policies stemming from this belief.
- **Racism** – in its simplest definition, the belief that race is the primary determinant of human traits and capacities and that racial differences produce an inherent superiority of a particular race. Racism consists of structures and cultures (institutional racism) and personal beliefs (individual prejudice).
- **Ageism** – stereotyping, prejudice or discriminatory practice of policies based on age.

- **Islamophobia** – a relatively new term used to refer to fear, prejudice or discrimination against Muslim people and Islam.
- **Heterosexism** – stereotyping, prejudice or discriminatory practice or policies that assume heterosexuals are superior to homosexuals.
- **Disabilism** – stereotyping, prejudice or discriminatory practice or policies based on the assumption that disabled people are inferior to non-disabled people.

Given the possibility of prejudice, stereotyping, discrimination and oppression, Bagilhole (2009: 29) argues that attempts to address equality and diversity are unified by key themes. These key themes are: aiming for equality for all; upholding social justice; challenging discrimination; making the best use of human resources; wanting services to be accessible to everyone; giving people a fair chance of getting jobs; and fair and equal legal obligations. Health and social care workers and students need to have an awareness and understanding of the issues connected with social differences in order to work in ways that promote, extend and include individuals and groups in equality. As a concept equal opportunities and diversity is seen as promoting fairness, justice, morality, impartiality and accountability (which are discussed in subsequent chapters).

The Equalities Review (2007: 16) defines equal opportunities and diversity thus: 'an equal society protects and promotes equal, real freedom and substantive opportunity to live in the ways people value and would choose, so that everyone can flourish'. For this society, barriers need to be removed and equality needs to be promoted so the whole of society can benefit. Bagilhole (2009: 53) argues this definition recognizes that it is not enough to treat people the same and that people may need additional support or resources to enjoy genuine freedom and fair access to opportunities. The enforcement agencies to ensure this position have previously been in the hands of a range of separate United Kingdom commissions but have now been subsumed into the Equality and Human Rights Commission. Working within a European (Bagilhole 2009) and globalized (Ritzer and Barnard 2008) context also has a bearing on equal opportunities and diversity legislation and enforcement.

The law and legislative framework is an essential part of promoting equality and diversity and challenging inequalities, discrimination and oppression. It contains the potential for challenging discrimination and oppression but is also part of the framework of dominance and subordination that maintains social order and inequalities. Legislation may be effective at anti-discrimination but rarely challenges wider structural concerns of oppression.

There are many conflicting interpretations on the various successes and failures of legislation to make a significant impact on oppressive practices. Thompson (2003) suggests legislation has a narrow legalistic focus to challenge discrimination and needs to be extended to cover various forms of oppression experienced by different groups. Bagilhole (2009: 223) suggests that for various reasons legislation has proved insufficient to eliminate inequality, discrimination and oppression but the law does have an important role to play as part of a wider project to challenge inequality.

Table 4.1 The most significant legislation in the areas of disability, race, gender, sexual orientation, religion or belief and age

1940s and 1950s	1944 and 1958 Disabled Person (Employment) Acts
	1948 British Nationality Act
1960s and 1970s	1962 Commonwealth Immigration Act
	1965 Race Relations Act
	1966 Local Government Act
	1967 Sexual Offences Act
	1968 Commonwealth Immigration Act
	1970 Chronically Sick and Disabled Act
	1970 Equal Pay Act (amended 1983)
	1971 Immigration Act (amended 1986)
	1975 Sex Discrimination Act
	1976 Race Relations Act
1980s and 1990s under Conservative government	1981 British Nationality Act
	1983 Equal Pay Act (amended)
	1985 Companies Act
	1986 Sex Discrimination Act (amended)
	1986 Public Order Act
	1988 Local Government Act
	1994 Sexual Offences Act (amended)
	1995 Disability Discrimination Act
	1996 Asylum and Immigration Act
	1996 Employment Rights Act
1990s and 2000s under New Labour government	1998 Human Rights Act
	1998 Belfast Agreement
	1998 Scotland Act
	1998 Government of Wales Act
	1998 Crime and Disorder Act
	1999 Immigration and Asylum Act
	2000 Sexual Offences Act (amended)
	2000 Race Relations (Amendment) Act
	2001 Sex Discrimination Act (amended)
	2002 Nationality, Immigration ND Asylum Act
	2002 Employment Act
	2003 Employment Equality (Sexual Orientation) Regulations
	2003 Employment Equality (Religion or Belief) Regulations
	2003 Sexual Offences Act
	2004 Asylum and Immigration Act
	2005 Disability Equality Act
	2006 Equality Act
	2006 Employment Equality (Age) Regulations
	2006 Racial and Religious Hatred Act
	2006 Work and Families Act
	2006 Government of Wales Act
	2007 Gender Equality Duty
	2008 Equality Bill

Adapted from Bagilhole (2009: 85)

These laws may look comprehensive but there exist 'old' and stubborn problems for equality and diversity such as the unequal pay of men and women, and assumptions about women being the main carers of children. New Labour, from 1997 onwards, attempted to consolidate and strengthen equality and diversity legislation and created a single equality commission to oversee equality and diversity issues. Hills *et al.* (2009: 16) suggests there was a broad and ambitious policy programme that attempted to tackle child and pensioner poverty, unemployment and worklessness, areas and neighbourhood deprivation, inequalities in health and educational attainment and inequalities by ethnic background. The complex and nuanced results suggest some improvement on inequality but remaining inequalities for the top and bottom members of society and with slow movement on key policy areas.

The European Union has also had a significant influence on equality and diversity directives although questions have been raised over the feasibility of driving forward initiatives and agendas for equality and diversity (Bagilhole 2009: 223). There are further difficulties in the heterogeneity of groups covered by equality and diversity legislation, the overlapping discrimination and oppression issues, future concerns such as an ageing population, increasing ethnic diversity, European expansion, new forms of migration, increasing disability, potential conflicts between disadvantaged groups and technological enhanced developments that impact on equality and diversity. The challenge for health and social care workers and students is to contribute positively to progressive changes to address inequality, discrimination and oppression, and make a real and significant change to disadvantaged groups and individuals.

CONCLUSION

This chapter has argued that equality, equal opportunities and diversity are difficult and contested terms. They have been used by different groups at different times to support and defend a range of positions. Prejudice, stereotypes, discrimination and oppression still give rise to significant barriers to promoting equality such as sexism, racism, disabilism, ageism, homophobia and Islamaphobia. The challenge for health and social care is to address these issues and problems.

SUMMARY OF MAIN POINTS

You should be able to:

- Recognize and discuss social difference and begin to apply this theoretical discussion to issues of class, gender, race and ethnicity, age, disability and sexual identity.
- Debate the notion of equality, inequality and equal opportunity.
- Discuss the consequences of prejudice, stereotyping, discrimination and oppression.
- Describe and discuss the human rights framework and identify relevant legislation and the European dimension.

MOMENT OF REFLECTION

Should everyone be treated the same?

1   Why do we need equal opportunities and diversity?
2   What are the significant barriers to promoting equality and respecting diversity?
3   How have approaches to equality and diversity changed historically?

MOMENT OF REFLECTION

Language: Appropriate language

The businessman has acted as chairman and was seen as the best man for the job to supervise the girls in the office who were typing the firemen's demands. Reflect on this sentence. What does it suggest to you?

Checklist of inclusive terms: Gender

Best man for the job	Best person for the job
Businessman/woman	Businessperson, manager, executive
Chairman/woman	Chair, chairperson, convener, head
Cleaning lady	Cleaner
Deliveryman	Delivery clerk, courier
Fireman	Fire-fighter
Forefathers	Ancestors
Gentleman's agreement	Unwritten agreement, agreement on trust
Girls, ladies (for adults)	Women
Husband/wife	Partner
Layman	Layperson
Man or mankind	Humanity, humankind, human race, people
Common man	Ordinary citizen, person
Manhood	Adulthood
Manpower	Human resources, labour force, personnel, workers
Miss, Mrs	Ms unless a specific preference has been stated – but do we need to use a title at all?
Policeman	Police officer
Righthand man	Chief assistant, lieutenant
Spokesman	Spokesperson, representative
Stewardess	Airline staff, flight attendant
Tax man	Tax inspector/tax officer
Waitress	Waiter, server
Workmanlike	Efficient, proficient, skilful, thorough

Checklist of inclusive terms: Disability

Normal	Non-disabled person
The disabled (not a homogenous group, separate from the rest of society; the focus is on disability as people's defining feature)	Disabled people (which emphasizes that people are disabled by the way society and the environment are arranged)
Handicap	Impairment, condition, difficulty
Epileptic (a medically imposed label is a stigma that only serves to undermine people's rights and abilities)	People with epilepsy
Mental handicap	Learning difficulties, learning disabilities
Mental age of ...	Severe or profound learning difficulties
Victim of ...	Person who has, person with ...
Wheelchair bound	Wheelchair user, uses a wheelchair, has impaired mobility
'Deaf' as a blanket term	Deaf people; hearing impaired person; some people in the deaf community prefer to use 'the Deaf' as a political term, emphasizing that they are a linguistic minority, *not* a disabled group
The blind	Blind or partially sighted person, person with visual impairment. Vague and cumbersome terms like 'visually challenged' serve little purpose
Invalid	Disabled person
An arthritic	A person with arthritis

Checklist of inclusive terms: Cultural diversity

Christian name	First name, given name
Ethnic group	Everyone belongs to an ethnic group whether they are, in a given context, members of an ethnic majority or ethnic minority. Use minority ethnic group and majority ethnic group according to context
Eskimo	Inuit
Immigrant	In the UK context, person coming from abroad to settle here. It is incorrect to use this term of British national or to distinguish black from white people
Minority languages	Community languages
Red Indian	Native American or use particular tribal name
Black	Use 'black people'. Black people refers to people of African, Afro/African-American, and Afro-Caribbean or South Asian origin (taken as a group). 'Black people' is often used as a political term to refer to the relative disadvantage and marginalization
Asian	The Asian community in the United Kingdom is not a homogenous group but is made up of communities drawn from several different countries, e.g. Pakistan, Bangladesh, India, and Kenya. There are several different languages spoken and also different religions followed. Opinion is divided among British Asians as to whether they consider themselves black. The term probably does not cover adequately other groups such as those of Middle Eastern origin, or those of mixed origins. It is best to state what groups are being discussed in a particular context
Third world	Developing world, majority world

REFERENCES

Abbot, P. (2006) 'Gender' in Payne, G. (Ed.) (2nd edition) *Social Divisions*, Basingstoke: Palgrave Macmillan.

Age Concern (2006) *How Ageist is Britain?*, London: Age Concern.

Anthias, F. (1998) Rethinking social divisions, *Sociological Review*, 46 (3), 505–35.

Anthias, F. (2001) The concept of 'social divisions' and theorising social stratification, *Sociology*, 35 (4), 835–54.

Bagilhole, B. (1997) *Equal Opportunities and Social Policy*, London: Longman.

Bagilhole, B. (2009) *Understanding Equal Opportunities and Diversity: The Social Differentiations and Intersections of Inequality*, Bristol: Policy Press.

Barnes, C. (1991) *Disabled People in Britain and Discrimination*, London: Hurst and Co.

Berger, P.L. (1967) *The Sacred Canopy: Elements of a Sociological Theory of Religion*, New York: Anchor Books.

Best, S. (2005) *Understanding Social Divisions*, London: Sage.

Braham, P. and Janes, L. (2002) *Social Differences and Divisions*, Oxford: Blackwell.

Butler, J. (1990) *Gender Trouble: Feminism and the Subversion of Identity*, London: Routledge.

Carling, A. (1991) *Social Division*, London: Verso.

Connell, R.W. (2001) *The Men and the Boys*, London: Allen and Unwin.

Connell, R.W. (2009a) *Gender: In a World Perspective*, Cambridge: Polity.

Connell, R.W. (2009b) *Masculinities* (2nd edition), Cambridge: Polity.

Davies, B. (1991) *Frogs, Tails and Feminist Tales*, Sydney: Allen and Unwin.

De Beauvoir, S. (1972 [1949]) *The Second Sex*, Harmondsworth: Penguin.

DHSS (1980) *Inequalities in Health*, London: DHSS.

Equalities Review (2007) *Fairness and Freedom: The final report of the Equalities Review*, London: Equalities Review.

Finklestein, V. (1980) *Attitudes and Disabled People*, New York: World Rehabilitation Fund.

Foucault, M. (1978) *The History of Sexuality*, London: Penguin.

Giddens, A. (2009) *Sociology*, Cambridge: Polity.

Hills, J., Sefton, T. and Stewart, K. (2009) *Towards a More Equal Society?*, Bristol: Policy Press.

Hunt, P. (1966) *Stigma: The Experience of Disability*, London: Chapman.

Macpherson, W. (1999) The Stephen Lawrence Inquiry, London: HMSO.

Marx, K. (1978 [1875]) *Critique of the Gotha Programme*, Moscow: Progress Publishers.

McEwan, E. (1990) *Age: The unrecognised discrimination*, London: Age Concern.

Oakley, A. (1974) *Housewife*, London: Allen Lane.

Oliver, M. (1990) *The Politics of Disablement*, Basingstoke: Macmillan.

Oliver, M. (1996) *Understanding Disability: From Theory to Practice*, Basingstoke: Macmillan.

Parekh, B. (1992) 'A Case for Positive Discrimination', in Hepple, B. and Szyszak, E.M. (Eds) *Discrimination: The Limits of Law*, London: Mansell Publishing.

Payne, G. (2006) (Ed.) *Social Divisions*, Basingstoke: Palgrave.

Pitt, G. (1992) 'Can Reverse Discrimination be Justified?' in Hepple, B. and Szyszak, E.M. (Eds) *Discrimination: The Limits of Law*, London: Mansell Publishing.

Plummer, K. (1975) *Sexual Stigma: An Interactionist Approach*, London: RKP.

Ritzer, G. and Barnard, A. (2008) 'Globalisation' in Barnard, A., Horner, N. and Wild, J. *The Value Base of Social Work and Social Care*, Milton Keynes: Open University Press.

Scott, J. (2006) 'Class and Stratification' in Payne, G. (Ed.) *Social Divisions*, Basingstoke: Palgrave, pp. 23–64.

Scott, S. and Jackson, S. (2000) 'Sexuality' in Payne, G. *Social Divisions*, Basingstoke, Palgrave Macmillan.

Shakespeare, T. and Watson, N. (2002) The Social Model of Disability: An Outdated Ideology?, *Research in Social Science and Disability*, 2, 11.

Shaver, P. and Hendrick, C. (Eds) (1987) *Sex and Gender*, London: Sage.

Siedman, S. (1997) *Difference Troubles: Queering Social Theory and Sexual Politics*, Cambridge: Cambridge University Press.

Smith, D. (1979) A peculiar eclipse: women's exclusion from men's culture, *Women's Studies International Quarterly*, 1, 281–95.

Stonewall. (2003) *Profiles of Prejudice: The Nature of Prejudice in England*, London: Stonewall.

Thompson, N. (2003) *Promoting Equality: challenging discrimination and oppression*, Basingstoke: Palgrave Macmillan.

Weber, M. (1979 [1925]) *Economy and Society: An Outline of Interpretive Sociology*, Berkeley: University of California Press.

Weitzman, L. (1972) 'Sexual Socialisation in Picture Books for Preschool Children', *American Journal of Sociology*, 77.

FURTHER READING

Braham, P. and James, L. (2002) *Social Differences and Divisions*, Oxford: Blackwell.

Miller, D. (1976) *Social Justice*, Oxford: Clarendon Press.

Thompson, N. and Mullender, A. (2004) *Promoting Equality: Challenging Discrimination and Oppression*, Basingstoke: Palgrave.

Webb, R. and Tossell, D. (1999) *Social Issues for Carers* (2nd edition), London: Arnold.

CHAPTER 5

INTRODUCTION TO SOCIAL POLICY

CHRIS TOWERS

OBJECTIVES

After reading this chapter you should be able to:

- Discuss the history of policy.

- Discuss the competing perspectives.

- Describe the traditional areas of social security, health, education, employment and housing.

- Discuss the difference between wants and needs.

After reading this chapter you will know the meaning of the following terms: Wants, needs, New Right, Socialism, Social Democracy, New Labour, social security, health, education, employment and housing.

There are four Moments of Reflection to work on throughout the chapter.

INTRODUCTION

Social policy as a field of study may or may not mean something to you. You might feel you have little knowledge of it or that it is remote to you and your life experiences. But chances are it does have significance for you in that social policies will have the potential to shape your choices whenever you need health care, housing, employment, child care or many other services.

Social policies are dynamic, they affect lives and will affect both the providers and the users of a range of health and social care services. This chapter introduces you to social policies. These may or may not be familiar to you but as a student of, or even a worker in, health and social care services it is vital to be acquainted with them. We need, therefore, to explore what they are and to show their significance.

We start this chapter with a few explanations of what social policy is before moving on to explore the various perspectives in social policy. There are different attitudes towards whom should provide for our welfare. People will have different values and beliefs. Governments and those that make policies will look at the world through different eyes. We compare and contrast those different perspectives. The chapter then looks at the vital issue of wants and needs. People will have differing needs from health, social care and other services. Whilst it is important to consider who should provide for them, be it government, charities, the family, etc., it is also vital to consider what should be provided. What do we 'need' in this society, just 'adequate' food, shelter and income or much more than that? We then consider policies in relation to some key areas of social policy; from social security to employment to education, health and personal social services. The chapter then has a section called 'finishing off', that features the final 'activity', one of many through the chapter, which will help you to reflect on the significance of social policies for people, services and society generally. We conclude with a summary of the main points from the chapter.

WHAT IS SOCIAL POLICY?

Everyone will probably encounter social policies at some point in their lives, either as workers and/or users of health and social care. Let us therefore outline a quite recent piece of social policy and show how it may affect you. Many people smoke cigarettes and others will know someone who smokes. Smoking affects our health and the decision to smoke can have an impact on many others, from friends and family to providers of health care. The Health Act 2006 was a piece of social policy that included provision for the outlawing of smoking in workplaces and enclosed public places. It relates to the smoking of tobacco or any other substance and related to manufactured cigarettes, hand rolled cigarettes and pipes. From 1 July 2007 those with responsibility for public spaces, from the small shop owner to larger employers, have responsibilities to place 'no smoking' signs. Businesses can be prosecuted if they fail to prevent smoking in a smoke free place and fail to display no smoking signs.

You are affected by the Health Act if you work in or around a hospital. There are smoking restrictions in place and these apply to patients as well as staff. Cigarette breaks are outlawed within the workplace if undertaken within confined spaces. The health care of patients is also affected, perhaps positively if there is evidence that the smoking restrictions lead to less use of tobacco. This may reduce incidents of various smoking related diseases.

The Health Act 2006 was an action of government, a law passed with the intention of promoting health, a vital part of people's welfare. The Act not only made provision for the outlawing of smoking in public or enclosed places but had other provisions attached to it. The legislation also introduced guidelines to control health care related infections and in particular those that people can acquire after visiting hospitals. It aimed to reduce infections by instigating more regulation through codes of practice. These guidelines affect those providing health care and those managing the provision of such care.

These plans and actions are part of the process of implementing social policies. Baldock *et al.* (2007) define policies as 'deliberate interventions by the state to redistribute resources amongst its citizens so as to achieve a welfare objective'. The no smoking and infections legislations are certainly 'deliberate intervention' and they are concerned with people's welfare. They penalise or at least restrict smokers in the interests of those who do not smoke. The infection related measures make deliberate the intention to improve the health and welfare of those entering hospitals.

But what of the other words in Baldock's definition? What does 'redistribution' mean and how can we understand what that means in practice? Let us turn to that word 'redistribution' shortly, but before then let us look at other aspects of social policies and how they may affect people's welfare.

Social policies will not only affect when or where people smoke or the quality of the health care they receive. They can also affect their access to the kind of housing they can access or how much income someone is entitled to when unemployed. They will affect how much they are paid at work. We have regulation such as the minimum wage or working tax credits, payable to those who take jobs when unemployed, allowing their income to be supplemented. Social policies affect people's ability to smoke where they wish or to not breath in smokers' fumes. They will also affect how much income someone has available to buy those cigarettes in the first place! When Baldock talks of 'redistribution' he means the business of moving resources, including money, from some groups to others or from some time of life to another. Giving benefits or credits to some and asking others to pay for them, redistribution simply means giving to some and taking it from others.

This may mean that people pay more in tax or national insurance to pay for unemployment benefits or other forms of welfare. It may mean that people 'pay in' through their working lives so that they are able to claim a pension in later life. Discussion around social policies and their aims draws some people to a 'Robin Hood' redistribution (Hills 2004). This is not necessarily 'robbing' some to pay others but distributing resources in certain ways so as to increase people's welfare. Social policies to some are about responding to inequalities in society by moving resources around in the name of fairness or equality. This could be considered 'social justice'. However, social policies are also about 'criminal justice' and Acts of Parliament designed to meet the 'needs' not only of people who commit criminal acts but of the wider community which needs protection.

Whatever the aims of social policy, it is a contentious subject. This is because issues of who pays for welfare always stir people's emotions. It brings up issues such as fairness, equality, the freedom to earn and spend our own money or to reach out to others in need. It is not only a contentious issue but it has practical significance for service users as it will relate to how health and social care can meet human needs. Social policies can of course be about Acts of Parliament, legislation passed with the direct intention of moving resources or providing services.

THE DIFFERENT PERSPECTIVES

There will be different ideas on the purpose of policies and how much government and others who make and implement policies should be involved in people's lives. It would be helpful, therefore, to outline some of the different perspectives in social policy but to see how far back attitudes go because some will have their roots in other times.

We can identify what may be called a so-called 'laissez faire' or liberal philosophy and outlook and this has its roots in nineteenth century social policies. The state or the government is said to have a minimum involvement in people's lives. UK social polices at that time were dominated by a system of welfare embodied in the 1834 Poor Law Amendment Act, in which the poorest were given welfare in workhouses. Only the most needy were given support. A stigma grew up around the workhouse for the poorest were often presumed to be idle and immoral.

The idea of less government involvement and minimum protection for only the poorest has shaped many later developments in social policy. The 1980s saw the development of the **'New Right'**, a political movement embodied in Margaret Thatcher who led the Conservative Party, elected in 1979. Welfare benefits were often conditional and in the 1980s benefits were withdrawn from young people who failed to take up the offer of a government training scheme. Social policy from this perspective sees government as a lawmaker and a rule maker but not necessarily there to offer extensive welfare support. Families and charities (part of the so called 'voluntary sector') are viewed as playing a significant part in the delivery of welfare.

There are other perspectives that may partly draw from the New Right or have their own concerns and ideals. **Socialists** see the relationship between the state and the individual in other ways. They are committed to reducing disadvantage with the government concerned with redistribution and reducing inequalities. **Social Democracy** tends to draw from these different perspectives, concerned to reduce inequalities through state involvement but acknowledging that the individual also has a responsibility to help themselves. Different perspectives tend to borrow from each other and also from the past.

When **New Labour** came to power in 1997 they talked about having a 'new contract for welfare' (DSS 1998). People were encouraged to seek their welfare through work not benefits. They wanted individuals to take responsibility and benefits to be conditional on some sort of effort to find work. They drew from the New Right in terms of talking about individual responsibility. They also drew from other perspectives when they stressed continued government support for people in need of welfare.

There are other perspectives, including feminist outlooks or ones concerned with the environment. The plans and actions of governments will be shaped to some extent by the nature of their ideals and visions for how welfare should be organised. These perspectives will shape not only policies but choices in health and social care, in the way services operate and the lives of service users and providers. See if you can trace the impact of social polices and also welfare ideologies in the case history of Sally and her choices (below).

MOMENT OF REFLECTION

Activity One: Sally and her choices

Sally, 35 years old, is a trained social worker who qualified 18 months ago from an English university. She has been looking for work for all that time but is struggling to find it. Whilst she did well on the course and shone on some placements, finding work has not proved so easy. She lives alone and has been drawing various social security benefits as she seeks work. There are opportunities all around the country and she sees many vacancies in *Community Care* magazine. She does not drive a car and this has restricted her chances of finding work. Lessons are very expensive and she cannot afford them. Sally would move away from her 'home' area but she has to look after her ageing mother and feels a commitment to her. She feels she has a 'right to work' and feels 'let down' and resentful of the fact that employers in inner city areas will not consider her application because of her lack of car driving. Sally also feels that she comes from 'the wrong side of town' as far as some employers are concerned and that she is stigmatised because of her background, her accent and where she comes from. She says that 'people from my part of town' don't always find it easy to find work even with qualifications and experience. Sally refuses to say more about this.

She also feels that benefits should be higher so that she can afford things like driving lessons. The job centre have 'recommended' that she goes on one of their government backed training schemes in information technology and that she may lose her benefits if she does not attend. Sally feels that she needs that time to look for work and would rather do things her way and look for work than 'waste time' doing an IT course. Many of her friends say that she has been unemployed 'long enough' and should take 'any job' going but Sally says that she only wants a job 'appropriate' to her skills and experience and that she will wait until such a post comes along. She feels, in any case, that she is 'better off' unemployed as a 'dead end' job would not only demoralise her but would not offer her any financial advantages.

What would the different perspectives say about Sally's choices?

WANTS AND NEEDS

Social policy is about choices, rights and responsibilities. It is also about need and meeting it, but there are different perspectives on what exactly is a 'want' and how this differs from a 'need'. Many people may argue that a place of shelter or basic standards of hygiene are essential needs as well as food, clothing and warmth. Others may argue that people have more complex needs and that items like the motor car, the mobile phone and money to take part in social activities are modern day needs rather than merely wants. Let us take some concrete examples of how issues of wants and needs will affect users as well as providers of health and social care.

You may, for example, be working as a social worker in a hospital and decide that the older person needs to return home as quickly as possible. They are, in your opinion, becoming too dependent on hospital services and as a result their ability to function at home will be impaired by staying in hospital. It will compromise their ability to remain independent. The doctors and medical staff are concerned about the health needs of the older person and say that they are at risk if they are discharged. They recognise that the woman 'wants' to go home but say that she 'needs' to remain in hospital for a while yet. The older person on the other hand agrees with the social worker and says she 'needs' to go home. Immediately there will be a tension between the workers and the older person with different needs being emphasised. The need to be 'safe' against the need for independence. Want and need will be defined differently and there will be a tension between these competing interests. Social policies will also define wants and needs differently. The Care (Delayed Discharges) Act 2003 encourages swift discharge from hospital in that it outlines that there should be financial incentives for local authorities to discharge patients and provide community care services to meet 'need' once back in the community.

Providers and users of health and social care will work with social policies that define exactly what people's wants and needs are. These needs may sometimes be interpreted as 'wants' by some of those involved whilst others see need in each situation. The 'need' for people to live in their own homes has been emphasised through many social policies. We can see this in the provisions of the 1990 NHS and Community Care Act. The Act arose from a report by Sir Roy Griffiths (DHSS 1988) which not only outlined a commitment to community care but suggested that social services should compete with private and voluntary groups to provide home based and community care (Baggott 2004). In other words, the aim was to ensure that people who had previously been cared for in institutions were now cared for in their own homes or in some sort of community setting. Social services were no longer seen as the main or sole provider of these services but they should work with other agencies to meet the aims of the Act. The legislation also stated that services should be 'needs led'. But what did this actually mean in practice?

The legislation actually referred to a number of different needs and these were defined as follows. A need for:

- information
- domestic assistance
- emotional support
- physical and/or nursing care
- financial support
- appropriate housing
- access to transport
- access to recreation, leisure or work.

You may want to reflect for a few moments on how far all of these can be defined as 'needs' or if any of them could be regarded as 'wants'. In doing so you are considering some fundamental issues in the delivery of welfare and the shape of social policies. It is important to consider the nature of need in order to assess if services are meeting it and to explore how far it is the government's responsibility to meet such need.

There are various theories on need, including Doyal and Gough (1991). They believe that people have two essential needs and these are for 'survival' and 'autonomy'. To achieve these two basic requirements other linked needs must be met including the need for protective housing, basic education, a so called 'non-hazardous' environment and nutritional food and water. Whilst they don't rank these needs in order, other theorists such as Abraham Maslow (1954) attempt to list human needs in a so called 'hierarchy of needs'.

Maslow suggested that people must first have their basic needs met, such as their physiological needs, the need for air, water and sleep, for example. Once these are met they can move on to more complex needs such as the need for safety and security. The suggestion is that the needs for love, for belonging and acceptance exist towards the top of a hierarchy and these are the things that people aspire to once the other more basic needs have been met.

Questions of need and how to define it are fundamental to understanding social polices and their consequences for the people who provide and use health and social care.

SOCIAL POLICIES: PAST, PRESENT AND FUTURE

Understanding today's social policies and how they affect health and social care will require some understanding of their history. If we look first at some of the key areas in social policy we can see how the past effects the present. We can cite the nineteenth century Poor Laws as influential for they established the idea of meeting the 'needs' of the poorest with only the very poorest worker receiving help in the workhouses. The so called 'principle of less eligibility' enshrined in the 1834 Poor Law Amendment Act will still shape polices today as many benefits and other services are means tested and people have to meet 'eligibility criteria'.

The Beveridge Report, written by William Beveridge in 1942, established a blueprint for welfare services that has shaped the development of what we call the 'welfare state', with free health care and a social security system. His identification of the 'five giant evils' of want (poverty), squalor, disease, ignorance and idleness led to a plan to rid society of these identified social problems. Let us then examine these histories in detail as we discuss contemporary issues in social policy.

POVERTY AND SOCIAL SECURITY

The system of social security in place in modern Britain has many of its origins in the Beveridge report, or to give it its full title 'The Report of the Inter Departmental Committee on Social Insurance and Allied Services'. This established the idea that the government should play a key role in combating poverty. People would pay national insurance through a working life time and thus qualify for social insurance benefits through times of sickness or unemployment. The subsequent legislation such as the Family Allowances Act 1945 and the National Insurance Act 1949 put in place a system of social security that still has strong relevance now.

These social policies have shaped the lives and choices of generations of people, offering financial security to some and yet leaving others to experience poverty. They are supposed to ensure that people do not live below a certain threshold of financial security. This may not be easy to ensure as 'poverty' and wants/needs can be relative to a person's situation.

Draw up your own list of what you feel you 'need' to live on (*see* Activity Two on page 71) and then see if the current levels of social security benefits[1] would suffice. You will need a weekly basket of food, you will need fuel of some sort and other items. Make up a list of what you consider to be essential needs and then work out the weekly sum of money, after housing costs, needed to meet that cost.

MOMENT OF REFLECTION

Activity Two: How much do I need to live on?

Item	Cost (weekly)

You may decide after undertaking this exercise that social security levels are either sufficient or not for you to live on. However this works out, issues of income, poverty and social security are familiar ones for users and providers of health and social care services. A knowledge of the rules and regulations plus some awareness of the lived experience of low income and poverty are all essential for anyone working in these services.

Governments have their own understandings of poverty, and benefit levels are set partly in response to those understandings. There are also issues of social exclusion and these have also been the concern of those making and delivering policies. But what does it mean to be socially excluded? This idea has in a sense been around for a long time. Richard Titmuss (1958) argued that it was the social security system itself that showed up the social divisions of society with some people entitled to private or tax subsidies whilst others received state welfare. Peter Townsend (1979) demonstrated some decades ago how families with low incomes cannot participate in the lives of the communities in which they live. Their exclusion happens because they cannot afford the things that make one part of a society.

However, it was the New Labour government, elected in 1997, that focused on the idea of social exclusion and promised to tackle it. They said that to be socially excluded is not just to experience problems with income. They identified housing related issues as well as problems in health, employment and access to social networks. They showed their commitment to this idea when they set up the Social Exclusion Unit in 1998. Social exclusion was defined as 'a shorthand term for what can happen when people or areas suffer from a combination of linked problems such as unemployment, poor skills, low incomes, poor housing, high crime environments, bad health and family breakdown' (Social Exclusion Unit 2002).

EMPLOYMENT

Employment is a key area for social policy and the 1997 elected government saw work as an important part of their strategy of tackling social exclusion. William Beveridge viewed employment as central to his plan and he aimed for 'full employment' (although he always accepted there would be *some* unemployment). Work also was a central element in New Labour's programme with its emphasis on 'welfare to work'. They introduced the 'New Deal' programme which gave special priority to getting 18–24-year-old young people who were claiming Job Seekers Allowance back into work (Baldock *et al.* 2007). They were given options including work or training experience. They were expected to accept one of the options with the understanding that work was the best form of welfare.

Social policies themselves are there to 'meet the needs for welfare and well-being within the population' (Alcock 2003). But plans for the New Deal just like any other social policies will not necessarily meet people's needs. Understanding social policies and the plans and actions of government will, however, require one to be critical of any easy notions that work is the best form of welfare.

MOMENT OF REFLECTION

Activity Three: Darren – work as welfare?

Darren is 21 years of age and lives with his girlfriend Karen in a flat. They have a young child of three years. He originally had a job through the government's 'New Deal' and this helped him, as he said, 'get used to work', and through it he found a job working more hours. His original job was as a care assistant but the hours were not substantial and he felt stressed with the job. He felt many of the older people at the home valued him, he felt part of the community there, but the money was simply not sufficient. He now does shift work at a bed factory and it involves working through the night. He has his 'dinner' at eleven at night just before he starts his shift, with some 'tea' at five in the morning, three hours before he finishes his eight hour shift. Food is not that great, mainly fry ups, egg and bacon, that sort of thing and he also 'snacks' on the job. But it is all he can get. He also admits to having a 'sweet tooth' and he worries about his teeth and decay and whether he can afford dental care now he is working. He has had bouts of toothache.

Karen stays at home and looks after their young child although does have a part-time job in a local health clinic in the afternoon. Darren gets home at about nine in the morning and sleeps until about 4pm, making it hard to care for his child. They therefore organise some child care for the period in the afternoon and Karen picks her daughter up so that she can join Darren at home in the late afternoon. They then have a few hours together before he is off to the bed factory for his 11pm start.

Darren feels like he's 'making the effort' and he feels a sense of respect for himself through working although he sees little of his friends who work 'regular hours'. When he does see them he is often tired and has to leave early to get to work. The couple claim working family tax credits and that helps.

Consider Darren's story and list ways in which work has and has not met his welfare needs.

EDUCATION

Education has always been a key area for social policy. The Beveridge Report identified 'ignorance' as one of the 'five giant evils' and the 1944 Education Act (also known as the 'Butler Act') established free education up to the age of 16 and set up a system of schooling organised through grammar, secondary modern and technical schools. The grammar schools were for the so called 'brightest' pupils who passed an examination at aged eleven, with those considered less able going to the other schools. This system courted controversy as to some it was seen as divisive. Education has always been a contested area of policy.

We have seen various education polices since then with raging debates about the curriculum, funding and issues such as loan and tuition fees in higher education. In 1988, the Education Reform Act introduced the National Curriculum with its systematic testing of pupils, league tables monitoring performance and more systems of inspection (Bochel *et al*. 2005). New Labour introduced key testing in primary schools and the so called 'literacy hour' as part of the 'national literacy policy' in England (Synder 2008).

Those working in health and social care will encounter young people who may or may not have had a positive experience of education. Education policies will have shaped their experience of schooling and may have given rise to issues of social exclusion.

The government promoted education as a key area of policy and it has talked of education in relation to issues of social exclusion.

However, many young people have not had a positive experience of education, despite the government's commitment to raising standards. Robert Winnett (2005) wrote in *The Times* about NEETS. These are a group of 1.1 million young people who are Not In Education, Employment or Training.

HOUSING

Anyone working within health and social care will also need to have an understanding of housing and the social policies that influence choices. Looking back into history we can note that the Beveridge Report not only suggested that 'squalor' was a social problem but that governments should do something to rectify it. Council housing on a mass scale was proposed but problems with housing remained. Poor housing, poverty and its effect on families and children were depicted in a film broadcast by the BBC in 1966 called 'Cathy Come Home', which brought issues of homelessness to public attention.

We have had various social policies since then that have attempted to respond to homelessness. The various Housing Acts, from 1977 through to 2002, have all emphasised the importance of 'intentionality'. In other words, help can only be granted if you are considered homeless not through your own intention or choice. Particular support is now offered to specific groups such as victims of domestic violence or those leaving children's homes or prisons.

Housing has also been linked to other social problems. The Social Exclusion Unit produced a report in 1998 entitled 'Bringing Britain Together: A National Strategy for Neighbourhood Renewal' which emphasised the need for action to improve 'deprived neighbourhoods' with not just problems in housing but a range of other social problems. There have been various other social policies related to housing need, from the 1980 Housing Act, which gave people the 'right to buy' their council house at a discount, to the 2004 Housing Act which included plans to free up empty houses for occupation.

HEALTH

Health is and has been a key concern of social policies. The National Health Service was founded in 1948 with its promise of health care free at the point of delivery. People can expect to receive this through a lifetime, paid for through national insurance contributions. There have, however, been growing concerns with the costs of health care and debates about rationing. The NHS Plan 2000 also promised to make health care more responsive to the individual needs of patients. There have also been concerns with the so called 'postcode lottery' whereby your ability to access treatment is dependent on which part of the country you live on, compromising the ideals of the NHS with its promise of equal access to health care.

THE PERSONAL SOCIAL SERVICES

Those working in health and social care will also be guided by a range of social policies concerned with what can be called 'the personal social services'. Those working with older people will work with a range of initiatives including the government White Paper *Our Health, Our Care, Our Say* (2006) which outlined the future of health and social care. Whilst there have been concerns to promote the well-being of those needing care, carers have also been given more focus and we had the Carers Recognition Act in 2005. People with disabilities can now seek protection from the law via the Disability Discrimination Act 2005 and there have been various Children's Acts since the Second World War with the most recent one being in 2004.

FINISHING OFF

Social policies will affect lives including the lives of those who seek help from health and social care. Examine now Stephen's choices, in the case study below. See if you can identify the effects of social policies on his life? There may be some general Acts of Parliament that have shaped choices or there may be some general plans and actions that have guided his life.

MOMENT OF REFLECTION

Activity Four: Stephen's choices

Stephen, a 25-year-old single man, wants a dentist and not having had an appointment with a dentist for some two years feels it is time to get a check up. He has had some slight twinges in his teeth and even if, perhaps, it is not toothache he needs it checked out. He is in low paid employment and earning just too much to qualify for housing benefit or any other welfare assistance. Stephen works as a care assistant and although he likes the job in many ways, the contact with people, he feels it hard work and his pay is low. He does not feel, in any case, that valued or recognised in his work as a carer and wishes the government would do more to recognise his work in terms of pay and conditions.

He lives in a privately rented flat and his rent takes up much of his income but it is hard to get cheaper rents in the area. If he lives too far out of the area he could not get to work. He often considers leaving this flat but he worries that trying to move may be problematic. Rents in the area are high and in any case he would have to find money for a deposit especially if he does not get all of his current one back when leaving the property.

Stephen has often felt that he would be better off in council housing. He knows, however, that it can be hard to access and perhaps he is not in a priority group, being a single man without dependents. He also has to pay for night classes but these will help him get a better job. He can't afford private dentistry and has to find an NHS dentist. He telephones at least four dentists in his area without being able to register. He feels frustrated that he can't find a dentist.

How have social policies shaped Stephen's life? Can you identify the ways in which they have influenced his work?

SUMMARY OF MAIN POINTS

You should be able to:

* Understand there are competing perspectives in social policy.
* Understand the historical contexts of social policies.
* Understand issues of poverty, housing and homelessness, educational attainment, unemployment and poor health.
* Understand social policies applied across a range of areas.
* Understand that anyone working in health and social care or any related field will need a working knowledge and understanding of the consequences of social policies.

NOTE

1 Jobseekers' Allowance is paid at different rates according to age. The rates that applied in 2009/10 were: £50.95 a week for under 25 year olds; £64.30 a week for over 25 years olds; £100.95 a week for couples, if over 18 years old. (http://afraser.com/welfare/jsa.html).

REFERENCES

Alcock, P. (2003) *Social Policy in Britain*, 2nd edition, Basingstoke: Palgrave.
Baggott, R. (2004) *Health and Social Care in Britain*, Basingstoke: Palgrave Macmillan.
Baldock, J., Manning, N. and Vickerstaff, S. (2007) *Social Policy*, 3rd edition, Oxford: Oxford University Press.
Bochel, H., Bochel, C., Page, R. and Sykes, R. (2005) *Social Policy: Issues and Developments*, Harlow: Pearson.
DHSS (1988) *Griffiths Report on Community Care*, London: DHSS.
Doyal, L. and Gough, I. (1991) *A theory of human need*, London: Macmillan.
DSS (1998) *A new contract for welfare: principles into practice*, London: The Stationery Office.

Hills, J. (2004) *Inequality and the State*, Oxford: Oxford University Press.

Kennett, P. (2004) *A handbook of comparative social policy*, Edward Elgar Publishing.

Maslow, A. (1954) *Motivation and personality*, New York: Harper.

Social Exclusion Unit (1999) *Bridging the gap: new opportunities for 16–18 year olds in education, employment or training. CM4405*, London: HMSO. [also online]. Available at: http://www.dfee.gov.uk/post16/br_white_exec.shtml

Social Exclusion Unit (2002) [online]. Available at: http://www.socialexclusionunit.gov.uk

Synder, I. (2008) *The Literacy Wars. Why teaching children to read and write is a battleground in Australia*, Allen and Unwin.

Titmuss, R. M. (1958) *Essays on the Welfare State*, London: Allen and Unwin.

Townsend, P. (1979) *Poverty in the United Kingdom*, Harmondsworth: Penguin.

Winnett, R. (2005) *Meet the 'Neets'. A new underclass, The Sunday Times,* March 2005 [online]. Available at: http://www.timesonline.co.uk/tol/news/uk/article438356.ece?token=null&offset=0&page=1 (Accessed 31 March 2009).

PART 2

STUDYING AT A HIGHER LEVEL IN HEALTH AND SOCIAL CARE: ARGUMENT, CRITICAL THINKING AND REFLECTION

SIÂN TRAFFORD

OBJECTIVES

After reading this chapter you should:

- Be aware of the expected development in writing skills from Level 1 to Level 3.

- Be able to put together a supported argument.

- Be aware of some of the pitfalls in arguments.

- Be able to implement strategies for critical reading.

- Be familiar with the concept of reflective practice.

After reading this chapter you will understand the key terms:
Argument, critical reading, critical literature review, reflective practice.

There is a Moment of Reflection at the end of the chapter.

INTRODUCTION

This chapter examines the skills necessary to develop a written argument. It addresses some of the problems to avoid when constructing an argument and the central elements of putting together an argument. It also explains how student work is expected to develop with each year of a University course, using the example of Bloom's taxonomy (*see* Petty 2004: 8). It then considers the link between critical reading and writing critically, before discussing how reflective writing can support and develop reflective practice.

There is an expectation that students' writing skills will increase in sophistication and complexity as they progress through their degree and that their work will display excellent critical analysis as well as effective, well-evidenced argument. To achieve this, students need to use the feedback they are given by tutors as a developmental tool that will allow them to implement improvements in their writing. If used conscientiously, feedback can help students to develop over their university careers through the six levels of learning identified by Bloom (Table 6.1): moving from learners with lower order skills, such as simply recalling facts, to learners with high order skills who can interpret, apply, analyse and eventually evaluate (*see* Petty 2004: 8).

Bloom's simple classification of skills can be helpful to students aiming to understand how their work is expected to develop as they progress from level 1 to level 3 because it demonstrates that learning, or rather understanding, becomes more complete as students progress through the skill levels. The higher order skills of analysis, synthesis and evaluation require students to think more deeply about a subject and to make connections between different parts of learning. These different parts of learning could be new learning, such as different parts of the same course, or they could be aspects of existing learning, such as knowledge accrued prior to university or learning acquired during work experience or volunteering opportunities. It is these connections that lead to understanding, which in turn leads to the deep learning necessary for a student to produce thoughtful, well-evidenced and well-argued work.

Table 6.1 Bloom's taxonomy of learning

Bloom's taxonomy		Direction of development
Evaluation	Make judgements, assess the value of ideas or theories, compare and discriminate between ideas, evaluate data	High order skills
Synthesis	Generalise from given knowledge, use old ideas to create new ones, organise and relate knowledge from several areas, draw conclusions, predict	↑
Analysis	Identify patterns, recognise components and their relationships	
Application	Apply methods, theories and concepts to new situations	
Comprehension	Interpret information in own words, grasping meaning	
Knowledge	Display knowledge of facts, recall of information	Low order skills

Adapted from Petty (2004)

DEFINING THE TERM 'ARGUMENT' AS USED IN ACADEMIC WRITING

In order to develop their proficiency at constructing written arguments, students need to be aware of what they are writing and what 'job' their writing is trying to do. The Adult Literacy Core Curriculum (DfES 2001) lists six different purposes of writing: to describe, to explain, to instruct, to inform, to entertain and to persuade. While academic writing may require the writer to describe, explain or even inform in certain instances, the most frequent task of a piece of academic writing is to persuade the reader of a certain point of view by means of a balanced and well-evidenced argument. Students and learners need to be able to recognise when their writing is being merely descriptive or explanatory instead of being persuasive and evaluative. It can help to consider whether the writing is 'drawing a picture with words' but not really drawing any conclusions or presenting a particular point of view, or whether it is really presenting an argument with persuasive reasons. For example, identify the purpose of the following sentence:

> Homeopathy is a widely practised alternative therapy which uses dilutions of substances to treat many conditions.

Is it a description or persuasion (in the form of an argument)? It is, of course, a description of what homeopathy is and does. There is no attempt to persuade the reader, for example, that homeopathy is an effective or ineffective therapy.

All too often, the term 'argument' is confused with the term 'quarrel' which is the difference of opinion between two opposing sides. However, the word 'argument' is derived from the Latin 'arguere' which means 'to make clear'. One contemporary definition is 'to debate, discuss and persuade by reason' (Pratchett 2000: 290), while Germov (2000: 39) defines argument as 'a set of propositions which are supported by evidence and allow logical conclusions to be made.' These definitions make it easier to understand what needs to be done in an academic essay. The writer wishes the reader to believe a certain opinion because of certain reasons or particular evidence (Fairbairn and Winch 1996). Without any reasons, the argument is merely an uninformed assertion. Consider the following examples:

> Trams are better for the environment.

> Health and social care workers play a valuable part in communities.

These are merely assertions because there are no reasons given for the statements. By adding the following, however, the assertions become reasoned arguments:

> Trams are better for the environment. They carry large numbers of passengers at a time and will, therefore, use less fuel per passenger than cars and ease traffic congestion.

> Health and social care workers play a valuable part in communities. They work with some of the most vulnerable members of society, providing practical and emotional assistance and empowering them to live independent lives.

It is as though 'because' has been inserted between the two sentences in each example. Posing the questions 'why' or 'how' can help to generate the evidence needed to support statements or assertions.

Argument in an essay, then, must consist of a clearly stated main idea or point of view supported by valid reasons and, usually, reliable evidence. Of course, to present an effective persuasive argument, the writer needs to demonstrate that opposing views have also been considered by discussing contradictory viewpoints and analysing the relevant supporting evidence, and then demonstrating why their argument is the stronger or more convincing. To return to the first example above, the opposing argument could be that trams, being powered by electricity, still use fossil fuels which are harmful to the environment, but are nevertheless cleaner and will therefore contribute to a decrease in air pollution.

ASSEMBLING AN ARGUMENT

Chapter 1, *Skills for study and practice* explained how the reader has to rely on punctuation to make sense of what has been written because of the lack of voice intonation, facial expression, and so on, which usually helps to express meaning during a conversation when working with people. Similarly, a written argument has to contain all the necessary steps to explain the development of the argument to the reader because, unlike a conversation, the reader cannot interrupt to request clarification of a particular point (Fairbairn and Winch 1996).

The final step of an argument is the conclusion, and this is built on a series of logical steps called premises, which are statements of facts or evidence. The poor construction of an argument can lead to confusion or even controversy. For example, consider these two statements:

> ASBOs are an individualised means of protecting the community from alarming or distressing behaviour.

> Therefore, ASBOs can discriminate against people with mental health problems.

The first statement is a premise and the second is the conclusion (adapted from Fairbairn and Winch 1996) although as they stand they appear to have little obvious connection. These statements form the basis of a legitimate argument but they require more 'steps' (premises) to allow the reader to follow the line of reasoning and therefore understand it fully. In its present form, it is simply not logical. Indeed, it is almost offensive, and the reader will not be able to see how one statement can lead to the other. The following statement inserted between the premise and the conclusion will add more information:

> ASBOs are issued to people who have perpetrated anti-social acts.

However, the connection is still not necessarily obvious so a further statement can be inserted:

> People with mental health problems can display challenging or what might be deemed anti-social public behaviour because of a misunderstanding of their mental health problems.

However, the final line of the argument still seems to be unconnected with the evidence that is being presented so additional explanation is needed:

> People with mental health problems can be more likely to get into trouble within their communities.

This explanation allows the reader to follow the line of reasoning and understand how the writer is able to draw the conclusion that follows:

> Therefore, ASBOs can discriminate against people with mental health problems.

These steps (premises) can now be assembled into a logical argument (see below). The writer is supplying the reader with enough information (evidence) to progress through each stage, and has communicated an argument about a sensitive issue:

> ASBOs are an individualised means of protecting the community from alarming or distressing behaviour and are issued to people who have perpetrated anti-social acts. However, people with mental health problems can display challenging or what might be deemed anti-social public behaviour because of a misunder-standing of their mental health problems. For this reason, people with mental health problems can be more likely to get into trouble within their communities. Therefore, ASBOs can discriminate against people with mental health problems.

Notice how certain words are added to give the argument 'cohesion' – that is, they act as 'glue' to link the sentences firmly together and to help the sentences to 'flow'. For example, *for this reason* refers back to the statement, made in the preceding sentence, that people with mental health problems can be misunderstood. Referring backwards and forwards to information contained in the paragraph connects the information and reminds the reader of the issues being discussed. Similarly the words *however* and *therefore* are 'signposting' the direction of the argument. *However* is indicating that a contrasting point is about to be made while *therefore* indicates that a conclusion is about to be reached.

When constructing an argument it is important that the premises are 'sound' – that is, care must be taken to ensure that they are not based on assumptions, false premises (incorrect steps) or flawed reasoning (assuming that because one thing is true, the other must also be true without considering alternative explanations). Consider the following example:

> City centres have become unpleasant places. The reporting of tripping and falling accidents in city centres has rocketed in recent years. This demonstrates that the fabric of city centres has deteriorated to an unacceptable degree.
>
> (adapted from Cottrell 2003)

The writers have made several errors in their argument. They have begun by asserting that city centres have become unpleasant places and concluded that the fabric of city centres has deteriorated to an unacceptable degree. This argument suggests that all city centres have become unpleasant places although no supporting statistics have been supplied, just a vague assertion (reporting ... has rocketed) and the opening argument could be deemed a false premise because the evidence given is inconclusive. The writer has not considered that the tripping and falling accidents could have been caused by people falling because of illness, clumsiness, vulnerability or even drunkenness, while the rise in reported cases could be because a reporting mechanism was only introduced relatively recently, or people are more empowered to challenge local authorities or even that there is the possibility of financial compensation which encourages people to report incidents. The writer has also not provided an explicit link between the 'tripping and falling' and the 'fabric of city centres', which makes the argument disjointed, even nonsensical, or forces the reader to make the assumption that broken paving stones are to blame. Moreover, only one type of accident has been considered and used to make a generalised conclusion from a limited sample. If other types of accident were to be examined (falling shop signs or roof slates, for example) the claim about the deterioration in the fabric of city centres might be strengthened.

CRITICAL READING, THINKING AND WRITING

In order to achieve an elegant, convincing, well-supported and well-researched argument, the material used to support it must, of course, be reliable. Critical reading is therefore a vital part of the process of creating good academic writing. It requires the reader to be objective about the writing and to consider the context (social, historical, political, and so on) in which it was written and who the audience was intended to be. Critical reading involves making judgements about how a text is argued, supported and put together. It involves assessing the perspectives that are being developed in relation to the subject matter and this allows the reader to determine the central claims or purpose of the text. It also requires the reader to distinguish which concepts are defined and used, the kinds of reasoning employed by the text, and invites examination of the evidence (the supporting facts, examples, and so on). Critical reading, then, requires more than just reading to discover information. It involves looking at how writers think about their subject matter, how they construct their arguments and how that is expressed in the language they use. For these reasons, critical reading is one of the most important ways to develop a good academic writing style.

Skilful critical evaluation of the evidence contained in literature is vital as health and social care policy and practice is underpinned by evidence. Students engage with the literature of a certain subject area by undertaking a critical literature review. This is a comprehensive review of sources (books, journals, *reliable* websites, and so on) covering a particular field of study and critical reading is essential to produce a thorough and successful critical literature review.

There are multiple and competing perspectives within health and social care and undertaking a critical literature review requires students to identify and evaluate these perspectives. Examining the strengths and weaknesses of an author's arguments allows the student to agree with or defend a given point of view, concede that a given point of view has limited merits or reject a point of view entirely because of inadequacies in the argument, such as assumptions, lack of evidence or lack of plausibility. It is also useful for the student to be aware of their own critical stance towards the literature; to identify their reasons for selecting a particular text or journal article and to recognise the strengths or weaknesses of their own critique of that text.

The key to thinking and reading critically is vigorous questioning, and the most effective way to do this is to employ Kipling's (1993 [1902]) 'Six Honest Serving Men'. These are the interrogative words 'what?', 'why?', 'when?', 'how?', 'where?' and 'who?'. They encourage thinking and provide reliable methods to discover facts, to probe, to make connections and to fulfil other tasks vital for reading, writing and thinking critically and, therefore, for writing academically. For example, establishing 'what?', 'who?', when?' and 'where?' will provide factual information which is useful for setting an issue in context, whether that is historical, political, social, and so on. 'How?' is helpful for probing issues to find out how they function while 'why?' is helpful for discovering the reasons behind a particular issue or event. It can help the questioner to establish cause and effect between an event and the resulting consequences.

Learning Development (2009) at the University of Plymouth has developed a 'Critical Thinking Model' and accompanying study guide which are available through the Learnhigher website. This model divides critical thinking into three phases: description, analysis and evaluation. Using Kipling's six questions for the first two stages, the model shows how skilful questioning can help students to progress through their writing from the descriptive stage (gathering information to introduce an issue and to provide a context or background) to the analytical stage (looking for reasons or causes and examining the implications and effects).

For the evaluative stage, however, which entails estimating the effectiveness, and therefore the value, of a particular strategy or action as well as requiring students to reflect on their own viewpoint, the model recommends questions such as 'what if?', 'so what?' and 'what next?'. There is, inevitably, some overlap between the analytical and evaluative stages, but 'what if?' and 'so what?' not only allow students to interrogate material for cause and effect but also encourage them to consider alternative situations with alternative outcomes. 'What next?' enables students to suggest possible solutions or recommendations for future action, should that be a requirement of the assignment.

The use of these deceptively simple questions can provide students with a powerful tool to discover essential contextual information, to determine causes, explanations or consequences or even to clarify their own opinion of a particular issue or event. This, in turn, will enable them to read critically, think analytically and write academically.

REFLECTIVE WRITING AND REFLECTIVE PRACTICE

Reflection is an invaluable tool for self improvement and is adaptable for study, professional practice, even for personal development. It is particularly valuable in health and social care professions because it develops professional practice by promoting learning and understanding. Bolton (2005: 4) explains that 'reflective practice can take us out of our own narrow range of experience and help us to perceive experiences from a range of viewpoints and potential scenarios'. To understand how it can do this, it is first necessary to explore what reflective practice is.

Bolton (2005: 5) asserts that reflective practice is not confession, neither is it merely 'an examination of personal experience'. Rather she maintains that it requires practitioners to question their actions and values from several viewpoints, and to do so with an open mind.

Similarly, Moon (2006: 37) considers the act of reflection to be 'a form of mental processing' and points out that it is usually reserved for problematic issues or events. She adds that, crucially, reflection would seem to be an attempt to gain insight into these issues and events by re-examining and reorganising existing knowledge and understanding.

To illustrate the process of reflection, the educational theorist David Kolb (1984) developed a cycle of learning, divided into four stages. The diagram below demonstrates these stages. The experience stage, which could be an event or incident or action, is followed by the reflective observation stage. The purpose of this stage is to reflect on the experience and its successes or failures. The next stage, abstract conceptualisation, is to consider these successes or failures, taking into account theory, available resources and so on. The final stage, active experimentation, is to plan amendments or adjustments to the experience, and then the cycle begins anew.

It is, of course, entirely possible to begin the cycle at any point. Indeed, it would be a wise precaution to approach some events by reflecting on past experiences, or by trying to find out as much as possible from other people's experiences, before proceeding through the abstract conceptualisation and active experimentation stages. Suppose, for example, a job interview was imminent. It is almost certain that an individual would reflect on past job interview experiences to find out which were successful and which were less so (Stage 2). Stage 3 involves asking *why* some were more successful than others. If the answers to some of these Stage 3 questions were 'I was better prepared because I knew more about the job and organisation' or 'I was more confident because I had had a practice interview', they might then research the position and organisation or seek help with CV writing and interview technique (Stage 4). Only then would they approach the concrete experience (Stage 1).

This process can be invaluable for learners too. They need to ask themselves what they are trying to achieve when reflecting or considering experiential learning. The ability to evaluate personal experience and learn from it is the main aim of these techniques and could be summarised as the point of education. Dennison and Kirk (1990) describe it as a change of behaviour and state that learners and practitioners should always be developing their knowledge through reflection and evaluation based on current theory, legislation and so on. Burnard (2002) talks about reflection as the personal learning which makes a difference to our self concept and that makes us more competent interpersonally.

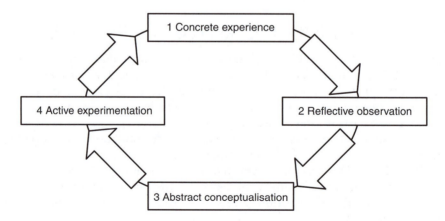

Figure 6.1 Kolb's cycle of learning

In a study context, for example, students could reflect on tutor feedback on their essays to improve their performance.

Stage 1 Concrete experience	*Describe and identify the actual event or activity:* assignment has lost marks for being descriptive and for poor referencing technique
Stage 2 Reflective observation	*Evaluate the experience (your work) for strengths and weaknesses:* what was successful, what went wrong
Stage 3 Abstract conceptualisation	*Identify how to make improvements:* mark could be improved by being more analytical and addressing the referencing conventions
Stage 4 Active experimentation	*Plan how to use this knowledge:* research the difference between descriptive and analytical writing; study the referencing conventions
Stage 1 Concrete experience	*Describe and identify the actual event or activity:* rerun the activity with the new knowledge incorporated into the next assignment

Professional practitioners can also implement Kolb's cycle to improve their performance.

Stage 1 Concrete experience	*Describe and identify the actual event or activity:* unsuccessful meeting between a social worker and a disengaged client with anger management issues
Stage 2 Reflective observation	*Evaluate the experience for strengths and weaknesses:* client disagreed with measures that were under discussion and lost his temper but a relationship was established
Stage 3 Abstract conceptualisation	*Identify how to make improvements using theory, guidelines and legislation:* client needs to feel part of the process and empowered
Stage 4 Active experimentation	*Plan how to use this knowledge:* build on relationship, include client in process, avoid them feeling something is being imposed
Stage 1 Concrete experience	*Describe and identify the actual event or activity:* subsequent meeting with client

The key, then, to effective reflection and reflective practice is to explore and analyse events, actions, thoughts, feelings and even values critically and honestly and then to put these reflections to use by action planning. The process helps to clarify how to establish the experience for review, identify areas for action and consider how to change actions or behaviour to improve performance. It is perhaps this staged cycle that makes reflective practice such an effective tool for personal, professional and academic development.

Techniques and tools for discussing personal experience and encouraging good reflection include keeping journals, a personal development portfolio, taking notes, summarising and gaining verbal clarification from a speaker at the time of the event. All of these techniques aid reflection by ensuring the evidence of the experiences is considered fully and that positive events are also reflected upon. It is also worth noting that, although reflective writing is usually in the first person, it must include theory or new knowledge with citation and referencing as evidence of the learning and development. Overall, reflection and experiential learning are powerful tools of expression that can assist students and professionals to continue developing and learning throughout their career.

CONCLUSION

This chapter has encouraged you to consider the progression of ideas in depth and sophistication through an undergraduate course of study. It discussed the increasing complexity and evaluation of Bloom's higher order skills. 'Argument' was defined and the support to evidence and assemble an argument was discussed. Critical reading, thinking and writing were discussed to allow you to develop higher order study skills. Finally, reflective writing and reflective practice was introduced to provide a vehicle for further and continuing skills development.

SUMMARY OF MAIN POINTS

You should be able to:

- Understand the expected development in writing skills.
- Be able to put together a supported argument.
- Be aware of some of the pitfalls in arguments.
- Be able to implement strategies for critical reading.
- Be familiar with the concept of reflective practice.
- Have an awareness of writing academically.

MOMENT OF REFLECTION

Consider the following terms. What do they mean?

**Assess   Analyse   Compare   Contrast   Criticise
Critically   Describe   Discuss   Evaluate   Examine
Explain   Illustrate   Interpret   Review**

Having made your choice of essay title, the first thing to do is look at the precise wording of the title and try to work out exactly what you are being asked to do. Apart from words relating to the content or topic, there are words which direct you to what you must do with that content. These so called **process** words include:

Assess – to determine the value; to evaluate.
Analyse – to examine in detail; to examine critically.
Compare – look for similarities and differences and reach a conclusion about which is preferable.
Contrast – set in opposition in order to bring out differences.
Criticise – give your judgement about the merit of theories and perspectives; back your judgement by a discussion of evidence or the reasoning involved.
Critically – to determine or decide or provide a judgement by argument.
Describe – give a detailed or graphic account of characteristics and features.
Discuss – investigate or examine by argument; sift and debate; give reasons for and against.
Evaluate – make an appraisal of the worth or value of something.
Examine – to weigh up; to test; to question.

Explain – make plain; interpret and account for; give reasons.

Illustrate – make clear by the use of concrete examples; use a figure or diagram to explain or clarify.

Interpret – expound the meaning of; make clear and explicit, usually giving your judgement.

Review – to examine again; to critically survey; to assess.

You must then decide what the relevant content is to include in your answer. What are the most important elements? What are the assumptions that lie behind the question and what are the implications that arise from it? By analysing (see above) the question you will give yourself a fair chance of selecting the relevant material as the basis for a good essay or exam answer.

REFERENCES

Bolton, G. (2005) (2nd edition) *Reflective Practice: Writing and professional development*, London : Sage.

Burnard, P. (2002) *Learning Human Skills: An experiential and reflective guide for nurses and healthcare professionals*, Oxford : Butterworth-Heinemann.

Cottrell, S. (2003) (2nd edition) *The Study Skills Handbook*, Basingstoke: Palgrave Macmillan.

Dennison, W. and Kirk, R. (1990) *Do, Review, Learn, Apply: A simple guide to experiential learning*, Oxford : Basil Blackwell.

Department for Education and Skills (DfES) (2001) *Adult Literacy Core Curriculum*, Nottingham: DfES.

Fairbairn, G. J. and Winch, C. (2006) (2nd edition) *Reading, Writing and Reasoning: A Guide for Students*, Maidenhead: Open University Press.

Germov, J. (2000) *Get Great Marks for your Essays* (2nd edition), Australia: Allen and Unwin.

Kipling, R. (1993 [1902]) *Just So Stories,* Ware: Wordsworth Editions.

Kolb, D. A. (1984) *Experiential learning: Experience as a source of learning and development*, US: Prentice Hall.

Learning Development (2009) *Critical Thinking*, Learnhigher, [online]. Available at http://www.learnhigher.ac.uk/learningareas/criticalthinkingandreflection/resourcepage.htm (Accessed 3 December 2009).

Moon, J. (2006) (2nd edition) *Learning Journals: A handbook for reflective practice and professional development*, Abingdon: Routledge.

Petty, G. (2004) (3rd edition) *Teaching Today: A Practical Guide*, Cheltenham: Nelson Thornes.

Pratchett, T. (2000) *The Truth,* London: Doubleday.

CHAPTER 7

HEALTH AND HEALTH CARE IN BRITAIN

BRIDGET HALLAM

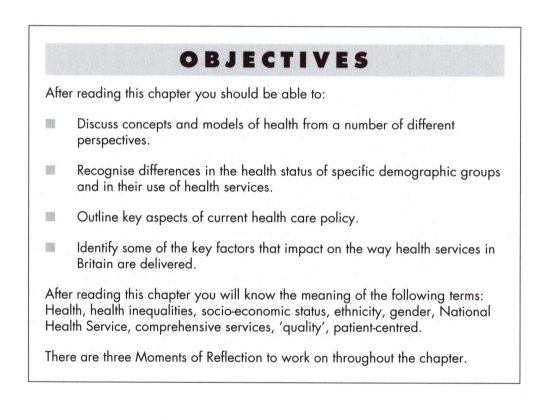

OBJECTIVES

After reading this chapter you should be able to:

- Discuss concepts and models of health from a number of different perspectives.

- Recognise differences in the health status of specific demographic groups and in their use of health services.

- Outline key aspects of current health care policy.

- Identify some of the key factors that impact on the way health services in Britain are delivered.

After reading this chapter you will know the meaning of the following terms: Health, health inequalities, socio-economic status, ethnicity, gender, National Health Service, comprehensive services, 'quality', patient-centred.

There are three Moments of Reflection to work on throughout the chapter.

Health, like the weather, is a favoured topic of conversation in Britain. Every day there are articles in magazines, news items and television dramas and documentaries featuring health and health care. When shopping, we are surrounded by advertisements for products that purport to improve or sustain our health and well-being. Health is vital to every living human being on earth, but what is it? People's ideas about 'health' and why it is important vary; different groups in society have different experiences of health and different approaches and attitudes to using health services. The organisation of health care services is complicated and seemingly ever changing. This chapter provides a brief introduction to ways of thinking about health, to the health experiences of different demographic groups and to key themes relating to the delivery of health services in Britain.

The chapter is split into two sections. The first begins by looking broadly at what we mean by the term 'health' before going on to explore health inequalities in relation to socio-economic status, ethnicity and gender. In the second section the focus shifts to look at issues relating to health care. It covers the organisation of the National Health Service (NHS), the issue of 'quality' and patient and public involvement in health as three key themes shaping health services in Britain.

CONCEPTS OF HEALTH

In 1948 the World Health Organisation published its definition of health as 'a state of complete physical, mental and social well-being and not merely the absence of disease or infirmity' (WHO 1948). Although sometimes criticised for being idealistic and unachievable, the definition remains useful in that it recognises health as a positive concept and an essential resource for living. However, it does not provide us with a clear definition of what this thing called health actually is and opinions on this vary.

Let us first consider how health is defined by 'ordinary' people, starting with your ideas.

MOMENT OF REFLECTION

Activity One

- Think of two people you would describe as being healthy. Who are they? How old are they? What makes you think they are healthy? Try to pick two people with different characteristics in terms of their age/gender/ethnicity/ social background.

- Use the characteristics that you have identified as being healthy to form your definition of health. How does your definition compare with that of the World Health Organisation?

- Have you put an emphasis on certain aspects of health?

COMMENTARY

Through this exercise you might have defined health as being physically fit, not getting ill very often or being able to recover easily from illness. Alternatively, you might have linked your idea of health to individual behaviour; not smoking or drinking alcohol, eating healthily, taking exercise and getting plenty of sleep. Other perspectives, often prevalent as people get older (Blaxter 1990), see health as a function – being able to do what you want to do – and recognise the importance of looking at the individual as a whole, not just their physical functioning. Your definition may have dimensions not mentioned here; this just reinforces the point that health is a contested concept and means different things to different people. There is no one definition that suits all.

Studies in recent decades have also identified that people's explanations of how health is achieved vary (Clarke 2010). For some, health is 'the luck of the draw', a feature of their genetic makeup, whereas for others it is something that can be worked for and achieved through effort.

By considering these different concepts of health it becomes clear that there may be several different models of health that attempt to provide an explanation and it is these that will be considered next.

MODELS OF HEALTH

The biomedical model

The Victorian era saw massive improvements in health and life expectancy in Britain as a result of broad public health measures such as the building of sewers, provision of clean water supplies and improvements in housing and education. However, the dominance of the medical profession, together with developments in medical technologies such as new drugs and surgery meant that a biomedical perspective increasingly dominated our view of health in Britain during the first half of the twentieth century. In this model, absence of disease or abnormality is fundamental to defining health, and ill-health results from bodily malfunctions, invasion by bacteria or viruses or through trauma. The body is seen as a machine to be 'fixed' or restored to health through the intervention of skilled medical professionals and the provision of specialist resources (Clarke 2010).

However, this model has been heavily criticised. McKeowan (1979 in Baggott 2004) highlighted the relatively limited contribution made by 'medical' interventions such as immunisation when compared with the impact of the earlier public health reforms such as those mentioned in the previous paragraph. The model can also be criticised for not taking into account the experiences of the individual and their mind and spirit alongside their physical being. Similarly it does not acknowledge the impact on health of social structures and environment. From these criticisms a number of alternative models have been proposed.

- A holistic model – argues that the body, mind and soul are indivisible and emphasises the need to focus on the 'whole' person, thus reflecting a client-centred approach to health.
- A behavioural model – stresses the responsibility that individuals have to support their own health and is often associated with health promotion.
- A social model – suggests that the causes of illness and disease lie not so much with the individual as with the way society is structured and the inequalities that this engenders. This model reflects many of the principles of the public health movement.

A biopsychosocial model

The truth is that all of the above models have a contribution to make to our understanding of health and illness but none in themselves gives the full picture. Acknowledging this and the limitations of the prevalent biomedical model, Engel (1977) proposed an alternative biopsychosocial model of health and illness which informs much of our thinking today. This model adopts a systems approach that recognises the interconnectedness of different factors that impact on health, and the fact that change in one part of the system (in this case the individual) will impact on all other parts of the system.

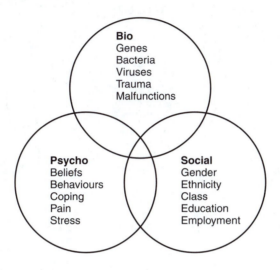

Figure 7.1 A biopsychosocial model of health and illness (adapted from Naidoo and Wills 2008: 105)

AN EXAMPLE

Mrs Fraser consults her doctor because she has been suffering from stomach pains, loss of appetite and feelings of nausea. At first sight these symptoms might suggest she has a stomach upset, perhaps caused by bacteria in something she ate. However, the doctor questions her a little further and finds that she has had these problems for a few weeks and that none of the other family members is ill.

When asked about her family Mrs Fraser explains that her husband was made redundant from work six months ago and is finding it difficult to cope with their change in circumstances. He spends a lot of time in the house watching television or sleeping and has become short tempered with her and their three children. The family are finding themselves increasingly in debt but she does not want to add to the pressure on her husband so is keeping the extent of their problems to herself. She has recently managed to find a job in a supermarket three evenings a week and enjoys this but does not finish until eleven o'clock at night. Despite the fact that she is very tired, she finds it difficult to get to sleep or, if she does, often wakes very early in the morning.

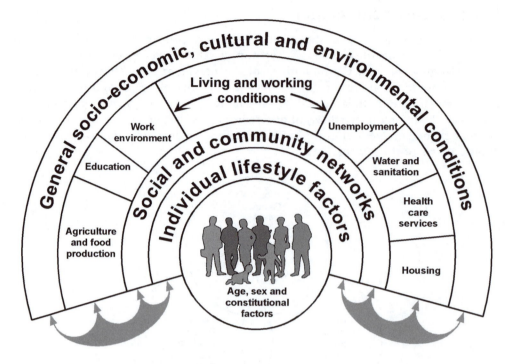

Figure 7.2 The main determinants of health
Source: Dahlgren and Whitehead (1993), reproduced in Dahlgren and Whitehead (2007)

Mrs Fraser may have a stomach upset but it is at least as likely, if not more so, that her family difficulties (the social factors) are understandably causing her stress (the psychological factors) and that the stress is leading to a rise in her adrenalin levels, resulting in her physical symptoms (biological factors).

It is clear then that health and people's experience of health and illness is influenced by a combination of factors as indicated by Dahlgren and Whitehead's (1993) 'Rainbow of Health' model which portrays the interrelationship between key determinants of health.

INEQUALITIES IN HEALTH

The Independent Inquiry into Inequalities in Health, commissioned by the Labour Government (Acheson 1998), explored a number of these determinants in some depth, focusing particularly on health inequalities. This next section looks at just three of these, socio-economic status, ethnicity and gender, before considering explanations that have been suggested to account for such inequalities.

Socio-economic inequalities

The link between socio-economic deprivation and poor health has long been recognised. The Black Report (DHSS 1980) highlighted inequalities in health that were wider in Britain than some other Western countries. At the time of its publication in 1980 the report did not receive wide acknowledgement from policy makers, however more recently the Acheson Report (Acheson 1998) reaffirmed the clear links between poverty and increased rates of mortality and morbidity. It has provided the stimulus for a huge and ongoing policy drive to reduce health inequalities. For more information on this and the progress made to date visit the Health Inequalities Section on the Department of Health (DH) website (DH 2009a).

But what is it that has so concerned the policy makers? In relation to mortality, we know that life expectancy has increased dramatically over the last one hundred years. In 1901 the life expectancy of newborn baby boys in the UK was 45 years and for girls it was 49 years. By 2006 it had reached its highest recorded level; a newborn baby boy could expect to live 77.4 years and a newborn baby girl 81.6 years (ONS 2009). However, although life expectancy has increased for all, these figures are not the same across all geographical areas.

There are very significant differences in the life expectancy of those living in some of the richest areas of Britain and those living in the poorest. Recent research (*see* Shaw *et al.* 2005) suggests men in the city of Glasgow have the lowest life expectancy in Britain and will live approximately eleven years less than their counterparts in East Dorset who have the highest. The figures are similar for women in Glasgow, who can expect to live nearly eight and a half years less than their peers in Kensington and Chelsea. What is of even greater concern is that despite the policy drive to decrease these inequalities, the gap between rich and poor remains (DH 2009b).

A similar pattern is seen if we consider infant mortality rates. Throughout the twentieth century, rates in Britain fell, as a result of improvements in housing, diet, sanitation and medicine and the availability of health care (Clarke 2010). However, studies continue to demonstrate clear inequalities when exploring the links between social class and infant mortality rates and social deprivation and infant mortality (Dorling *et al.* 2008).

Patterns of morbidity also show that those living in deprivation and who are unemployed or working in manual occupations have significantly higher levels of self-reported ill health and long-standing illnesses and higher rates of consultation for a range of conditions including high blood pressure, accidents and mental health difficulties (Acheson 1998).

In 2001, in an effort to address socio-economic health inequalities, the Government published two national Health Inequalities targets as follows:

Starting with children under one year, by 2010 to reduce by at least 10 per cent the gap in mortality between manual groups and the population as a whole.

Starting with health authorities, by 2010 to reduce by at least 10 per cent the gap between the fifth of areas with the lowest life expectancy at birth and the population as a whole (DH 2001).

Some progress has been made but it is unlikely that these targets will be achieved by 2010 and they have been criticised for focusing too specifically on socio-economic inequalities and not addressing other inequalities relating to age, ethnicity and gender (House of Commons Health Committee 2009).

Ethnicity and inequality

There are also inequalities in the health status of people from black and ethnic minority (BME) groups. Bangladeshi and Pakistani men and women report higher rates of poor health and limiting long-term illness than the majority of the population, while Chinese men and women report lower rates (Sproston and Mindell 2006). Similarly, the incidence of some diseases such as cardio-vascular disease and diabetes in South Asian and African Caribbean communities is much higher than in the general population (Sproston and Mindell 2006). The infant mortality rate in ethnic minority groups is also higher overall, particularly in Pakistani and Caribbean groups where it is twice as high as the white British population (ONS 2008). However, it is important to note that there are variations in health within different ethnic groups as well as between them and one criticism of these statistics is that they tend to cluster different groups together under a broad banner such as South Asian, which does not give the accurate information needed to develop culturally relevant services (Nazroo 1997).

The trends might to some limited extent be the result of genetic or behavioural differences but the explanation is more complex than this. As with the majority population, people from BME groups experience inequalities in health related to their socio-economic circumstances (Nazroo 1997). Additionally, there is evidence suggesting that other factors, 'including the experience of racial discrimination or cultural insensitivity in the provision of health care' (Kings Fund 2006: 4) might also play a part in determining health. For example, although surveys on the prevalence of mental illness show relatively little difference between groups in the community, people from BME communities are far more likely to be diagnosed with a serious psychotic illness and to be admitted to psychiatric hospital care than their white British counterparts (Baggott 2004). Another important concern is that stress resulting from exposure to racism in the community can itself be a cause of physical and mental illness although limited research has been done in this area (McKenzie 2003).

In 2005, the Department of Health published its Race Equality Scheme for 2005–8 (DH 2005). This outlined the strategies already in place and identified a number of priorities to address some of the inequalities in health outlined above. However, a report from the Healthcare Commission in 2009 (now the Care Quality Commission) highlighted that, overall, BME patients continue to report less positive experiences of health care services than the majority population. Of particular concern is access to services, provision of information and involvement in decisions about care (HCC 2009a) themes that have been echoed in previous studies. As we will see later in the chapter, these aspects of care are central to modernising health services in Britain. Despite their inclusion for action in the DH Race Equality Scheme, the report also highlights discrimination towards BME staff in the NHS and ineffective systems of data collection to support effective planning, delivery and monitoring of services. It seems there is still a lot to be done before these inequalities are eradicated.

Gender and inequality

We saw in an earlier section that women generally live longer than men. Men are more likely than women to die prematurely from heart disease as well as having higher mortality from lung cancer and from injuries, poisoning and suicides (Doyal *et al.* 2003). Some health needs, for example the need for maternity services, are sex specific, as are treatments for cancers such as prostate and ovarian cancer. However, genetic and hormonal influences also have an impact on the course of diseases such as TB and coronary heart disease, where differences in outcomes for men and women would not at first sight be expected (Doyal 2001). Overall, more men than women in Britain report their health to be good with women reporting higher levels of ill health than men, particularly anxiety and depression and in later life arthritis and rheumatism (ONS 2004).

Gender, as defined through the roles and expectations placed upon men and women by society, also has an impact on health. For example, eating disorders are more common in women than men and violence towards women is a significant cause of death and morbidity, not only in Britain but across the world. Stereotypical 'male' behaviour leads to men's greater exposure to violence and murder, and challenges to male identity that come from unemployment and deterioration of traditional industries have led to higher levels of suicide (Doyal 2001). Men are also more likely than women to experience illness related to behaviours such as smoking and drinking alcohol (ONS 2004). However, as women's health related behaviours become more similar to men's it seems likely that these differences will reduce.

With regard to accessing health services, surveys suggest women make more use of GP services and have more admissions to hospital than men. There is also evidence that the services accessed and received by men and women may be influenced by their gender. Doyal *et al.* (2003) suggest women may find it more difficult to access health care as a result of transport difficulties or caring responsibilities whereas men can be reluctant to access services for fear of appearing weak. They also suggest that health professionals may make different diagnoses and offer different treatments for the same conditions in men and women. In order to address these differences they recommend changes to the way health services are shaped including more research into gender differences in health, improved access to health care in workplace and community settings and increased sensitivity to gender by professionals, particularly in relation to health promotion (Doyal *et al.* 2003).

EXPLANATIONS FOR INEQUALITIES IN HEALTH

As noted earlier, determinants of health do not operate in isolation from one another. Similarly, inequalities in health interact; a combination of factors relating to gender, ethnicity, socio-economic status and age contribute to the inequalities we see. However, knowing this does not fully explain why these factors should lead to inequalities.

MOMENT OF REFLECTION

Activity Two

Think back to the preceding sections on inequality. What explanations are put forward to suggest reasons for the inequalities outlined there? You may have other suggestions too.

COMMENTARY

A number of different ideas have been put forward to explain inequalities in health. Some argue that inaccuracies in data collection and misinterpretation of statistics lead to wrong conclusions being drawn, but this does not seem likely to account for the significant inequalities we see (Baggott 2004). Biological and genetic factors have their part to play as do individual health behaviours, which may be linked to gender, social and cultural expectations and pressures (Clarke 2010). However, there is also clear evidence that inequalities in health are linked closely to the wider societal inequalities in income, educational achievement, child poverty, unemployment, housing and crime that are seen across geographical areas and between different groups in society (Acheson 1998; Marmot 2009).

Despite interventions across government departments, limited progress has been made in reducing these wider inequalities and thus inequalities in health (DH 2009a). The Government has commissioned a review to explore the way forward in terms of tackling the wider determinants of health. This will explore all aspects of health including the delivery of health care services.

HEALTH CARE IN BRITAIN

The delivery of health care in Britain is complex. Some is provided through the private and the voluntary sectors although the majority is publicly funded through taxation which pays for our National Health Service (NHS). It is care provided through the NHS that will be the main focus for the rest of this chapter. The aim is to give you an overview of key aspects of NHS health care services and some of the principles that are shaping the way they are delivered.

THE NATIONAL HEALTH SERVICE

Health care services in Britain, as we are familiar with them today, really started to develop with the inception of the NHS in 1948. Prior to that the provision of services was haphazard and largely dependent on who you were, where you lived and how rich you were. After much debate and negotiation between politicians, local authorities, doctors and other key stakeholders, the NHS finally came into being on 5 July 1948.

It was founded on three core principles:

* Services should be free to all at the point of delivery.
* There should be equity of access to services for all.
* Services should be based on clinical need, not the ability to pay.

These have remained at the heart of British health policy, although there have been ongoing criticisms about inequity of access depending on where people live; the so called postcode lottery (Appleby and Gregory 2008). Similarly, recent debates about whether people should be allowed to fund drugs not available on the NHS whilst remaining as NHS patients have centred on the principle that all should be treated based on their need rather than ability to pay (Pollock *et al.* 2009).

Nevertheless, for many years and despite several administrative reorganisations and policy changes, the NHS operated in a broadly similar way to the system originally introduced in 1948 (for a full history of health policy and reforms from 1948 to the present *see* Rivett 2009 online). However, through the 1980s and the 1990s the NHS came under pressure. Following devolution in 1999, Scotland, Wales and Northern Ireland developed their own systems of NHS care and in England, increased public expectations, criticisms about standards, the challenges of meeting demand and limited funding prompted the launch of a huge programme of modernisation published as the NHS Plan (DH 2000). The Plan introduced a number of additional principles that have helped to shape the health services we now see in England.

These principles underpin health care across Britain. In order to give you a brief insight into the way services have developed in recent years, it is the system in England that will provide the focus for the rest of this chapter and just three principles: the provision of comprehensive services, an emphasis on quality and a patient-centred NHS.

COMPREHENSIVE SERVICES

The NHS provides a huge range of services to meet the very disparate needs of patients, including those who are healthy, helping them remain so, as well as those who are sick. Services are delivered in a wide range of settings from acute hospital trusts through to patients' homes. The NHS Constitution (DH 2009c: 5) sets out the rights of patients in terms of accessing these services. However, understanding who is responsible for what in the NHS can be difficult, so here is just a brief outline of some of the main components of the NHS in England.

The Department of Health and Strategic Health Authorities

The overarching responsibility for the strategic direction of health care lies with the Department of Health, whilst Strategic Health Authorities manage the NHS in their respective areas. There are ten Strategic Health Authorities in England. Together with the Department of Health they are responsible for developing and overseeing the implementation of policy and strategy for health and health care, setting standards and ensuring the effective delivery and quality of health services.

Primary care

Primary care is care delivered outside hospital settings and is usually the first port of call for most people requiring health care services. Primary Care Trusts (PCTs) are the organisations responsible for ensuring the delivery of effective, accessible health care services including commissioning hospital services for the populations they cover. They control 80 per cent of the NHS budget and employ general practitioners (GPs), community nurses and health visitors, dentists, pharmacists and many other health professionals. Newer services such as NHS walk-in centres and the telephone advice service NHS Direct, designed to make primary care more accessible, are also primary care services.

Secondary care

Where health needs cannot be met by primary care services, more specialist and emergency services are provided by hospitals; this is called secondary care. NHS trusts are the organisations that manage most secondary care through hospitals. Other areas of secondary care such as acute mental health services and ambulance services are managed by separate Mental Health and Ambulance Trusts.

Additionally, the Department of Health has given some NHS Trusts increased freedom to decide how they will run their services and spend their money, the plan being that they will be able to more effectively meet the needs of their local population. These Trusts are called Foundation Trusts. There have been criticisms of Foundation Trusts relating to lack of clarity about how they are managed and the suggestion that they will create a two-tier system of hospital care (Davidson 2004). Having said this, the Trusts are expected to, at a minimum, meet the standards and targets expected of all other NHS Trusts. It is vital that all health care services, wherever and however they are delivered, are safe and of good quality hence the principle outlined in the NHS Plan (DH 2000: 4) that:

> The NHS will work continuously to improve the quality of services and to minimise errors.

It is this principle that will be considered next.

IMPROVING THE QUALITY OF SERVICES

When talking about quality it is easy to assume everyone has the same view of what quality is but this is not necessarily the case. Consider an example far removed from health care.

MOMENT OF REFLECTION

Activity Three

You wish to eat out in a restaurant with friends. What factors might you take into account when choosing the restaurant and deciding whether or not the meal you have had is of good quality? Take into consideration all aspects of the eating out experience.

COMMENTARY

There are lots of things you might have considered here before even getting to the restaurant including its location, reputation, the availability of parking, the amount of money you wished to spend, the type of food you wanted to eat and whether or not it was a special occasion. Similarly, you would not judge the quality of your experience simply on the standard of the food that you ate. Factors such as the atmosphere of the restaurant, cleanliness, friendliness and competence of staff, ability to meet special dietary requirements, time you had to wait for your meal and value for money would all be relevant. These might have more than exceeded your expectations but if you contracted food poisoning as a result of your meal you would be unlikely to judge it a high quality experience.

It is the same with health care; there are many aspects of the service, from the cleanliness of the hospital to the competence of the surgeon and the friendliness of the receptionist that impact on a patient's experience and all need to meet high standards in order to ensure high quality provision. This is the focus for the NHS approach to quality today but it has not always been so.

Until the 1980s the issue of quality in health care was relatively low profile; people accepted the services they were given and were expected to be grateful for them! Systems of medical and clinical audit were management tools with the emphasis being on workload and financial targets rather than outcomes. This changed significantly in 1998 with the publication by the Department of Health of 'A First Class Service' (DH 1998) which outlined a framework for quality in the NHS and in 1999 the Health Act placed a statutory duty of quality on health care organisations.

This Framework of Clinical Governance was introduced in all NHS environments as a means of not only ensuring that services are safe and meeting the required standards but also of ensuring that those working in the NHS continue to look for ways to improve services. The expectation is that all who work in a health care setting, from the cleaners and porters through to the Chief Executive will take responsibility for the standard of service provided. Additionally, the Department of Health has put in place National Service Frameworks for a number of important areas of health and social care including services for older people, mental health services, coronary heart disease and cancer, their purpose being to set clear standards and eliminate the variations in care so often seen in the past.

Despite these initiatives and the setting of targets for many aspects of care (which in themselves have caused heated debate) failures in quality are still not uncommon (*see* HCC 2009b) and it is therefore vital that the quality of health care provision is systematically assessed. Inspection and regulation of all health services is carried out by the Care Quality Commission (CQC) which is also responsible for checking standards of adult social care. Where standards fall below what is expected the CQC can impose fines, give public warnings or even close down areas of care.

For health services to meet or exceed the expected standards they need to be based on good evidence. The National Institute for Health and Clinical Excellence (NICE) is an independent organisation which provides guidance to all interested parties, not just health practitioners, on care and the treatment of specific health problems, the use of new drugs and other technologies, and the best ways of promoting health. The input of NICE is not unproblematic – they provide advice based on a whole range of criteria including cost-effectiveness, not simply the efficacy of interventions and this leads to tensions when some treatments or drugs are not recommended for use in the NHS (Walker *et al.* 2007).

A PATIENT-CENTRED NHS

Another significant change in NHS health care over recent years has been a refocusing of services to put patients' interests to the fore. This might seem obvious but for a long time services were organised to meet the needs of the service providers so, as part of the modernisation agenda, the NHS Plan (DH 2000) set out a strategy to increase patient and public involvement. Patient-centeredness impacts on many different areas of health care including having choice about how, when and where care is accessed. The NHS Constitution outlines patients' rights regarding the choices they have about their care and also, just as importantly, their rights to information about the available choices so that they can make informed decisions about their care (DH 2009c).

Some of this information comes from Patient Advice and Liaison Services (PALS) which have been set up in all trusts to provide confidential advice and support. They aim to resolve concerns where possible, to signpost to more specialist sources of information and to advise patients, carers or members of the public who wish to make complaints. PALS provide feedback from these stakeholders to health care providers to help them improve their services.

A patient-centred NHS is not just concerned with individual patients; it also means actively participating with patients, carers, communities and the public. The Health and Social Care Act 2001 gave all NHS organisations a legal duty to consult with patients and the public when they are planning services and considering changes to services. A number of different approaches have been taken to fulfil this duty including having lay members on the governing bodies, involving local authorities in inspecting health services and monitoring changes, patient surveys and forums and developing local involvement networks (LINks) to enable patients and the public from all communities (including those often excluded) to have a voice and effective representation so that they are able to have an influence on shaping health and social care services.

Despite these initiatives, a recent report from the Health Care Commission (HCC) (now part of the CQC) highlights a significant lack of progress in patient and public engagement stating 'Those in the poorest health, in vulnerable circumstances or experiencing discrimination, often found it more difficult than others to engage with health services' and 'few trusts could demonstrate that people's views routinely influence their decision making' (HCC 2009c: 5). In response to this the Department of Health has published a new vision of Patient and Public Engagement (DH 2009d) to support progress in this key agenda.

CONCLUSION

This chapter has provided you with a brief snapshot of some of the factors that combine to shape our understanding of health and health care in Britain. It has focused particularly on inequalities in health as a key issue that concerns the British public and remains a challenge for those providing health services. It has provided an insight into how health services are organised and explored two of a number of themes that are high on the health policy agenda. Suggestions for wider reading given below will develop the themes considered and introduce others in a lot more detail than is possible in one chapter.

SUMMARY OF MAIN POINTS

You should be able to:

- Discuss concepts and models of health from a number of different perspectives.
- Recognise differences in the health status of socio-economic, ethnicity and gender groups and in their use of health services.
- Outline key aspects of current health care policy.
- Identify some of the key factors that impact on the way health services in Britain are delivered.

SUGGESTED READING

Acheson, D. (Chair) (1998) *Independent Inquiry into Inequalities in Health Report*, London: The Stationery Office.
Baggott, R. (2004) *Health and Health Care in Britain*, Basingstoke: Palgrave Macmillan.
Clarke, A. (2010) *The Sociology of Health Care* (2nd Edition), London: Pearson Education Limited.

USEFUL WEBSITES

Department of Health website – gives access to a huge range of information and publications relating to all aspects of health and health policy:
http://www.dh.gov.uk

NHS Evidence – an electronic library for health that links to all sorts of health related online resources:
http://www.library.nhs.uk/default.aspx

National Health Service History Website – provides a regularly updated and comprehensive review of developments in the NHS since its inception:
http://www.nhshistory.net/

REFERENCES

Acheson, D. (Chair) (1998) *Independent Inquiry into Inequalities in Health Report*, London: The Stationery Office.

Appleby, J. and Gregory, S. (2008) *NHS spending, Local variations in priorities: an update*, London: King's Fund.

Baggott, R. (2004) *Health and Health Care in Britain*, Basingstoke: Palgrave Macmillan.

Blaxter, M. (1990) *Health and Lifestyle*, London: Routledge.

Clarke, A. (2001) *The Sociology of Health Care* (2nd Edition), London: Pearson Education Limited.

Dahlgren and Whitehead 1993, reproduced in Dahlgren, G. and Whitehead, M. (2007) *European strategies for tackling social inequities in health: Levelling Up Part 2,* Copenhagen: World Health Organization Regional Office for Europe [online]. Available at: http://www.euro.who.int/socialdeterminants/publications/publications

Davidson, A. (2004) Stormy Weather for Labour's NHS Reforms, *Canadian Medical Association Journal,* January 20, 170 (2) [online]. Available at http://ecmaj.com/cgi/content/full/170/2/187 (Accessed 1 December 2009).

DH (Department of Health) (1998) *A First Class Service: Quality in the New NHS,* London: The Stationery Office.

DH (2000) *The NHS Plan: a plan for investment, a plan for reform*, London: The Stationery Office.

DH (2001) *Tackling Health Inequalities: consultation on a plan for delivery* [online]. Available at http://www.dh.gov.uk/prod_consum_dh/groups/dh_digitalassets/@dh/@en/documents/digital asset/dh_4053524.pdf (Accessed 18 November 2009).

DH (2005) *Race Equality Scheme 2005–2008*, London: Department of Health.

DH (2009a) *Health Inequalities* [online]. Available at http://www.dh.gov.uk/en/Publichealth/Healthinequalities/index.htm (Accessed 20 November 2009).

DH (2009b) *Tackling Health Inequalities: 10 years on* [online]. Available at http://www.dh.gov.uk/prod_consum_dh/groups/dh_digitalassets/documents/digitalasset/dh_098934.pdf (Accessed 20 November 2009).

DH (2009c) *The NHS Constitution: the NHS belongs to us all* [online]. Available at http://www.dh.gov.uk/en/Publicationsandstatistics/Publications/PublicationsPolicyAndGuidance/DH_093419 (Accessed 2 December 2009).

DH (2009d) *Putting patients at the heart of care: The vision for patient and public engagement in health and social care* [online]. Available at http://www.dh.gov.uk/prod_consum_dh/groups/dh_digitalassets/documents/digitalasset/dh_106042.pdf (Accessed 3 December 2009).

DHSS (Department of Health and Social Security) (1980) *Report of the Working Group on Inequalities in Health* (The Black Report), London: DHSS.

Dorling, D., Gregory, I., Norman, P. and Baker, A. (2008) Geographical trends in infant mortality: England and Wales, 1970–2006, *Health Statistics Quarterly,* Winter No. 40, 18–29.

Doyal, L. (2001) Sex, gender, and health: the need for a new approach, *British Medical Journal,* 323, 1058–60.

Doyal, L., Payne, S. and Cameron, A. (2003) *Promoting gender equality in health*, Manchester: Equal Opportunities Commission.

Engel, G. L. (1977) The Need for a New Medical Model: A Challenge for Biomedicine, *Journal of Interprofessional Care,* 4 (1), 37–53 [online]. Available at http://dx.doi.org/10.3109/13561828909043606 (Accessed 17 November 2009).

HCC (Healthcare Commission) (2009a) *Tackling the challenge: Promoting race equality in the NHS in England* [online]. Available at http://www.cqc.org.uk/_db/_documents/Tackling_the_challenge_Promoting_race_equality_in_the_NHS_in_England.pdf (Accessed 19 November 2009).

HCC (2009b) *Investigation into Mid Staffordshire NHS Foundation Trust,* [online]. Available at http://www.cqc.org.uk/_db/_documents/Investigation_into_Mid_Staffordshire_NHS_Foundation_ Trust.pdf (Accessed 3 December 2009).

HCC (2009c) *Listening, learning, working together? A national study of how well healthcare organisations engage local people in planning and improving their services,* [online]. Available at http://www.cqc.org.uk/_db/_documents/Engaging_patients_&_public_national_report.pdf (Accessed 3 December 2009).

Hicks, J. and Allen, E. (1999) *A Century of Change: Trends in UK Statistics Since 1900,* Research Paper 99/111, London: House of Commons Library.

House of Commons Health Committee (2009) *Health Inequalities: Third Report of Session 2008–2009,* London: The Stationery Office Limited [online]. Available at http://www.publications.parliament.uk/pa/cm200809/cmselect/cmhealth/286/286.pdf (Accessed 18 November 2009).

King's Fund (2006) *Access to health care for minority ethnic groups* [online]. Available at http://www.kingsfund.org.uk/research/publications/briefings/access_to_health.html (Accessed 18 November 2009).

Marmot, M. (2009) *Forward to Tackling Health Inequalities: 10 years on* [online]. Available at http://www.dh.gov.uk/prod_consum_dh/groups/dh_digitalassets/documents/digitalasset/dh _098934.pdf (Accessed 20 November 2009).

McKenzie, K. (2003) Racism and Health, *British Medical Journal,* (326), 65–6.

Naidoo, J. and Wills, J. (2008) *Health Studies: an introduction* (2nd edition), Basingstoke: Palgrave Macmillan.

Nazroo, J. (1997) *The health of Britain's ethnic minorities: findings from a national survey,* London: Policy Studies Institute.

ONS (Office for National Statistics) (2004) *Focus on Gender* [online]. Available at http://www.unece.org/stats/gender/publications/UK/Focus_on_Gender.pdf. (Accessed 19 November 2009).

ONS (2008) *Large differences in infant mortality by ethnic group* [online]. Available at http://www.statistics.gov.uk/pdfdir/imeth0608.pdf (Accessed 18 November 2009).

ONS (2009) *Life Expectancy: Life Expectancy Continues to Rise* [online]. Available at http://www.statistics.gov.uk/cci/nugget.asp?ID=168 (Accessed 17 November 2009).

Pollock, A., Price, D. and Arthur, M. (2009) *Response to the Department of Health's consultation on guidance for NHS patients who wish to pay for additional private healthcare,* Edinburgh: Centre for International Public Health Policy, Edinburgh University.

Rivett, G. (1998) *From Cradle to Grave: fifty years of the NHS,* London: King's Fund [online]. Available at http://www.nhshistory.net/bookdata.htm (Accessed 30 November 2009).

Rivett, G. (2009) *National Health Service History Website* [online]. Available at http://www.nhshistory.net/ (Accessed 30 November 2009).

Shaw, M., Smith, G. D. and Dorling, D. (2005) Health inequalities and New Labour: how the promises compare with real progress, *British Medical Journal,* (330), 1016–21 (30 April).

Sproston, K. and Mindell, J. (Eds) (2006) *The Health Survey for England. The health of minority ethnic groups,* London: The NHS Information Centre.

Walker, S., Palmer, S. and Sculphor, M. (2007) *The Role of NICE Technology Appraisal in NHS Rationing* [online]. Available at doi:10.1093/bmb/ldm007 (Accessed 3 December 2004).

WHO (1948) *Preamble to the Constitution of the World Health Organization as adopted by the International Health Conference, New York, 19 June – 22 July 1946,* signed on 22 July 1946 by the representatives of 61 States and entered into force on 7 April 1948, Official Records of the World Health Organization, (2), 100.

CHAPTER 8

KEY THEMES IN HEALTH AND SOCIAL CARE

CHRIS RING

OBJECTIVES

After reading this chapter you should be able to:

▪ Understand some recent developments in legislation and policy in relation to the planning and delivery of social care and community health services.

▪ Understand how these are realised in meeting the needs of two service user groups.

▪ Understand the importance of the social context and multi-professional working, as critical success factors.

▪ Apply these insights to critique contemporary developments in health and social care.

After reading this chapter you will know the meaning of the following terms: Health care, social care, outcomes, quality of life, personalisation, safeguarding and interprofessional working.

There are five Moments of Reflection to work on throughout the chapter.

INTRODUCTION

This chapter examines how social policy and practice respond to emerging health and social needs, and the outcomes experienced by individuals and groups. The practical challenges associated with three key policy aims: improving outcomes, providing individualised care, and protecting adults and children from harm, are illustrated using experience in areas of particular practice, such as mental health care and young people in care.

Focusing on service users' experience and observed outcomes in these settings, we examine how professionals working within current policy and practice frameworks contribute to the impact of health and social care services, and the conditions for success.

THE NATURE AND PURPOSE OF HEALTH AND SOCIAL CARE

Any definition of the term 'health care' is liable to be problematic: while it is easy to list services and procedures universally agreed to be health care, its boundaries are ill-defined and disputed. This matters, because organising public systems of care demands the allocation of resources and responsibility between organisations, in ways that enable social policy to be effectively implemented. In much of the UK, government has distinguished the purposes and processes of 'health' and 'social' care, allocating responsibility to different public bodies – health and local authorities – using a variety of labels for these in different eras. A working definition of health and social care is therefore critical for anyone needing to understand or work within either of these sectors.

Health care may be broadly understood as any individual or population-based intervention seeking to remedy the causes and effects of physical or mental ill-health, or injury, and/or to promote good health. Our society recognises these aims as valid ends in themselves. However, achieving them also assists people's other needs to be met – this is arguably the principal purpose of social care.

They may remain unmet for a variety of reasons other than ill-health. Social or family circumstances and functioning, poverty, or maladaptive behaviour are some of the important factors which render people of all ages 'in need'.

Social care and other policy programmes (welfare benefits, education) have evolved in order to address issues such as these, which are generally not amenable to health interventions. The range of issues involved makes the boundaries of these programmes fluid; social care is distinguished firstly by its focus on the relation between the individual and society, and a remedial or 'prosthetic' approach, which first seeks to help develop individuals' and families' capacity to manage their lives, and second, provides alternative care in areas where they continue to require this.

In the consultation document preceding publication in 2006 of proposals for the future of adult social care, this was defined as:

> the wide range of services designed to support people in their daily lives and help them play a full part in society.
>
> DoH (2006) *Independence, Wellbeing and Choice*

Examples of social care included home care, day centres, residential and nursing homes, and practical help to assist individuals overcome barriers to social inclusion. Social care services were defined primarily in terms of their purpose, rather than the detailed form of services, envisaging the increasing replacement of current forms of services with those more able to meet their desired ends. These would include 'support in managing complex relationships and emotional distress', and might be provided in a variety of ways, particularly through more individually tailored ('personalised') support.

Applying these working definitions to a specific example will help to appreciate the distinction between health and social care. Take Sheila, a working age adult woman with two children under ten, who has developed multiple sclerosis. Sheila is likely to:

- Require drug treatment and possibly physiotherapy – health care.
- The skills and equipment available from an occupational therapist (arguably health or social care).
- Practical support and advice – in the form of a home care or a personal assistant, help to apply for appropriate benefits, and to make other adjustments desired, to enable her and her family to maintain their normal activities and participation in society (broadly social care).

This example illustrates how, given a range of needs presented by a serious and usually progressive illness, 'health' and 'social care' services can complement and combine to achieve good outcomes which include maximising well-being, preventing deterioration, and enabling the person to make the best of the abilities they retain.

The 'modernisation' of health and social care services following the election in 1997 of the Labour administration, and major subsequent policy developments in health and social care have led to radical and continuing reorganisation. In the remainder of this chapter we will examine the nature and impact of these changes, with a particular emphasis on the experience and outcomes for people receiving them.

PROVIDING CARE – KEY FEATURES OF EMERGING SYSTEMS

A focus on outcomes

From the 1990s onwards, increasing attention has been paid in developing social policy and practice to their intended outcomes, and to the lived experience of people using services. Outcomes are the intended result of receiving a service; for example, medication (health care) to treat multiple sclerosis may seek to reduce the pain or muscle spasm associated with the illness; if successful, it has achieved its (intended) outcome. The services of a personal assistant to help Sheila get her children off to school (social care) enables her to maintain her role as a parent – achieving its outcome of enabling her to continue to play a full part in society.

The intended outcomes of current health and social care policy are summarised in *Our Health, Our Care, Our Say* (DoH 2006a), and include (for social care):

- improved health and emotional well-being
- improved quality of life
- making a positive contribution
- choice and control.

Fewer specific health outcomes were proposed, but include reductions in childhood obesity and in teenage pregnancy. Overall, there is a strong emphasis on prevention and early intervention, in both health and social care. Further development of policy and practice will focus clearly on outcomes such as these – demonstrated by the Care Quality Commission in its final report (CQC 2009).

While it is hard to dispute the value of a focus on outcomes, it presents additional challenges to those seeking to improve and justify policy and practice. Both the measurement of outcomes, and their attribution to specific interventions (services), demand much more effort and critical scrutiny than monitoring compliance with recommended practice – a focus on process.

A process approach – for example, time taken to complete a comprehensive needs assessment – continues to be the chief means of assuring service quality at local level. The establishment of National Service Frameworks for a number of conditions during the past ten years has provided useful standards of care and treatment, providing a means of focusing efforts to improve the quality of care, and standards to audit this against.

Increasing commitment is now being given to outcome based monitoring, in the form of PSA (Public Service Agreement) targets – set between local authorities/partnership and government, capturing progress towards key policy objectives. For example, PSA15 relates to the proportion of people with mental health problems in employment, addressing an important priority for mental health policy in both health and social care domains.

MOMENT OF REFLECTION

Consider the value of using outcome measures such as 'quality of life' to assess the impact of health and social care services. What does 'quality of life' mean to you? Is it really 'measurable'? Do you know of any approaches to doing this?

AN EMPHASIS ON LIVED EXPERIENCE

Changing public expectations of health and social care, recognition by organisations and their staff of the critical contribution of the patient/service user to the success or otherwise of treatment and care, and changes in the broader political climate towards a consumerist paradigm for public services, have led to a marked emphasis on improving people's experience of using health and social care services. The following developments reflect this:

- The involvement – at every level – of patients and service users in the planning, management, and oversight of systems of care.
- An increasing emphasis, at an individual level, on obtaining feedback from patients and service users on their experience of care. Examples include the NHS Patient Surveys in a wide range of clinical care areas (Care Quality Commission 2009).
- The development of standards for care and care settings which reflect features valued by patients and service users, such as the quality of the care environment, respect by staff, information and flexibility. Services are increasingly audited against these standards, which contribute to overall performance ratings.

Associated with this is an increasing attention to the voices of both service users and those providing informal care (carers), through the increasing development of advocacy services, and to their wishes – specifically in the form of the Mental Capacity Act (2005).

The latter lays down procedures to be followed regarding anyone requiring health or social care, or assistance to manage their finances. They must be fully involved in any decisions made, and where they cannot participate fully in these decisions, those acting on their behalf must act in their best interests and accommodate their wishes as far as possible.

PROTECTING PEOPLE FROM HARM – SAFEGUARDING

Child abuse and child protection have been long-standing concerns of social care (and especially social work). The statutory framework and associated policy and procedures (DES 2003) have been extensively developed, but it remains impossible to guarantee that every child will remain unharmed.

A series of enquiries have followed a number of child deaths during the last two decades, for example Laming (2003, 2009). Recommendations have been implemented to varying degrees and further changes seem likely. But social change, wider societal attitudes and the challenges of this type of work are likely to limit the scope to reduce the risk of a small number of children experiencing serious abuse, from which some will die. However, this must be viewed in the context of the very large numbers of children identified as at risk, who are subject to timely and effective protection measures, involving challenging work involving numerous agencies. Their successes receive little public attention, but failures are subject to intense critical scrutiny.

In addition, very large numbers of children, while not exposed to significant abuse, remain 'children in need' – liable to impaired health and development for a wide variety of reasons. Many of these are 'looked-after children', where the local authority has parental responsibility (a social care function); they also require high standards of education and health care for them to attain their potential – which they often fail to do.

More recently (from the 1990s), it has also become apparent that the circumstances of many adults rendered them vulnerable to mistreatment and neglect. While the most shocking instances of this emerged initially in care settings, the extent and prevalence of abuse at the hands of family members has become increasingly apparent. Detailed guidance – 'No Secrets' – was issued some years ago (Department of Health and Home Office 2000), making local authorities lead agencies in coordinating an effective multi-agency response to cases of suspected abuse, and was followed by additional guidance 'Safeguarding Adults' (Association of Directors of Social Services 2005). However, research has revealed that substantial numbers of adults living at home have continued to experience abuse – most commonly in the form of neglect or financial exploitation (O'Keefe *et al.* 2007). The limited legal powers available to prosecute and prevent abuse of adults has led to calls for legal measures equivalent to those in force to protect children – so far with very limited effect.

The continued widespread abuse and harm experienced by vulnerable people of all ages has therefore become a key theme in health and social care. While the 'safeguarding' programmes outlined above seek to address these, some of the developments envisaged below (the 'personalisation of social care') seem likely to increase the risks of abuse.

MOMENT OF REFLECTION

Can you remember any examples featured in the media of the abuse of vulnerable people either in institutional settings, or their own homes, or in the community? See if you can find details of these.

RECOGNITION OF THE VALUE OF FAMILY RELATIONSHIPS AND INFORMAL CARING

The care and support provided by family members and friends to adults and children are increasingly recognised as a crucial component of the outcomes overall health and social care provision. The new Carers Strategy (DoH 2008a) promises recognition, training, and support for them – perhaps recognising that they will be become increasingly important given rising numbers of people requiring care, and constraints on public finances.

ESTABLISHING NEW SYSTEMS OF CARE

You may have realised from what you have already read, that these policy aims allow for a wide range of organisational arrangements and practices to achieve them. While these must deliver (among other outcomes) effective safeguarding, choice and control, and improved outcomes , this may be accomplished in a variety of ways.

We will go on to look at how the skills, knowledge and attitudes of different professions and occupations, and the assets of people who use services and their families, will be applied to these aims. We will consider how these are being reorganised and managed to deliver the new 'personalised' (person-centred) services, and scrutinise the extent to which these are or can achieve some of their intended outcomes – focusing on enhanced choice and control, and improving quality of life.

It may strike you that this omits attention to other important goals, for example, prevention, and to other factors likely to influence their attainment.

MOMENT OF REFLECTION

Establishing new systems of care?

In selecting the above outcomes for attention, what important aspects are omitted? (There are no right/wrong answers – select one, and explain why.)

PUTTING PEOPLE FIRST? – PERSONALISATION IN PRACTICE

Placing the individual and their needs at the centre of social care practice has become an increasingly dominant theme during the last decade, and an explicit approach to achieving this was outlined in the White Paper 'Independence, Wellbeing and Choice' (Department of Health, 2006).

- Proposals for the new 'personalised' services were outlined early in 'Transforming Social Care' (DoH 2008b). A strategic shift was proposed towards prevention/early intervention, to promote independence and well-being.
- A multi-agency approach – while social care would lead, the involvement of other public agencies – health, housing and transport – and the private and voluntary sectors, was conceived as critical.
- Choice and control – conceived as the essence of personalisation – were to be achieved increasingly through self-assessment and selection, and procurement and control of services by the consumer.
- Direct payments (cash made available to the service user for social care) and Individual Budgets (combining a number of income streams) are envisaged as critical vehicles to enable to exercise choice and control.
- Local authorities, acting in partnership with other commissioners and providers, are responsible for development of an appropriate range of services available to purchase.
- The social work role would change from assessment and gatekeeping, to advocacy and brokerage. Indeed, the proposal envisages extensive workforce development, including formation of a 'Social Care Skills Academy'.

Personalisation was defined as 'the way in which services are tailored to the needs and preferences of citizens. The overall vision is that the state should empower citizens to shape their own lives and the services they receive'.

Much of the drive to deliver this focused on developing individual budgets and 'self-directed support'. However, it is clear that personalisation, as defined above, requires much more than this.

PROFESSIONAL AND INTER-PROFESSIONAL WORKING

While some human needs may be met by discrete health or social care interventions – minor surgery, or home care services – to understand and address many people's situations demands a combination of services, provided by two or more agencies. Partnership working has become one of the major policy developments for health and social care. Organisations therefore require formal or informal arrangements for this – these may involve shared procedures; agreements to share/combine resources; working arrangements and mutual understanding – all of which allow practitioners, service users and other parties to cooperate effectively.

You may already be aware of some of the organisational arrangements facilitating inter-agency working, such as the 'Single Assessment Process' (for older people).

Leathard (2003) has outlined a number of models for inter-professional working, and many examples exist of how this can be successfully achieved.

However, many barriers exist to consistently achieving high-quality inter-agency working. Differing agency priorities, confused or highly risky situations, practitioners' limited knowledge, skills or willingness to cooperate, or their different perspectives, can all compromise the achievement of good outcomes, and even fail to prevent serious harm or loss of life.

The further development of person-centred care envisages new patterns of service, with a wider variety of providers. Current experience of multi-agency services, exemplified in the case examples below, suggest that further progress in this direction will not be easily achieved.

MOMENT OF REFLECTION

What examples of serious harm occur to you, resulting from failures in inter-agency or inter-professional working? Try and find out details, and lessons which can be learnt from these.

Let us now examine the ways in which the changes outlined above are being incorporated into current practice, and consider their likely impact. The following (fictional) case examples illustrate this.

Experiencing care – mental health

Tony Jones, a 35-year-old single white British man, developed a recurring schizophrenic illness in his mid-20s. Three years ago, he returned to living in a highly supported group living setting, after an earlier attempt to live more independently had broken down, due to exploitation of his good nature, and invasion of his property by 'friends' he made on the estate where he lived. He now wishes to live more independently, make new friends with 'normal' people, find a life partner, and pursue his interests in gardening and creative writing. However, social anxiety, partly consequent on his early experiences, prevents him from pursuing these plans; and he has become increasingly withdrawn during the past six months and is prone to periods of despair and suicidal thoughts.

Mike, Tony's care coordinator, believes that significant improvements in his quality of life are attainable, given the increasing flexibility of arrangements offered by 'personalisation'. These entitle Tony to an Individual Budget to meet his agreed needs, and plans are made for him to move to a flat of his own. Combining funding from several sources, the budget will provide him with practical help and personal support at home, and supported access to community facilities to pursue his outside interests. He is assessed as having the mental capacity to recognise the risks associated with his move, but develops strategies with Mike to minimise these. Tony agrees with his 'care team' that they will use the 'Outcomes Star' to monitor their success (or otherwise) in making the changes to his life that he wants.

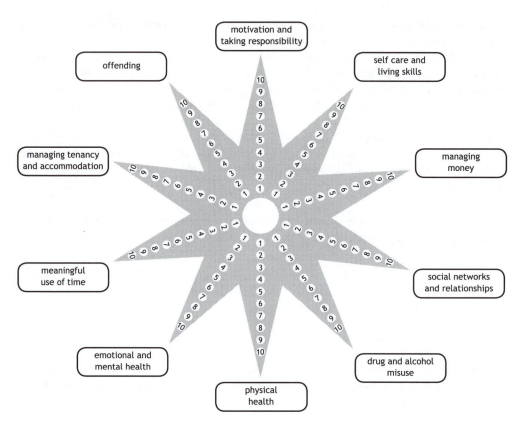

Figure 8.1 The Outcomes Star
Reproduced with permission Triangle Consulting/London Homeless Action (2009)

The Recovery Star is one of a family of Outcomes Star tools for supporting and measuring change when working with vulnerable people. It consists of ten defined scales underpinned by a model of change. For details and to download the stars go to www.outcomesstar.org.uk

His move to a flat of his own with floating support is managed by a partnership between a housing association and a voluntary agency, and funded through 'Supporting People' and a range of benefits. An individual budget combining these income streams allows him to employ (via the agency) a personal assistant, Ian. Because Ian got to know Tony before his move, he was able to support him during this, when Tony initially became very anxious during the six weeks. Help from Ian (in the form of anxiety management training and support with benefits applications), combined with a temporary increase in his medication, helped Tony become much more settled. He now attends an adult education course in creative writing (with Ian), who is also helping him to develop confidence in social situations outside his home – including volunteering on an allotment project.

Four months later, Tony reports that he feels better, is able to manage many (not all) routine household and personal care tasks, and Ian confirms this. Mike and Tony's GP agree there is significant improvement from their perspective. Use of the 'Outcomes Star' shows improvements in his mental health, independent living skills, and involvement in work and learning. So far he has not made friends outside his home in the way he had hoped, but still wishes to do this and is hopeful of success.

COMMENTARY

This example illustrates many of the positive features of the emerging forms of service, referred to above, which are beginning to become apparent (Spandler and Wick 2006). These include:

- The service user increasingly 'calls the shots'. Tony has identified changes he would like to make (living more independently, pursuing new interests and making friends). Health care (medication and anxiety management) and social care (benefits advice and sharing community activities) are a means to these ends – which Tony has chosen. The Outcomes Star is an effective and user-friendly way of measuring progress towards these objectives.
- An individual budget is the key to providing the flexible and person-centred care and support that Tony receives. While creative writing and gardening are available in mental health provision, an individual budget provides him with the flexibility of support to access these in the mainstream settings, where he is more likely to make new friends.

MOMENT OF REFLECTION

Can you identify features of practice in this case study, which exemplify (or contradict) any other key themes referred to above? In what ways is practice compatible with these?

EXPERIENCING CARE – LOOKED-AFTER CHILDREN

Concern about the quality and outcomes of children 'looked after' by local authorities has been apparent during the last two decades. Reviews by Sir William Utting in 1991 and 1997 of the widespread abuse and failures experienced by children in the 'care system', was followed by successive policy initiatives. These include 'Quality Protects' (1998), a programme aimed at improving outcomes for looked-after children, particularly through promoting fostering over residential care as a form of accommodation; the Children (Leaving Care) Act 2000, aiming to improve care leavers' notably difficult transition to adulthood; and *Care Matters* (Department of Children, Schools and Families, 2007) which identifies a number of priorities for action, including improvements to physical and mental health, standards of foster care, and support to care leavers.

Being 'looked after' as a young person

Sarah is a young woman with an Afro-Caribbean heritage, aged 15. She is four months into her second fostering placement, having been placed in local authority care 18 months ago when her mother (a single parent) was admitted with an overdose associated with long-standing depression and alcohol misuse. Sarah is still in regular contact with her mother. Her attendance at school has been poor, and her mock GCSE results suggest she is unlikely to pass in more than two subjects. When not attending school, she has been associating with other young people and was recently cautioned for shoplifting small items.

Her social worker (Diane) has begun to develop a trusting relationship with Sarah, who reports that she is being bullied, accused of being 'mental' (by association with her mother), and stigmatised for being 'in care' because of this. Sarah is drinking regularly with 'her mates'; they share a common experience of unhappy homes, disaffection from school and its associations, and an attraction to music and lifestyles reflecting their alienation from mainstream society. Sarah's present foster parents (Mary and Steve) are in their 40s, also Afro-Caribbean, have professional backgrounds and two children: David (19) lives away, but Dawn (18) is still at home – she is friendly with Sarah, but regards her as 'weird' and 'moody', and sometimes loses patience with her. Sarah's foster parents have high expectations of their children; while recognising her troubled background, they too sometimes become exasperated with her moodiness and brushes with the law, and are discouraging association with her 'fellow outcasts'.

However, Diane is encouraging Sarah to explore aspects of school that she finds difficult and those she enjoys. Recognising the positive features of Sarah's attachment to her peer group, she introduces her to a young carers' group; with Sarah and her foster parents they start to explore Sarah's divided loyalties between her two 'families'. Together they develop ways to support Sarah in her wish to maintain contact with her mother, affirming the importance of this role for her.

Diane also encourages Mary and Steve to nurture Sarah's self-esteem, affirming her positive achievements, helping her pursue the subjects she does enjoy, and to talk about the ups and downs of her schooldays. Diane also starts to develop a Pathway Plan with Sarah and puts her in touch with a Connexions adviser, who will explore what Sarah might do when she has done her GCSEs, whatever the results might be.

COMMENTARY

Features of Sarah's situation illustrate common concerns about the welfare of children and young people today. We examine three of these below, illustrating how social policy and practice is being developed in response.

Poor outcomes – Sarah's background, behaviour and poor mental health, and a predisposition to misuse alcohol, render her very unlikely to attain all five outcomes of 'Every Child Matters': staying safe; being healthy; enjoying and achieving; making a positive contribution; achieving economic well-being – the measures referred to above all address these concerns head on. 'Quality Protects' (1998) invested considerable resources in developing fostering as an alternative to residential care for looked-after children; The Children (Leaving Care) Act, set out clear duties of local authorities to provide after-care and personal support to care leavers (hence Diane's development of a Pathway Plan, and identification of a personal adviser). *Care Matters* (2007) focuses both on the foregoing and on improving mental and physical health, and on educational outcomes. In supporting the fostering relationship, and encouraging Sarah to focus on positive aspects of school and to look beyond this, Diane is contributing to improving Sarah's future prospects.

The importance of informal caring – Sarah's relationship with her birth mother is affecting her formal status (a looked-after child), has shaped her attachments and the person she is, and is significantly affecting her relationship with her peers. Social work practice has increasingly grappled with practical and ethical challenges associated with state intervention in the parent–child relationship. The recently published Carers Strategy (Department of Health 2008a) identifies support to young carers as a major concern. Diane's recognition of the importance to Sarah of maintaining a relationship with her mother and the increasing availability of young carers' groups, allow for the reality of such relationships in the life of many young people.

Inter-professional working – this example suggests how outcomes may be improved when social work, health, education and other professionals work together with young people. The ways in which they help include:

- Helping children and young people negotiate the challenges they face (particularly by representing their interests to large bureaucracies which they have to learn to deal with to survive).
- Drawing in and coordinating resources which no one agency can access, for example careers advice, mental health care, peer support.
- Providing a system which (when it works well) is robust enough to provide and be accountable for consistent support – complying with the requirements of the Children (Leaving Care) Act.

CONCLUSION

These examples demonstrate ways in which health and social care services are adapting in response to changing policy aims – in particular those which focus on improving outcomes, and making services more person centred. The case studies exemplify good practice that offers real prospects of improving the lives of people in need.

But to do so demands staff with a wide range of skills and knowledge, with access to significant resources, and who work within organisations and a culture which supports these ends.

This is often not the case. And the changes envisaged by current policy, particularly relating to personalisation, and those currently being considered – for example, for the future funding of social care – will place additional demands on welfare systems. Reflecting on these issues can help you make sense of a wide variety of initiatives and processes observed in practice, and focus on those which promise to improve the lives of people in need – which is what this book is all about.

SUMMARY OF MAIN POINTS

You should now:

- Understand some of the recent developments in legislation and policy in relation to the planning and delivery of social care and community health services.
- Understand how these are realised in meeting the needs of two service user groups.
- Understand the importance of the social context and multi-professional working, as critical success factors.
- Apply these insights to critique contemporary developments in health and social care.

APPENDIX: DISCUSSION OF MOMENTS OF REFLECTION

Quality of Life

Although this term is widely used in the media and in political and other discussions and debates, most of us would be hard put to define it clearly. You might associate many different words and phrases with it – happiness; freedom from anxiety, poverty and want; particular lifestyles; and particular environments. Many of these have positive associations and appear to be intrinsic to a (high) quality of life, or to be strongly associated with it. The appeal of the term is its value in summarising the overall (desired) outcomes of many public and commercial services. Health and social sciences and economics, where most work has taken place to develop and apply measures of quality of life, have tended to distinguish two components, each comprising several elements: objective conditions, for example physical safety and adequate nutrition; and subjective experience, for example, self-esteem and rewarding relationships. This work also confirms how quality of life is influenced by material circumstances and these variations can be expressed in quantitative terms. A wide variety of measurement tools have been developed, mainly for work in health care, for example, the Lancashire Quality of Life Scale (Oliver *et al.* 1996) is a comprehensive tool that has been used for service evaluation. But you may feel that such developments offer a spurious accuracy to experiences that cannot be quantified.

Abuse in institutional settings

Recent examples publicised in the media include physical abuse of older people in residential care and degrading treatment of people with learning difficulties (the latter was featured in a TV programme made by an undercover reporter – 'MacIntyre Undercover'). Others have been public enquiries (for example Flynn (2006) into the care of adults with learning difficulties by Cornwall NHS Trust), or have followed complaints by victims, often many years later (for example, children abused in residential care). Abuse of people in their own homes is also widespread and subject to media coverage, for example, 'Britain's Homecare Scandal' (BBC 2009), and systematic surveys (O'Keefe *et al.* 2007).

Establishing new systems of care

It may have struck you that focusing on outcomes such as 'quality of life' is appealing, but neglects the realities of everyday practice, where it is difficult in some situations to ensure that even basic needs are met. Resources are increasingly an issue – you may have thought of the current problems of staffing health and social care services in some parts of the country, or of the likely impact of the recent economic crisis on public services.

Failures of inter-professional working

Lord Laming's report into the death of Victoria Climbie (2003) highlights extensive shortcomings in inter-professional working, and earlier enquiries, for example into the 'Care and Treatment of Christopher Clunis' (Ritchie *et al.* 1994) revealed similar failures in mental health care.

CASE STUDY: TONY

Another feature of this situation is the risk of harm, and the need to manage this – 'safeguarding'. Ian and Tony have considered this. Ian is supporting Tony in managing his social anxiety and is monitoring the situation for possible signs of abuse.

REFERENCES

Association of Directors of Social Services (2005) *Safeguarding Adults*, London: ADSS.

BBC (2009) Britain's Homecare Scandal, *Panorama* April 2009, London: BBC Productions.

Care Quality Commission (2009) *The State of Social Care in England 2007–2008*, London: HMSO.

Department of Children, Schools and Families (2007) *Care Matters: Time for Change*, London: HMSO.

Department of Education and Skills (2003) *Every Child Matters*, London: The Stationery Office.

Department of Health and Home Office (2000) *No secrets: guidance on developing and implementing multi-agency policies and procedures to protect vulnerable adults from abuse*, London: Department of Health.

Department of Health (2006a) *Our Health, Our Care, Our Say*, London: HMSO.

Department of Health (2006b) *Independence, Well-being and Choice*, London: HMSO.

Department of Health (2008a) *Carers at the Heart of 21st Century Families and Communities*, London: HMSO.

Department of Health (2008b) *Transforming Adult Social Care, LAC (DH) (2008) 1*, London: HMSO.

Flynn, M. (2006) Joint investigation into the provision of services for people with learning disabilities at Cornwall Partnership NHS Trust, *Journal of Adult Protection*, 8 (3), 28–32.

Laming, H. (2003) *The Victoria Climbie Inquiry: Report of an enquiry*, London, HMSO.

Laming, H. (2009) *The Protection of Children in England – A Progress Report*. London: The Stationery Office.

Leathard, A. (2003) Models for Interprofessional Collaboration in Leathard, A. (Ed.) *Interprofessional Collaboration*, Hove/New York: Brunner Routledge.

O'Keefe, M., Hills, A., Doyle, M., McCreadie, C., Scholes, S., Constantine, R., Tinker, A., Manthorpe, J., Biggs, S. and Erens, B. (2007) *UK Study of Abuse and Neglect of Older People: Prevalence Survey Report*, London: NatCen.

Oliver, J., Huxley, P., Bridges, K. and Mohamed, H. (1996) *Quality of Life and Mental Health Services*, London: Routledge.

Petch, A. (2009) How Successful so far have Individual Budgets been, *Community Care*, 2 July 2009, 32–3.

Ritchie, J., Dick, D. and Lingham, R. (1994) *The Enquiry into the Care and Treatment of Christopher Clunis*, London: HMSO.

Spandler, H. and Wick, N. (2006) Opportunities for Independent Living using Direct Payments in Mental Health, *Health and Social Care in the Community*, 14 (2), 107–15.

Triangle Consulting/London Homeless Action (2009) *What is the Outcomes Star?* [online]. Available at http://www.homelessoutcomes.org.uk/About_the_Outcomes_Star.aspx (Accessed 19 November 2009).

CHAPTER 9

PHILOSOPHICAL AND POLITICAL DEBATE IN HEALTH AND SOCIAL CARE

ADAM BARNARD

OBJECTIVES

After reading this chapter you should be able to:

- Discuss the purpose of philosophy and learning to philosophise.

- Examine a range of schools of political and moral philosophy.

- Consider moral problems and political dilemmas.

- Appreciate freedom, authority, rights and social justice in health and social care.

After reading this chapter you will know the meaning of the following terms: Freedom, authority, rights, justice, liberalism, socialism, social democracy, conservatism, New Right, New Labour, utilitarianism, deontology, virtue.

There is a Moment of Reflection at the end of the chapter.

INTRODUCTION

This chapter will allow you to develop analytical skills that will enable an examination of political and philosophical issues, which impact upon health and social care, by introducing key philosophical, political and ethical theories. It starts with a consideration of philosophy and the purpose of philosophical inquiry for health and social care. This opens the discussion to various aspects of philosophical inquiry of the moral concepts of rights, responsibility, freedom, authority and power.

Having cleared the ground for some of the central concepts of philosophy, political philosophical schools are examined. This is not intended to be exhaustive but represents key political philosophies that have informed, shaped, impacted upon and continue to inform the theory, policy and practice of health and social care.

When asked why people want to study or work in health and social care, they often reply, 'it's because I want to make a difference', 'I want to put something back', 'I want to help change things', 'I had a good experience involving health and social care' or 'I'm interested in what makes people tick'. Health and social care also involve the 'big' questions about life and death, what responsibilities and duties we have to ourselves and others, what type of society we could or should live in. This chapter reflects upon some of these motivations and attempts to provide a more sustained reflection of these questions. In order to do this, the chapter examines the questions of politics, philosophy and ethics to health and social care.

PHILOSOPHY AND LEARNING TO PHILOSOPHISE

This chapter takes the philosophical position that welfare in health and social care is a normative, moral and political debate. Political and moral issues concern the right and wrong ways to exercise political power, and normative judgements consider the best way to deliver welfare. This leads to debate around the claims of justice that can be made on citizens and on the state (Plant 1991: 2). There are a multitude of competing perspectives in philosophy, political philosophy and moral philosophy. The aim of the chapter is not to include an exhaustive review of these positions but to provide a crash course to the main, and most influential debates, that have influenced and shaped health and social care. If philosophy is defined as the love of wisdom, we can use wisdom to justify the provision of welfare in health and social care. It can also provide us with a basis from which to make decisions about welfare entitlements and provide principles to moral conceptions such as rights and justice. Philosophy allows us to provide justified true beliefs about the propositions we are talking about and provides a basis for action and organisation for basic needs. Philosophy also allows us to investigate political notions and ideas about how we should shape and deliver health and social care. Thompson (2000: 64) suggests philosophy has been seen as being elitist, difficult, obscure and abstract, but can illuminate key debates in health and social care and make a positive role in facilitating high standards of professional practice.

POLITICAL PHILOSOPHY

Politics is about power, and conflict and its resolution at all levels of society (Hoffman and Graham 2009: 1). Politics is experienced at an everyday level, for example thinking about right and wrong, justice and injustice. Politics, understood as political activity and political thought, is also fundamental in shaping the delivery of health and social care. Power is often seen as something that limits what people can do such as force, constraint, subordination or coercion, but power can also be generative and facilitate or generate action. Lukes (2005) argues there are three dimensions of power. The first identifies power as decision making, the observable open act of making choices. The second dimension is that power is exercised to exclude certain issues from discussion and decision and issues are kept off the agenda. The third dimension is when people 'express preferences that are at variance with their interests' (Hoffman and Graham 2009: 7), that is they make decisions against their interests. Antonio Gramsci (2007, 1996, 1992) would suggest this is to do with 'hegemony', where people agree or give a popular consensus to political action and decisions that are not always in their best interests. With hegemony, dominant ideas achieve a 'consensus' through the agreement of the population. Many policies and practices within health and social care could be helpfully viewed from the perspective of hegemony, for example a range of issues such as welfare, provision, euthanasia, migration, and care for adults and children. Recent years have seen the growth of political thought and action to prioritise different interests of different groups. For example, service users' voices and interests have recently gained a level of political power to be able to articulate their needs and interests. Power is linked to further political philosophical concepts of freedom and authority.

FREEDOM

Isaiah Berlin (1991) suggested there are two types of liberty, a negative and a positive theory of liberty. Negative liberty is freedom 'from' interference or the absence of external restrictions or constraints on the individual. Positive liberty is freedom 'to' do things or ability to be one's own master, to be autonomous or to flourish. In health and social care much of this debate about freedom has taken place between the idea of 'paternalism', the provision of welfare to support and protect individuals and groups, and autonomy or the self-determination and self-ownership to make free choices (Fitzpatrick 2008: 97). This then has consequences for debates around protection from harm (for example, banning smoking or legalising drugs), choice (for example, where to send your child to school), relationships (who should care for older people), and 'big' moral and political questions such as abortion and euthanasia (Fitzpatrick 2008). Philosophical and political debate around freedom is implicit in much health and social care. For example, how much freedom should people who use health and social care have to do what they want compared to how much protection from harm they should have? Debates surrounding freedom are linked to questions of authority.

AUTHORITY

Heywood (2007: 328) suggests authority is the right to exert influence over others by virtue of an acknowledged obligation to obey. Weber (1922) suggested authority is established in three senses by charismatic, traditional and rational–legal authority. Charismatic authority is based on the charisma of an individual involved; traditional authority stems from things having always been done that way; and rational–legal authority is derived from a framework of laws or rules, very like a bureaucracy. For political decisions, authority needs to be legitimate or it accepted that political authority is rightful and, therefore, that those subject to it have a moral obligation to obey. Habermas (1975) suggests a legitimation crisis for political authority can come about economically when the economy performs badly, rationally when the decision-making process is seen as unjust, or motivational when political priorities and interests change. For health and social care, a legitimate authority needs to be in place at a government level, through the service organisation and at individual professional levels. Services need to be seen to be delivered by people in authority (in that they hold a recognised and respected position) and people who are an authority (so they are experts in the field) to deliver authoritative health and social care services. Freedom and authority are central to questions of 'rights' as rights can define the freedom we can enjoy and who has the authority to do what.

RIGHTS

Heywood (2007: 339) suggests rights are a 'broad ideological disposition that is characterised by sympathy for principles such as authority, order, hierarchy and duty'. Human rights are entitlements to treatment that a person enjoys by virtue of being a human being. Human rights are universal, they apply to everyone and are not contingent on being a member of a state or culture. Human rights have been criticised, as they place great moral weight on individual autonomy at the expense of considering welfare and community. Hoffman and Graham (2009: 416) suggest there are three issues to do with rights: the types of rights; the nature of the holder of rights; and conflicts between rights. Rights can carry costs for others and can be internally complex. For example, what does a right to marry provide? Do children and animals have rights? Does a right to life override a right to resources? Miliband (2005: 40) suggests the eighteenth century saw individuals granted civil rights (equality before the law), the nineteenth and twentieth centuries brought political rights (equality of the franchise or vote), and the early twentieth century increasing social rights based on principles such as equality of access to education, health care and housing. Marshall (1950) had established this vision of civil, political and social rights some 50 years earlier. Social rights are the most difficult to establish and maintain as debate about what counts as full participation in society is not a clear or uncontested discussion. Rights have been criticised for being 'nonsense on stilts' (Bentham 1962: 510) as they do not consider the consequences of action and create a philosophy of isolated, atomistic individualism rather than broader notions of welfare (for example, 'it is my right to ...' rather than 'we have a right to ...'). Legally, the Human Rights Act (1998) has made a significant contribution to codifying and collecting a set of rights together (Hoffman and Rowe 2006). Rights have also been central to debates in health and social care. For example, service users' rights, patients' rights, the right to services or the right to withdraw treatment all add to the debates and discussion on the nature or rights, who holds them and which rights have priority. The satisfaction of rights, however defined, is seen as central to ideas of justice. A just society is one where sets of rights are satisfied.

JUSTICE

The final political and moral philosophical concept in this chapter is justice. There are a host of debates surrounding justice and it is fair to argue justice has been the cornerstone of philosophical debate for millennia. Justice can be defined as the satisfaction of rights or 'a moral standard of fairness and impartiality' (Heywood 2007: 33). Justice has also been strongly linked to ideas of redistribution or desert ('share stuff out' or 'keep what you have earned'). Social justice is the 'notion of a fair or justifiable distribution of wealth and rewards in society' (Heywood 2007: 33). Significant recent debate has been around justice as fairness.

Rawls (1971) claims that the principles of justice were those that would be chosen by individuals located behind a veil of ignorance so they would not know their own abilities, identities, histories or social position. Using their capacity to reason, most individuals would favour a situation where everyone had the ability to participate and inequalities would favour the least well off. Rawls provides a liberal theory of justice that sees it as fairness but one that allows inequalities to exist if they work for the disadvantaged.

Miller (1976) suggests three principles to justice: 'rights, deserts and needs'. Rights are straightforward – an individual receives justice according to rights being satisfied within the rules and regulations of their society – for example, we have a right to vote as a citizen in England. Deserts are the rewards that people can gain because they deserve them or because they are based on merit. For example, people are selected for employment 'based on merit' because they are the best person for the job (Bagilhole 2009: 45). This principle of selecting people on merit is enshrined in equal opportunities and diversity legislation such as the Sexual Discrimination Act or the Equal Pay Act. There are two related issues to the principle of deserts. First, just because there is a legislative and legal framework to protect groups from unequal treatment does not mean this always translates into reality and many have argued that merit is a justification for powerful groups to maintain their position and power (Parekh 1992: 276). For example, women should receive the same pay as men for the same job but all kinds of research suggests this is still not happening (Equalities Review 2007). The second issue surrounds positive action or discrimination. Pitt (1992: 282) suggests 'positive action is not committed to the preference of a less qualified candidate'. The Equality Bill 2008 suggests that in the future, when selecting between two equally qualified candidates employers will be able to choose one of them on the basis of the under-representation of disadvantaged groups in their organisation (Bagilhole 2009: 45). The third principle is that of 'needs', where individuals and groups are entitled to things they lack or are necessary to them. Again, this is not without difficulty as who defines 'needs'? For example, disability groups have suggested that a health and social care professional's definition of need can be different from that of an individual person with a disability.

Freedom, authority, rights and justice are central to the theory, policy and practice of health and social care and have, arguably, framed much of the debate around health and social care services and provision. These moral questions, dilemmas and debates have also been informed by and are central to political philosophical questions that have underpinned dominant political ideologies. Liberalism, socialism and conservatism are discussed to provide a flavour or orientation to key debates on the political questions of health and social care.

LIBERALISM

As a political ideology liberalism has a long history often associated with 'classical liberalism'. Historically significant events are associated with liberalism such as the English 'Glorious Revolution' of 1688, the American War of Independence 1776, the French Revolution 1789 and it has become the dominant ideology of the industrialised West. Hoffman and Graham (2009: 176) argue the 'emergent democracies' of Eastern Europe are attempting to establish a form of liberal democracy.

There are variations with this ideology. Classical liberalism is a tradition within liberalism that seeks to maximise the realm of unconstrained individual action, typically establishing a minimal state and reliance on market economics. The idea of freedom of the individual is a key liberal political idea. The market is a system of economic exchange between buyers and sellers controlled by impersonal market forces (Heywood 2007: 49). In liberalism, the market is seen to have authority in providing the necessary goods and services. For example, private finance initiatives have used the market to provide schools and hospitals, built by private finance but for public need. Modern or neo-liberalism is seen as a tradition within liberalism that provides a qualified endorsement for social and economic intervention as a means for promoting personal development. Key thinkers in a liberal tradition are Hobbes, Locke, Mill and latterly Rawls. Liberalism has a fundamental commitment to freedom as the defining feature of its ideology. This commitment to freedom and liberty leads to various 'rights' having been formulated as part of liberalism's ideology.

Liberalism has the features of being individualist, egalitarian, universalist, and meliorist. Being individualist is the assertion of the primacy of the individual over any social collectivity, community or society. It is egalitarian as it considers all men (and it is men) equal and to have the same status which is not to be interfered with by legal or political order. It is universalist as it is characterised by a unity of humans; we all have the same worth across histories and cultures. Finally, it is meliorist as social institutions and political arrangements should serve humans in a constantly improving and progressive way. Liberalism has a commitment to the autonomy of the individual or the idea that the individual is primary and more important than any form of social collective. Individuals should be afforded the greatest freedom to allow them to flourish, to have personal freedom of choice, and to protect individual rights and freedoms.

SOCIALISM AND SOCIAL DEMOCRACY

Socialism has a rich history reaching back into the nineteenth century. Socialism as a philosophy is unified by its opposition to capitalism and its attempt to provide a social alternative to the exploitative conditions of capitalism. Humans are seen as social and creative creatures unified by a common humanity and perverted by capitalism away from cooperation towards competition. Equality is the central value of socialism and the necessary condition for social cohesion, stability and satisfying material need. There are a host of traditions that fall into a broad socialist camp, for example Marxism and social democracy. Socialism has been used in a variety of ways for a variety of groups but will be used here to indicate a philosophy based on the core ideas, values and theories of community, cooperation, equality, class politics and common ownership. Socialism carries with it the idea of a revolutionary transformation of society whilst social democracy implies a gradual change to humanise capitalism.

Health and social care has been strongly influenced by socialist ideas. Arguably, the whole establishment of the welfare state, the value of social justice, and health and social care services facilitating the equalisation of resources is driven by the political philosophy of socialism. Held (1987: 125–6) provides an accessible discussion of the defining features of socialism.

As an ideology, social democracy emerged in the early to mid part of the twentieth century as a result of Western socialist political parties adopting parliamentary strategies and revising socialist goals (Heywood 2007: 129). Rather than abolishing capitalism, social democrats sought to humanise it and stand between the market economy on one hand and state intervention on the other. Arguably, the establishment of the welfare state owes much to social democracy, as an attempt to socialise and humanise the effects of capitalism on inequality and poverty, and use the state to redistribute wealth through welfare, provide social security and a 'cradle to grave' provision of health and social care services. For example, the National Health Service is a testament to the strength and influence of social democratic ideals and goals. The post-war years from 1945 represent a golden age of social democratic welfare provision. However, since the 1970s and 1980s, social democracy has struggled to retain its electoral and political impacts (Heywood 2007: 130) in the face of neoliberalism and conservative administrations. Conservatism, similarly, has a long and rich tradition and was the dominant government administration during the 1980s.

CONSERVATISM

It is an interesting paradox that conservatism's basic credo is to conserve that status quo or that which exists. However, conservatism's ideological make up is a hybrid and changeable (Hoffman and Graham 2009: 197). Margaret Thatcher was a conservative but had a hybrid ideology that included nationalism and liberalism to such an extent that it was seen as a new conservative ideology of 'Thatcherism' (Hall 1998; Gamble 1988).

For conservatives and their desire to conserve, progress must be careful, tentative, respectful of past practices, pragmatic and go with the conservative view of human nature (Hoffman and Graham 2009: 197). They are against any large scale or rapid social change. There are unifying themes in this political ideology even if there are wide variations between specific writers and political parties. Pragmatism, conservatism, fallible humans and pessimism form the defining features of conservatism.

If rationalism is the analysis of social and political problems with an attempt at solutions, conservatives favour adopting pragmatism to find a solution. Conservatives fear radical experiments as we cannot fully predict all the consequences of our actions. Edmund Burke, fearful of the radical political experiment of the French Revolution in 1789, advocated a conservative position to defend the existing order of things.

Human beings are seen as limited in their ability to understand their own position and the complexity of society. Humans also are imperfect and will always have shortcomings. For these reasons conservatives reject 'visionary politics' (Hoffman and Graham 2009: 197) or revolutionary, radical politics. Conservatism's pessimism about the fallibility of human kind means that the provision of welfare and health and social care is at best paternalistic and at worst absent, with change being careful and tentative and the expense seen as unjustified. Conservatives are strongly supportive of institutions as the distillation of previous wisdom, a way of restricting people's fallibility and a source of allegiance.

Conservatism provides an idea of unity and strength at the level of the nation state and moral virtues and identity, law and order, family, and Britishness are key conservative themes. Early conservatives see welfare as primarily based on charity, later conservatives see a commitment to state welfare through paternalism (for example, Harold Macmillan's Tories or 'Wet' Conservatives). Recent conservatism has led to the protection of consumer rights and extension of individual rights. For example, Thatcherism during the 1980s was critical of large scale, social democratic health and social care provision and prioritised individual consumer choice. This has consequences, for example poverty is seen as something to be tackled when it presents a threat to social order.

The 'New Right' is a term that has been used to describe a range of ideas such as demands for tax cuts, limited immigration and the extension of the market into health and social care. Heywood (2007: 88) contends that the New Right is a marriage between two contrasting ideological positions. The first is classical liberal economics, particularly the free market ideas of Adam Smith, that are seen as a way to challenge the large state bureaucracies and inefficient spending of social democratic welfare. The second is the neoconservative focus upon order, authority and discipline. The New Right was dominant through the 1980s and early 1990s until electoral success from the 'Third Way' or New Labour government in 1997 (Miliband 2005).

NEW LABOUR

The Third Way, as Heywood (2007: 136) suggests, is shrouded in debate and confusion as it has taken many different forms in different countries. There are a number of unifying themes that have emerged from the Third Way. A belief in the 'old' socialist ideals of overthrowing capitalism is no longer seen viable and the influence of neoliberalism has led to the Third Way's acceptance of a 'dynamic market economy'. For example, the UK's Labour Party jettisoned its commitment to common ownership contained in Clause IV of its constitution. New Labour's departure from this fundamental aspect of socialist political ideology has seen moves towards 'earned citizenship', where health and social care provision is ordered by sets of rights to which we are entitled but that have sets of duties attached – the 'rights and duties' approach on domestic issues has been a central plank of New Labour's mainstream appeal (Goodhart 2005). The idea of a conditional entitlement to health and social care fits uncomfortably with the egalitarian socialist ideals.

Health and social care has been influenced by the range of ideological positions and political philosophies. Neoliberalism has underpinned health and social care services through the introduction of markets such as Private Finance Initiatives to build schools and hospitals. Conservatism, particularly the form associated with Thatcherism, has prioritised the individual consumer over ideas of collective welfare. The Third Way of New Labour has attempted to balance the demands of a dynamic market economy with ideas of social justice and tackling poverty, to uneven success (Hills *et al.* 2009). The ongoing political philosophical debate will inform, shape and impact on the future of health and social care. Implicit and associated with political philosophy are those normative questions about ethics and moral philosophy.

ETHICS

Ethics is a branch of philosophy with a long and rich history and tradition. It reaches far back in time to the ancient Greeks but also allows discussion of those pressing contemporary questions. This chapter is not exhaustive in what it covers but attempts to provide a flavour of some of the political and philosophical resources available to those who are interested in this area of health and social care. Those who would like to go further and perhaps add a more nuanced understanding can make use of the referenced reading at the end of the chapter. The final discussion will cover three main ethical philosophies that have contributed to and informed health and social care theory, policy and practice.

CONSEQUENTIALISM

Consequentialism, based strongly on the liberal political tradition of liberalism and utilitarianism, is concerned with the outcomes, results or consequences of actions and how far actions promote intrinsic goods like happiness or pleasure. Actions are right in as far as they promote happiness for utilitarians. The strength of consequentialism is its intuitive appeal. It makes sense to say those things are good that promote happiness. There are problems with this approach. For example: what counts as happiness?; how can you measure it?; it uses a crude calculation that does not allow for individual differences or preferences – is this the same between peoples, cultures and societies?; what duration do you count? It is an unrealistic ethics, and are there other motivations for ethics? Most difficult, the idea of consequences promoting happiness can lead to atrocities rather than the greater good. Finally, consequentialism considers individuals as moral saints who do not have a moral obligation or special responsibilities to others. For example, should we give all our money to charity or do we have a special responsibility to family? By example, if you are given a test of your courage to execute one of your party in order that the rest can go free, consequentialism would suggest you should on a simple calculation, but most people would consider individuals have 'integrity' (Smart and Williams 1973: 98–117) or a special responsibility to the group (Sidgwick 1981).

Utilitarianism and consequentialism have been used to promote the idea of public welfare. Actions that lead to an overall aggregate of happiness are morally right actions (Goodin 1995; Bailey 1997). This moral perspective is often contrasted with deontology and Kantian ethics.

DEONTOLOGY

Deontologists, such as Kant (1991), reject consequentialism and utilitarianism, arguing it is principles that justify certain actions; that is those things that come before or precede actions, not the consequences. Kant's ethics have received sustained examination (O'Neill 1989; Baron 1995) and he provides a different basis for ethics, 'the ground for of obligation must be looked for, not in the nature of man nor in the circumstances of the world in which he is place, but solely *a priori* in the concepts of pure reason (Kant 1991: 55).

With reason as the capacity to make decisions, people make moral laws from ethical principles or maxims. A hypothetical imperative is when you do something to achieve something else, or 'if ... then' decisions (Fitzpatrick 2008: 46), such as 'work hard to succeed'. These are instrumental goods or using one thing to achieve another. Intrinsic goods are those that are good in themselves such as human well-being or flourishing or happiness. This leads to Kant's famous formulation of the categorical imperative in the *Groundwork*: 'I ought never to act except in such a way that I can also will that my maxim should become a universal law' (Kant 1991: 67). As such, Kant provides a universal ethical theory that the way we act should be generalised to everyone, and everyone should have a duty to uphold this universal moral law.

Fitzpatrick (2008: 46) argues that Kant's identification of the capacity to reason, and the demand to recognise others' rationality, leads him to a second formulation of the categorical imperative to 'act in such a way that you always treat humanity, whether in your own person or in the person of any other, never simply as a means, but always at the same time as an end' (Kant 1991: 9). In a 'kingdom of ends' we would all recognise each other's ability to reason, act according to universal laws of morality and treat each other with respect (for our reason and duty to laws). This has the derived principle of 'respect for others' that has become central to health and social care. Commentators, such as Fitzpatrick (2008: 47), argue that this 'is the core of what for many is the most persuasive model of liberalism: one based on the freedom of rational beings to observe the laws and duties of universal reason in a moral and social system of mutual respect'.

There are many criticisms levelled at Kant's ethics (MacIntyre 1985: ch. 14). It is too formal and rigid; it is abstract and too distant from everyday life; it is emotionless, treating individuals as moral robots; it requires an unquestioning duty to morality rather than being moral; and it excludes consequences. Kant is also seen as too universalist, too rational, too Western (Fitzpatrick 2008: 86). Deontology is strong on individual autonomy, but poor on social justice. It is an atomistic ethics that requires a reasoning subject or individual who has an emotionless obedience to the rules. Focusing on universal laws ignores consequences to try to militate against certain undesirable effects. Kant's emphasis on the kingdom of ends means that there will always be a presumption in favour of the individual's sovereignty, their inherent moral worth, an important point whenever the actual consent of agents is difficult to obtain (Fitzpatrick 2008: 87), such as in end of life decisions.

VIRTUE ETHICS

Driver (2007: 136) suggests dissatisfaction with utility and Kant over their abstract and emotionless ethics has led commentators to consider the agent or actor rather than their actions or principles. Aristotle sees virtue as leading to *eudaimonia* or human well-being. Aristotle's virtue ethics have been characterised as the 'doctrine of the mean' where virtues lie between two vices or extremes. For example, bravery lies between cowardice and foolhardiness, and temperance lies between gluttony and abstinence. For Aristotle, the ends of actions are moral if they fulfil the functions of human nature, the good being a flourishing of human potential, and virtue ethics updates this position. MacIntyre (1985) has made a significant contribution to contemporary virtue ethics.

It has been argued that virtue ethicists overemphasise common humanity, do not provide a guide for action and deny contemporary findings in psychology (Driver 2007: 150). The relationship of social justice can also be problematic for virtuists. Virtues change over time and place. The strength of virtue ethics is in the indeterminancy of moral decisions against the calculus of utilitarians and the moral imperatives of Kantians.

Each of the above theories offers indispensable insights while there remain genuine differences and difficulties for all of them. Ethical decision making is hard to achieve unless everyone is given equal consideration in some space that is important in the particular theory. It is difficult to see how an ethical theory can have general social plausibility without extending equal consideration to all at some level. For us to able to debate philosophically and politically we need a necessary condition of equality (in some form and at some level) to consider things ethically.

CONCLUSION

Having considered various philosophical positions we can conclude that health and social care need an orientation and sensibility for freedom, authority, rights, justice and responsibilities. What considerations of philosophy and politics provide for the health and social care worker and student are the ability to reflect upon the complex and challenging situations presented by health and social care and to engage with the very air we breathe of philosophical, political and ethical debate.

SUMMARY OF MAIN POINTS

You should be able to:

•   Appreciate the ways in which fundamental principles of philosophy and politics can be defended by rational argument and applied to health and social care.
•   Discuss the relationship between philosophical and political concepts and their application to health and social care.
•   Understand the complex relationship between public, social and political philosophies.
•   Debate the concepts of rights, responsibility, freedom, authority and power.

MOMENT OF REFLECTION

Make a list of the strengths and weaknesses of socialism, social democracy, conservatism, liberalism and New Labour. Which do you see as the most effective for health and social care? Why?

REFERENCES

Bagilhole, B. (2009) *Understanding Equal Opportunities and Diversity: The social differentiations and intersections of inequality,* Bristol: The Policy Press.

Bailey, J. (1997) *Utilitarianism, Institutions, and Justice,* Oxford: Oxford University Press.

Baron, M. (1995) *Kantian Ethics Almost Without Apology,* London: Cornell University Press.

Bentham, J. (1962) *The Complete Works. Vol. II.* Edited by Bowring, J., New York: Russell and Russell.

Berlin, I. (1991) Two Concepts of Liberty in Miller, D. (1991) (Ed.) *Liberty,* Oxford: Oxford University Press, pp. 33–57.

Driver, J. (2007) *Ethics: The Fundamentals,* Oxford: Blackwell.

Equalities Review (2007) *Fairness and Freedom: The final report of the Equalities Review,* London: Equalities Review.

Fitzpatrick, T. (2008) *Applied Ehtics and Social Problems: Moral questions of birth, society and death,* Bristol: Policy Press.

Gamble, Andrew. (1988) *The free economy and the strong state: the politics of Thatcherism,* Basingstoke: Macmillan Education.

Goodhart, D. (2005) Britain's Glue in Giddens, A. and Diamond, P. (Eds) *The New Egalitarianism,* Cambridge: Polity Press.

Goodin, R. (1995) *Utilitarianism as Public Policy,* Cambridge: Cambridge University Press.

Gramsci, A. (2007) *Prison Notebooks. Vol. III* (Trans. Buttigieg, J.A.), New York: Columbia University Press.

Gramsci, A. (1996) *Prison Notebooks. Vol. II* (Trans. Buttigieg, J.A.), New York: Columbia University Press.

Gramsci, A. (1992) *Prison Notebooks. Vol. I* (Trans. Buttigieg, J.A.), New York: Columbia University Press.

Habermas, J. (1975) *Legitimation Crisis* (Trans. McCarthy, T.), London: Heinemann Education.

Hall, S. (1998) *The Hard Road to Renewal: Thatcherism and the crisis of the Left,* London: Verso.

Held, D. (1987) *Models of Democracy,* Cambridge: Polity.

Heywood, A. (2007) (4th edition) *Political Ideologies,* Basingstoke: Palgrave.

Hills, J., Sefton, T. and Stewart, K. (2009) *Towards a More Equal Society?,* Bristol: The Policy Press.

Hoffman, D. and Rowe, J. (2006) *Human Rights in the UK: An introduction to the Human Rights Act 1998,* Harlow: Pearson Longman.

Hoffman, J. and Graham, P. (2009) *Introduction to Political Theory,* Harlow: Pearson Education.

Fitzpatrick, T. (2008) *Applied Ethics and Social Problems: Moral questions of birth, society and death,* Bristol: Policy Press.

Kant, I. (1991) *Groundwork of the Metaphysics of Morals,* London: Routledge.

Lukes, S. (2005) (2nd edition) *Power: a radical view,* Basingstoke: Palgrave.

MacIntyre, A. (1985) *After Virtue: A study in moral theory,* London: Duckworth.

Marshall, T. H. (1950) *Citizenship and Social Class,* Cambridge: Cambridge University Press.

Miliband, E. (2005) 'Does Inequality Matter', in Giddens, A. and Diamond, P. (Eds) (2005) *The New Egalitarianism,* Cambridge: Polity Press.

Miller, D. (1976) *Social Justice,* Oxford: Clarendon Press.

O'Neill, O. (1989) *Constructions of Reason,* Cambridge: Cambridge University Press.

Parekh, B. (1992) 'A Case for Positive Descrimination', in Hepple, B. and Szyszak, E.M. (Eds) *Discrimination: The Limits of the Law,* London: Mansell Publishing.

Pitt, G. (1992) 'Can Reverse Discrimination be Justified?', in Hepple, B. and Szyszak, E.M. (Eds) *Discrimination: The Limits of the Law,* London: Mansell Publishing.

Plant, R. (1991) *Modern Political Thought,* Oxford: Blackwell.

Rawls, J. (1971) *A Theory of Justice,* Oxford: Oxford University Press.

Sidgwick, H. (1981) *The Methods of Ethics,* Indianapolis, IN: Hackett.

Smart, J. J. C. and Williams, R. (1973) *Utilitarianism: For and Against,* Cambridge: Cambridge University Press.

Thompson, N. (2000) *Theory and Practice in Health and Social Care,* Milton Keynes: Open University Press.

Weber, M. (1922) *Economy and Society,* New York: Bedminster.

CHAPTER 10

RESEARCH IN HEALTH AND SOCIAL CARE

KRISTAN HOPKINS-BURKE

OBJECTIVES

After reading this chapter you should be able to:

- Discuss principles of quantitative and qualitative research.

- Understand questionnaire design.

- Understand quantitative and qualitative techniques for data analysis.

- Be able to compare different research methodologies and their application in health and social care.

- Evaluate and use research in health and social care.

- Discuss research ethics in health and social care.

After reading this chapter you will know the meaning of the following terms: Quantitative, qualitative, methodology, method, evidence-based practice, research design, experiments, natural experiments, surveys, questionnaires, observation, case studies, action research, grounded theory, narrative, content analysis, ethics.

There are five Moments of Reflection to work on throughout the chapter.

INTRODUCTION

In recent years it has become increasingly important for students and practitioners in the field of health and social care to develop their knowledge and skills of research. This requires an ability to evaluate, use and critique other people's research. Closely linked to this has been increased government pressure on the public sector to engage in research that seeks to continually monitor and improve its practice. More broadly, this is part of the quality assurance programme and the 'audit' society (Hopkins-Burke 2008) and the impact of the Research Governance Framework for research in health and social care (DoH 2005, 2001).

However, it may still be helpful to distinguish between those involved in the *production* and those involved in the *consumption* of research. Practitioners in the field of health and social care, for example, midwives and nurses, social workers and the police, may or may not actually do research, but there is still a need to develop their 'research literacy' (Hek and Moule 2006) *particularly* within the climate of evidence based practice. Furthermore, it is argued that the failure of practitioners to make use of the available research evidence – in the drive towards evidence based practice – can, in part, be explained by a lack of research appraisal skills (Hopkins-Burke 2008). It is the aim of this chapter to provide the reader with an introduction to some of the key issues in relation to social research with particular reference to the field of health and social care.

EVIDENCE BASED PRACTICE

Since the 1990s there has been a rapid expansion in the adoption of evidence based practice for health and social care. It is argued that 'evidence based practice means basing intervention on proven effectiveness derived from empirical research' (Gray and Mcdonald 2006: 7). In the past, decisions made in practice relied less upon the influence of research and more upon previous knowledge gained in training, opinion (or prejudice), and information gained from more experienced colleagues (Trinder and Reynolds 2000). Advocates of this approach argue that practice should be based on the most up to date, valid and reliable research, while ironically, critics argue that there is 'no *evidence* that evidence based practice actually works' (Hek and Moule 2006: 5). Furthermore, it is argued that the 'ontological and epistemological assumptions' of evidence based practice, particularly in social work, are 'inappropriate' and too narrow (Gray and Mcdonald 2006). While some writers see professional accountability as a good reason to embrace evidence based practice (Rosen *et al.* 1999) others argue it is too restrictive (Trinder 2000b; Webb 2001). A good example of this criticism is provided by Williams and Garner (2002) who review the value of an evidence based approach to psychiatry. The authors argue that the emphasis upon 'the evidence' is restraining clinical practice and that a degree of professional consensus is necessary.

Examination of the current debate highlights its contested and political nature. Within the criminal justice system for example, evidence based practice has been directly linked to the 'what works' agenda (Hopkins-Burke 2008). However, critics question this 'so called' *objective* application of rigorous scientific research findings to the phenomenon of offending behaviour (Bateman and Pitts 2005), arguing that the process actually entails subjectivity in the selection of research findings which is far from objective.

The rise of evidence based practice represents a cultural shift from the previous often unspoken orthodoxy of 'trusted professional judgement based practice' (Davies *et al.* 2000; Hek and Moule 2006; Trinder 2000a) to that of research informed practice. Other terms used are 'what works evidence' (Hudson and Sheldon 2002 cited in Trevithick 2005). The concept of evidence based practice which has its origins in medicine, has come to take on very specific meanings. In social work, for example, it is equated with 'current best evidence' or 'technically better research' as opposed to the medical equivalent of 'clinical experience' or 'clinical practice' (Trevithick 2005: 54). It is important for students and practitioners to understand that knowledge is acquired in different ways and not all knowledge carries the same status. Within social work for example, meta-analyses which aim to identify, appraise and synthesise contradictory research (Glasziou *et al.* 2001) are advocated by some (Sheldon 2000) while others argue for a combination of methodologies (Ferguson 2003). The biggest critique of such systematic reviews (meta-analyses), however, comes from 'scientific realism' which argues that 'what works' in one context may not apply to another. Therefore, it is important that researchers identify not only 'what works' and for whom but in which contexts it does or does not work (Pawson and Tilley 1994, 1997).

In summary, proponents of evidence based practice point to improved outcomes for service users, greater credibility and enhanced accountability. Sceptics are more critical of the methods employed, for example experiments which they contend are inappropriate to the study (and complexity) of human life (*see* Chapter 17 by Raithby and Ring).

WHAT IS RESEARCH?

There are as many definitions of research as there are ways to do research. However, a defining characteristic of research is that it is systematic and disciplined. It relies upon scientific as opposed to anecdotal evidence. There is also a strong empirical tradition in that researchers typically collect primary data in the form of observations and experiments. The aim is to produce findings which are both valid (measures what it claims to measure) and reliable (reproducible or consistent) although sometimes there is a trade off between the two. The key point is that research is organised, systematic and verifiable.

TYPES OF RESEARCH

It is helpful to distinguish between research in the social and research in the natural sciences. Within the scope of this chapter, we are concerned with *social* research, which can be defined as 'any research that investigates human behaviours and social life' (Berg 2004 cited in Hansen 2006: 10). Within the social sciences there are close connections between the theoretical approach of *positivism* and the natural sciences. Basically, the fundamental tenet of positivism is the belief that the social sciences can and *should* appropriate the methods of natural science, otherwise known as the scientific method. The quantitative methodological approach of the social sciences shares this view.

Quantitative methodology

From the point of view of the quantitative researcher, objective reality exists and is capable of being measured and methods such as social surveys are thought to be capable of measuring this. The most common methods associated with quantitative research are experiments – particularly randomised controlled trials within the health and social care setting – social surveys and questionnaires. The defining feature of this methodological approach is that the data is numeric or is at least capable of being analysed numerically. In addition, researchers often utilise existing data – data collected for other purposes – otherwise known as secondary sources. There are a range of secondary sources which can be utilised, for example, hospital records, letters, case notes and official statistics. Moule (2005) describes the use of diaries in a study which explored health care students as a community of learners (cited in Hek and Moule 2006: 92).

A number of factors are contributing to a growth in the use of secondary sources. First, recording practices within health care have generally increased (Hek and Moule 2006). Second, an EU Directive (2004) has made primary research within the NHS extremely difficult. All research applications now have to be processed through local, regional and multi-regional ethics committees which are sanctioned by law. Third, there has been an explosion in the availability of large-scale datasets online, for example, the UK Data Archive and the National Centre for E-Social Science. Fourth, the rise of evidence based practice has necessitated the collection of evidence to inform policy changes in health and social care. Finally, the ethical governance framework for both health and social care has made secondary research rather than primary empirical research more attractive.

Qualitative methodology

From the point of view of the qualitative researcher, objective reality is a fluid commodity and less amenable to precise measurement. The emphasis is therefore upon the way that knowledge is socially constructed. The methods of natural science are deemed inappropriate to the study of social life. The most common methods associated with qualitative research are observation, particularly in natural settings, and indepth and unstructured interviews, for their ability to capture and express the subjective viewpoints of participants. A good introduction to ethnography is provided by Hammersley and Atkinson (2007). This highlights the importance of *reflexivity* to the approach. For a more recent introduction to qualitative research, particularly for those researching in health care, Hansen (2006) provides a comprehensive overview.

The dichotomy between quantitative and qualitative research

Over the last century there has been a rigid divide between those social scientists who favour quantitative and those who favour a more qualitative approach (Kelle and Erzberger 2004). More recently, this has been overshadowed by the emergence of a new approach known as mixed methods research (Tashakkori and Creswell 2007). This is particularly true of research in health and social care where there has been a huge expansion within the literature on 'how to' do mixed methods research (Creswell 2003), but also an increase in the area of published research (Caracelli and Greene 1993; Saks and Allsop 2007; Tashakkori and Teddlie 2003). There is now an online journal dedicated to this enterprise called the *Journal of Mixed Methods Research*. In a recent article, the question was posed as to whether mixed methods research should be conceived as a distinctive methodology (Greene 2008) and it has also been referred to as 'the third research paradigm' (Onwuegbuzie & Leech 2004 cited in Burke Johnson and Onwuegbuzie 2004: 15).

Within the field of social work, where qualitative methods have tended to dominate, some writers are also advocating the use of mixed methods research (Shaw 2000). Within the literature, however, the difference between mixed methods and triangulation is ill-defined. Kimchi *et al.* (1991) identify six different types of triangulation: *theory*, *data*, *methods*, *investigator*, *multiple* and *analysis triangulation*. Edwards and Talbot (1999) define it as a three-point perspective on a phenomenon. This may involve the use of several *methods*, *participants* or *researchers*. From the above definitions, it is difficult to see how triangulation and mixed methods differ.

Triangulation is often referred to as a technique that uses multiple sources to get at the *same* phenomenon which can help with data validation (Gomm 2008). Indeed, when triangulation was first articulated by Denzin (1989) it was defined as 'the combination of methodologies in the study of the *same* phenomenon' (cited in Burke Johnson *et al.* 2007: 114). It is important to note the emphasis upon the *same* as opposed to a number of different phenomena.

The work of Burke Johnson *et al.* (2007) helps to elucidate the distinction between mixed methods and triangulation. In the early days of triangulation, sources could be triangulated '*within-method*' or '*between-method*'. Denzin (1989) argued for the latter as it meant you were not restricted to one methodological approach, therefore reducing the potential for bias. However, in contrast to triangulation, mixed methods research *always* incorporates data from a quantitative and a qualitative perspective which is not a stringent requirement of triangulation. Triangulation seems to be more about combining sources in order to validate findings – or not – as the case may be.

An example of this approach to health and social care research is provided by Burr (1988) a study exploring critical care family needs. While the quantitative data was useful in devising the Critical Care Family Needs Inventory (CCFNI), the qualitative data helped to provide a complete picture of the family needs that the CCFNI alone had missed. The usefulness of triangulation to health care evaluation research is further explored by Ammenwerth *et al.* (2003).

Mixed methods research is, therefore, when a researcher (or team of researchers) employs a range of methods to answer *different* questions as opposed to the use of multiple sources to answer the same question. In this instance, the method(s) best suited to the research question(s) will be used. Within a large project this might involve interviewing, alongside analysis of documentary evidence and a questionnaire. The researcher might conduct indepth interviews to learn more about a particular issue which may then help to generate a suitable questionnaire. This is particularly useful when engaged in exploratory research of a new topic. Nicolson *et al.* (2005) utilised mixed methods in their study of practitioners in neonatal nursing. They collected data using both quantitative and qualitative methods, including a survey, interviews and focus groups.

It would seem that mixed methods has become a methodological paradigm replacing the dualism of the quantitative and qualitative divide. However, some researchers continue to argue against mixing the two. It is argued that the different theoretical underpinnings make data validation difficult (Gomm 2008). This issue remains unresolved.

MOMENT FOR REFLECTION

Activity – Quantitative/qualitative and mixed methods research

Find a research paper within a reputable journal, for example, the *British Journal of Social Work*. Select a paper that uses quantitative methods (or is largely quantitative in its approach) and another which is qualitative, preferably on the same topic. Compare and contrast these papers thinking about the design, aims and outcomes of the research. Identify the limitations of each. Would a mixed methods research design be favourable?

METHOD AND METHODOLOGY

It is important to understand the difference between 'method' and 'methodology'. Research method refers to the 'tools of the trade' – the specific techniques employed to gather data, for example, a postal questionnaire or an interview schedule. However, methodology is rooted at a deeper level – the way in which knowledge is produced and reality created – tied up in questions of *epistemology* and *ontology*. Epistemology is a branch of philosophy which concerns itself with the science of knowing and how to investigate the social world, whereas ontology is about existence itself and the nature of reality. Before the birth of mixed methods research, selection of a methodology was a primary consideration. However, today researchers have more freedom to select method(s) best suited to the research question(s). Of course, research does not take place within a vacuum and there are always other considerations which impact upon such choice. The research student is usually limited by external factors such as time and money. Similarly, Edwards and Talbot (1999) have written a survival guide for the hard-pressed researcher who is constantly trying to juggle paid employment with research and sometimes family life as well. Seale (1999) reviews a number of different paradigms including positivist, naturalistic, constructivist and postmodern. He argues that the search for quality – particularly in qualitative social research – was part of a modernist phase which could be partly explained by the need to justify quality to funding bodies. He argues for a pragmatic approach to research which sensitises practising researchers to the strengths and weaknesses of different types of research without constraining them:

> [what] I would like to see is some sense of there being a community of social researchers who have respect for the strengths of a variety of positions within that community, appreciating the need also to develop research skills taken from a number of genres (quantitative, as well as qualitative, in fact), in much the same way as artists learn how to paint, draw or sculpt in a number of different styles.
>
> (Seale 1999: 476)

DATA COLLECTION TECHNIQUES
Quantitative research

Quantitative research is a deductive (rather than inductive) approach which begins with a hypothesis (a hunch or a tentative theory), moves on to collect data and then in the light of the data/findings makes a decision about whether to accept or revise the theory. It is deductive therefore, because it moves from the general to the particular. It is the scientific method par excellence. Before we move on to consider different techniques it is important to consider research design.

Research Design

Cross-sectional designs involve collecting data at one point in time. Many descriptive surveys employ this type of design. Longitudinal designs involve collecting data at different points in time whereas the pre-test/post-test design – extremely common to evaluation research – collects data at two points in time 'before' and 'after' the intervention. All good research is planned. A research design is essentially a 'blueprint' for how you will proceed and needs to consider a number of issues including theoretical, practical and ethical. Many writers identify stages in the research process from selecting a topic, reviewing the literature, narrowing and refining the research questions, right through to data collection, analysis and writing of results (Bell 1997; Hansen 2006). How to write research proposals has also received wide attention (Punch 2006) along with how to conduct literature reviews (Fink 2005). Aveyard (2008) has written a book on conducting literature reviews in the field of health and social care.

Experiments

The experimental method is probably the best method for studying causality. For this reason, it is hugely popular in health care research (Gomm *et al.* 2000b). The randomised controlled trial (RCT) is considered to be the 'gold standard' in health care research and is essentially an experiment that takes place in a practice setting. However, there are a number of ethical issues raised by RCTs, for instance, holding back a treatment thought to be beneficial to participants is considered unethical. Sibbald and Roland (1998) provide a helpful review of such trials and their usefulness to health research. They argue that:

> it remains an ideal that all new health care interventions should be evaluated through randomised controlled trials. Given that poor design may lead to biased outcomes, trialists should strive for methodological rigour and report their work in enough detail for others to assess its quality.
>
> (Sibbald and Roland 1988: 201)

The experiment is the method par excellence for studying the relationship between independent and dependent variables. The former are, as their name suggests, 'independent' (causal) whereas, the latter are 'dependent' (effect). An independent variable is therefore likely to precede the dependent variable temporally. The main objective for the researcher is to isolate variables in order to explore their interaction. Researchers typically exercise a high degree of control when using this method which helps them to rule out the influence of extraneous factors.

The experiment usually involves two groups – an experimental group and a control group. The experimental group generally receives some kind of treatment – a drug for example – while the control group does not. In a double blind study (the gold standard) neither the researchers nor the participants know which group receives the treatment. The double blind study is therefore considered to be superior.

Researchers who conduct experiments usually want to test a hypothesis (deduction) and they employ statistical methods to measure outcomes. The most critical aspect of the design of an experiment is that other variables are controlled for. Researchers need to be certain that any change brought about in the dependent variable is caused by the independent variable alone. Equally important to the design of the experiment is *randomisation*. This refers to the way in which participants are selected for inclusion in the study. Aside from the issue of representativeness, it is vital that differences between people allocated to either group are similar. It is easy to control for known differences between participants, for example, age or gender, but it is argued that random allocation will help take care of unknown factors as well. A famous experiment was of course 'obedience to authority' (Milgram 1974) more recently recreated by Burger (2009) who made changes to the design of the study to meet current ethical standards.

OBEDIENCE TO AUTHORITY – MILGRAM (1963, 1965, 1974)

A series of studies were conducted to explore whether people were capable of committing atrocities (such as the holocaust) as a result of following instructions. Participants were told that they were taking part in a study concerned with the effects of punishment on learning. They were assigned to the role of teacher rather than learner (an actor) and told to administer electric shocks to the 'learner' (strapped in a chair in a connected room) each time an incorrect answer was given. The shocks ranged from 15 to 450 volts. In reality, no electric shocks were administered but the participants believed they were. The experimenter encouraged participants to continue even when the learner was heard to protest, scream in pain and demand to be released. As the shocks increased the learner would bang on the wall and eventually there was no response. Many participants began to resist at this point and would refuse to continue but the experimenter would use a number of verbal prods to request they continue. In the first round of experiments, 65 per cent of participants managed to administer shocks all the way up to 450 volts.

OBEDIENCE TO AUTHORITY – BURGER (2009)

In the more recent version of this experiment Burger was able to replicate Milgram avoiding some of the ethical difficulties. Respondents were screened to avoid including anybody who might have reacted negatively. Respondents were informed that they could withdraw at anytime and still receive their payment of $50. Burger informed participants immediately after the experiment (no time delay) that no shocks had been administered. The experimenter was a trained psychologist and was instructed to end the experiment if the participant was to show signs of stress. Importantly, the experiment did not allow a participant to administer an electric shock beyond 150 volts. Burger found similar results to Milgram but his interpretation differs. He argues that factors other than people being 'inherently evil' can explain this response. Power is a key factor as is having little time to 'think'.

MOMENT OF REFLECTION

Video clip: http://www.youtube.com/watch?v=BcvSNg0HZwk

Watch this video. How do you think you would respond in this situation? What do you think were the main ethical problems with the original study? To what extent did Burger's replication overcome them?

Natural experiments

Natural experiments are experiments in the social world that occur naturally as opposed to those artificially created within the confines of the research laboratory. Such experiments are also sometimes referred to as 'quasi' or 'field' experiments. Ethics play a major role in determining what we can or cannot do. If events happen naturally, researchers can intervene to examine the relationship between variables (Gomm 2008). Statistical analyses and tests are really a way of controlling for variables post-hoc in order to measure their influence.

Surveys and questionnaires

Questionnaires and social surveys are the most commonly used tool within the social sciences. It is possible to collect large quantities of data from geographically dispersed populations which can be analysed numerically. Two common fallacies are first, social surveys and questionnaires are the same, second, questionnaires are easy to create.

SURVEYS

A social survey is more than a questionnaire. A social survey is a research design that can include questionnaires but may also include other methods such as documentary analysis and interviewing. The classic text on surveys was written by Moser and Kalton (1958, 2001). This provides a historical overview of the origins and development of the social survey. However, other sections focus upon questionnaire design (and scales), as well as sampling techniques. More recently, Fink (2006) provides detailed guidance on the design, implementation, analysis and presentation of survey data for researchers of the twenty-first century.

Basically there are two types of surveys, 'descriptive' and 'correlational' although some writers prefer to call them 'descriptive' and 'analytic' (Gray 2004). The former, as the name suggests, aim to provide a comprehensive overview of a phenomenon, for example, a patient satisfaction survey. They aim to provide a snapshot at a particular point in time. A descriptive survey as the name suggests would therefore make use of descriptive rather than inferential statistics. A good introduction to descriptive statistics is provided by Rugg (2007). A general approach to survey analysis, interpreting figures and cross-tabulation tables is provided by Procter (1994). The strengths and weaknesses of quantitative research designs – in relation to bereavement research – are explored by Walker (2005) who argues that the methodological limitations of such designs can jeopardise the validity of findings.

Correlational surveys move beyond the level of description to explore relationships between variables. Referring back to our previous example, instead of reporting the number and percentage of patients who were satisfied with their experience as in or out-patients, the analysis would go further to explore how this connected with their previous experience, the nature of their condition or some other variables. The researcher would need to make use of inferential statistics not only to describe but also to infer relationships and, more importantly, to infer back to the population from which the sample was drawn, assuming a probability sample was used. An excellent introduction to some of these terms and concepts, for example 'statistical significance', is provided by the work of Rugg (2007).

QUESTIONNAIRES

A questionnaire is an instrument we can use to ask questions of our respondents. Questionnaires are generally perceived to provide *objective* information and as such they have been widely used or abused (Boynton 2004). When creating questionnaires it is vital that they are objective, valid and reliable. In general, questionnaires tend to score more highly on reliability (consistency of response) than validity (measuring what you intend to measure). If the questionnaire to be administered is for self completion, for example, it is important that the questions are unambiguous and that each respondent interprets them in the same way otherwise you are not comparing like with like and risk threats to validity. This is why piloting is so important. It is also important to avoid leading questions and double-barrelled questions (Oppenheim 2001). In a recent study by Gleeson *et al.* (2008) the attitudes of medical students towards abortion were explored, which involved surveying 300 medical students. This study highlights the breadth that such an approach can achieve. For those working in health and social care, a key text has been produced by Bradburn *et al.* (2004) which provides guidance on social and health questionnaires.

While there is choice about how to administer questionnaires – by hand, by post, face to face, online – response rates do tend to be low. This obviously has detrimental effects on the success of a study. A study by Booth *et al.* (2003) which sampled social workers and occupational therapists, achieved a mere 27 per cent response rate. When response rates are this low, representativeness is questioned.

MOMENT OF REFLECTION

Activity – questionnaire design

Devise a questionnaire with at least twelve questions (a mix of open and closed questions). Ask a friend, family member or colleague to complete it. Did they interpret the questions in the way you intended? What problems did you identify? Think about the questions in terms of validity and reliability. How could the questionnaire be improved?

QUALITATIVE RESEARCH

Qualitative research is inductive rather than deductive. It therefore moves from the particular to the general – the particular being the observations from which the theory is generated rather than tested. However, the distinction between induction and deduction is never really this clear cut in practice. In the case of *grounded theory*, for example, there is an iterative process between the data and the theory which means that induction involves elements of deduction and vice versa (Bryman 2008). Moreover, a researcher may initially start out with exploration of a problem that, in turn, leads them to formulate a hypothesis (induction). However, if they later devise a hypothesis for testing, they would be involved in deduction. So, the two are not mutually exclusive and it is easy to see how they may complement each other in mixed methods research designs.

In the past, qualitative research has been considered a soft science lacking in rigour and low status. It is rather ironic, therefore, that qualitative research has also been associated with feminist theories. Feminist theories have challenged traditional notions of research, highlighting their political nature. The term research 'participant' is preferred to that of research 'subject'. The methods preferred are those that render the relationship between researcher and participant more equal. Methods such as focus groups and in-depth interviews are preferred because of their ability to tap into the subjective experiences of participants. Within criminology, for example, a new approach emerged in the 1970s and 1980s known as 'feminist criminology'. This was largely attributed to the work of Smart (1977). There have been disagreements as to whether this really did comprise a new methodological approach (Gelsthorpe and Morris 1988), but what is clear is that it was a reaction against a traditional *male* or 'malestream' criminology that neglected, marginalised and stereotyped women.

The perception of qualitative research as unscientific was largely the result of a perceived inability to generalise from the specific to the general but also a lack of transparency with respect to how such research is conducted (Bryman and Burgess 1994). There was also the difficulty of being able to replicate research given the argument that it was overly subjective (Bryman 2008). Qualitative researchers found themselves under increased pressure to prove their worth (Seale 1999), especially in the pursuit of government funding.

Nevertheless, many writers have argued in defence of the approach and many solutions and justifications have been offered to counter this. The use of multiple researchers involved with the collection and analysis of data is said to increase inter-coder and inter-researcher validity. Grounded theory became an important analytic technique which made use of 'theoretical sampling' and employed systematic negative case analysis. The constant comparative method has also been advocated as a way of testing the general applicability of findings beyond the specific, for example in case study research (Flyvbjerg 2006).

In general, the status of qualitative research has grown in recent years as more and more practitioners have perceived its value to their practice. This is particularly true of health care settings where research and evaluation have become commonplace. Government pressure to conduct research, to evaluate practice and to listen to the consumer voice has been important in this development (Hansen 2006).

OBSERVATION

The technique of observation provides researchers with an opportunity to observe people, firsthand, in their natural surroundings. This is sometimes referred to as *naturalism* in contrast to positivism (Hammersley and Atkinson 2007). There are two types of observation: participant and non-participant. The latter is considered to be unobtrusive since the researcher observes from a distance and does not get involved. This method is particularly useful if you are interested in people's behaviour and interactions as opposed to their perceptions. The main problem with observational research is the fear that the presence of an observer may influence the behaviour of respondents in some way. This is known as the Hawthorne effect.[1] However, it is generally felt that the more time one spends with a group the less impact the researcher's presence will have upon them. That is, over time, the researcher is less likely to influence their behaviour.

There are different ways to conduct observational research, including the more structured variety whereby a researcher makes use of an observation schedule. Interestingly, while observational research quite clearly fits within the qualitative tradition, when a researcher employs an observation schedule, they are quite clearly engaged in a counting exercise. Hence, they are collecting data that is quantifiable. The purpose of a systematic observation schedule is to eliminate the possibility of researcher bias by making the data collection process more objective. What is observed is therefore dictated by the items included in the schedule. This is similar to when a researcher is engaged in a content analysis of secondary sources, for example newspaper reports. Great importance is placed upon what gets included in the schedule (Denscombe 2007). Once the data has been collected (observation) or the analysis has been completed (content analysis) it is very difficult to go back and start again if something important has been missed. Also, despite being *objective*, it is clear that subjectivity plays its part in what is selected for inclusion in the schedule.

Observation research can be time consuming but it is particularly useful if you are trying to understand the views of participants. Barker (1984) studied a sect for almost seven years in her attempt to understand recruitment to the Moonies. The method originates from anthropology and was adopted by sociologists of the early twentieth century who introduced terms such as 'field work' and 'field studies' (Hansen 2006). Observation and participant observation are used by researchers from a range of disciplines doing ethnographic research. The method is central to qualitative research and a number of studies exist in the area of health and social care (Leininger and McFarlane 2002; Grbich 2003). An interesting example is found in the work of Hughes (1989) which explored decision making by reception clerks working within a district general hospital. This was a traditional 'participant observation' study which explored the relationship between bureaucratic rules and decision making within a health care setting.

Studies highlight the difficulties involved in gaining acceptance from the group (Lofland and Lofland 1984), establishing and maintaining good field relations, the researcher's role and role conflict (Lawton 2001), and the recording of field notes (Fetterman 1998). There are examples whereby researchers have observed secretly, otherwise known as 'covert observation' (Humphreys 1970), itself a violation of the ethical principle of informed consent. It is hard to imagine anybody being given permission to conduct covert research within the current climate of ethics committees.

A strength of observation research is the recognition that there is a difference between what people say and what people do (Lambert and McKevitt 2002). This is not necessarily to imply that people are deceitful because in some instances they are simply at the mercy of poor memory recall. Whether this matters or not depends upon your research perspective because, obviously, if you are trying to get at the 'truth' the accuracy of such details is important. However, if you are interested in the account (the narrative or story) this is less important. The technique of observation provides researchers with in-depth, holistic accounts of situations as they happen *in situ* and are central to qualitative research. Researchers who conduct case studies within their own organisations will invariably employ observation of one kind or another.

MOMENT OF REFLECTION

Activity – Unobtrusive observation

Go to a public place such as a shopping precinct and spend a short time observing interactions between people. Can you observe any patterns in their interactions? Can you classify any of this behaviour? What do you notice about the way people negotiate space as they move around?

CASE STUDIES

The case study is highly appropriate to research in health and social care settings because of its association with small scale research. It involves the intensive study of a single case, whether this is an individual, an organisation or a setting. It is important at the outset of the study to identify the *unit of analysis*. Some argue that the case study is very much part of the qualitative tradition (*see* Creswell 2007) while others argue they can be used either quantitatively or qualitatively (Bryman 2008; Yin 1994, 2003). The defining feature of a case study is its focus upon 'complex social phenomenon' (Applebaum and Patton 2003) which provides a 'holistic' view.

Typically, a case study will utilise a range of different methods that suggest a natural 'fit' between the case study and mixed methods research. For example, Sidell (1995) researched the perspectives of the elderly in relation to health and illness. A range of methods were utilised including qualitative interviews and official statistics. To learn more about the case study approach consult the work of Yin (1994, 2003) who differentiates between descriptive, explanatory and exploratory case studies and is an authority on this approach. A good overview is also provided by the work of Gomm *et al.* (2000a).

The major criticism of this method is the argument that you cannot generalise from a single case (Lincoln and Guba 1985). However, Flyvbjerg (2006) drawing on the work of Stake (1995) and Ragin and Becker (1992) presents a very good argument for why the case study is equally important to the project of science. He argues that the distinction between quantitative and qualitative research is spurious and provides further support for research that is driven by problems rather than hegemony. The analogy is made between Popper's 'black swans'[2] and the case study. We need the case study (the black swans) to be able to falsify results. Indeed, negative case analysis is central to qualitative data analysis. The strength of large-scale research from which you can generalise – assuming probability sampling is used – is its breadth. In contrast, the case study offers depth and is the natural complement.

> Good social science is problem driven and not methodology driven in the sense that it employs those methods that for a given problematic, best help answer the research questions at hand.
>
> (Flyvbjerg 2006: 242)

Case study research is useful for those researching within their own organisations and for those engaged in small-scale research. It is a popular approach that has close connections with action and practitioner research.

ACTION RESEARCH

Action research – coined by Kurt Lewin in the 1930s – is basically an approach that emphasises research for *change*. It is very often associated with qualitative research but not necessarily so. Like evaluation research it is problem driven. The process of research is cyclical: *action–reflection–change–action–reflection*. It is particularly relevant to practitioners who are keen to develop and improve their practice, indeed it was first developed within the context of education.

> The key features of action research ... it is concerned with improvement; it is a cyclical, reflective process and it is a participative process.
>   (Kember 2000; Patton 1990 *cited in* Benson and Blackman 2003: 44)

Another name given to action research is practitioner research – when practitioners conduct research into their own practice – which is not the same as when the researcher is an 'outsider' (Edwards and Talbot 1999). Hockley and Froggatt (2006) conducted two action research projects that aimed at developing knowledge about end-of-life care for older people in care homes. This is an excellent example of action research within a health care setting. The researchers highlight its relevance in their reflections on the study.

Like case studies, data collection methods for the action researcher are varied but an important tool is the *reflective diary*. Different kinds of notes are recorded in a reflective diary, for example, what happened and when, how you responded, your emotions at the time and what you plan to do next. The diary therefore helps with both data collection and analysis. There are obvious similarities between the reflective diary and the recording of observation field notes. However, self reflection is central to action research, which is designed to bring about change and improvement to practice. This again is a technique that is highly suited to those researching within their own organisations, especially those subject to continuous change (Edwards and Talbot 1999).

Action research, like qualitative research more generally, is sometimes associated with feminist research. This is particularly true with respect to restoring the power imbalance between researchers and researched. There is less concern about the views of the researcher influencing the response of the participants because in actual fact your views as a researcher are an important part of the research. Dick (2004) provides a review of the scope of action research ranging from *appreciative inquiry* (AI) through to 'work based learning' and participatory research. A recent participatory action research (PAR) project was conducted by Van der Velde *et al.* (2009) which explored the mental health needs of immigrants and refugees.

DATA ANALYSIS TECHNIQUES

Grounded theory

Grounded theory, originally popularised by the seminal work of Glaser and Strauss (1967), is an inductive approach that requires researchers to rid themselves of any preconceptions and immerse themselves in the data. It has become 'the most widely used framework for analysing qualitative data' (Bryman 2008: 541). Borreani *et al.* (2004) conducted a review of a number of published medical journals and discovered that grounded theory was the most frequently used methodological approach. Within health and social care, a grounded theory approach offers a number of attractions:

1   The emphasis upon the views of those being studied.
2   The clearly articulated framework for 'how to' do grounded theory.
3   Their inductive nature which is thought to render them apolitical.

(Hansen 2006: 64)

The basic idea is that the theory emerges from the data and therefore remains *true* to the data. It is characterised by 'theoretical sampling' and 'theoretical saturation'.

> Almost like a detective, the researcher follows a trail of clues. As each clue is followed up it points the research in a particular direction and throws up new questions that need to be answered. Sometimes the clues can lead the researcher up blind alleys. Ultimately, though, the researcher should pursue his or her investigation until the questions have been answered and things can be explained.
>
> (Denscombe 2007: 25)

Grounded theory was originally developed by Glaser and Strauss (1967), who could not agree. Glaser (1992) went on to criticise Strauss (1987) and Strauss and Corbin (1990, 2008) for advocating an overly prescriptive approach. Strauss and Corbin (1990, 2008) developed a systematic approach introducing the notion of 'theoretical sampling' and the constant comparative method (whereby data is compared with emerging categories). More recently, Charmaz (2006) has developed a social *constructivist* approach to grounded theory. Creswell (2007) argues in favour of the interpretive approach of Strauss and Corbin (1990, 2008) especially for the novice researcher because of its systematic nature. Bryman (2008) argues that the term grounded theory is sometimes treated as synonymous with induction but this is incorrect. However, it is important to be aware of the different approaches to grounded theory. Data analysis is characterised by the interlinking of codes and higher level categories: open coding (breaking the data into units), axial coding (deducing relationships between categories) and selective coding (the integration of categories to produce a theory).

It is not simply about 'describing', it is about 'analysing', understanding, interpreting and ultimately generating theory. The data does not simply 'speak for itself' or 'tell a story' as in the narrative approach of phenomenology. Analysis is iterative (repeated cyclically) being refined in each cycle. This continues until 'theoretical saturation' is reached. The main criticism of this approach is that it fragments the data and the question is asked about how researchers know when they have reached theoretical saturation. However, in its favour it tries to minimise the effect of researcher preconceptions.

Narrative

Those who favour the analysis of textual data using a narrative approach are more interested in the 'story' as opposed to establishing the truth. The focus is upon the way that people represent themselves through narrative (Silverman 2006). The approach therefore has close connections with discourse and conversation analysis and is informed by social constructivism as opposed to positivism. Different types of data can be suited to narrative analysis, for example life and oral histories (Plummer 2001). See the work of Silverman for an account of more structuralist approaches.

Content Analysis

Content analysis is firmly rooted within the quantitative tradition although depending upon the perspective of the researcher it can be used more qualitatively. It can be applied to various kinds of 'documents' such as text, film, TV or radio. It can also be applied to primary or secondary data. Two defining features of this technique are the importance of being 'objective' and 'systematic'.

> Content analysis is an approach to the analysis of documents and texts that seeks to quantify content in terms of predetermined categories and in a systematic and replicable manner.
>
> (Bryman 2008: 275)

It should be noted that it can be rather time consuming. Essentially the researcher is involved in a process of 'counting'. A set of *categories* is devised and the researcher counts the number of instances that fall into each category. The researcher therefore requires both a coding schedule and a coding manual. The categories need to be precise to enable different researchers to arrive at the same results and this establishes inter-coder reliability. It is therefore considered to be a reliable and valid measure. In practice, therefore, a researcher needs to go through a number of steps beginning with clarifying and narrowing the hypothesis. A checklist is produced to identify the variables and to aid the counting process. The unit of analysis is very important because the researcher needs to identify the boundaries of the analysis. If you were conducting a content analysis of newspaper articles over a ten year period for example, you might be comparing the number of times that a particular phrase is used in one paper compared to another. Within the context of health and social care a recent study by Pastrana *et al.* (2008) used discourse analysis to explore definitions of palliative care. The study highlighted the importance of semantic and ethical differences to understanding the concept. A more qualitative study which also used content analysis, explored difficulties faced by residents in training within a hospital setting and the delivery of 'end of life care' (Luthy *et al.* 2009).

The main advantages of this technique are that it is unobtrusive (hence, non-reactive) and useful for historical comparisons. However, it is criticised for being simplistic and it is not very good at answering the why questions. An approach that tries to overcome this simplicity is semiotic analysis, which tries to get at the underlying message of the text and to distinguish between 'surface' and 'deeper' meaning.

Quantitative Analysis

The strength of quantitative analysis lies in the breadth of the data, rather than the depth, and the ability to generalise beyond those studied to a wider population. While planning is vital to the successful completion of any research project, this takes on particular importance when engaged in the collection and subsequent analysis of quantitative data. Levels of measurement of variables studied will determine what you can and cannot do with the data. It is important to understand the difference between variables which are *nominal, ordinal, interval/ratio*. This is because some techniques of analysis are suitable to variables at the highest level of measurement (interval/ratio) but not to those at the lowest (nominal). Therefore, if you want to measure statistical association between two or more variables but fail to ask these questions at the correct level of measurement, you may find yourself stuck. If only you had asked the question in a different way!

When conducting qualitative research it is quite usual for the research to evolve over time and even change direction. As new questions emerge the research can take a different direction. There is a dialectical interplay between data collection and analysis. Early findings and preliminary analyses may determine what to ask/explore next; this is particularly true of 'theoretical sampling'. In a quantitative research design, however, the stages of data collection and analysis are more clearly demarcated. Data analysis does not start until all the data has been collected. Levels of measurement determine what you can and cannot do with your data and it is essential to get this right at the start. A useful explanation of this approach and some of the common terms is provided by Rugg (2007) or Davies (2007).

In general, data analysis will take the form of numbers and percentages, frequency and cross-tabulation tables. It is important when reading tables that you understand the difference between valid and cumulative per cents. Generally, researchers will want to employ statistical tests to measure the statistical significance of findings. When reading published research, you will find numerous references to *p values*. It is important to have a basic understanding of statistical significance and *p values* without necessarily being a master of all statistical tests. All statistical tests rest on the theory of probability.

Whether measuring difference or association, all statistical tests are using the theory of probability to deduce how likely it is that these findings could have arisen by chance. The less likely it is that your findings have arisen by chance, the greater confidence you can have in your findings. Researchers talk of confidence intervals. A *p value* which is less than 0.05, for example, means we can be 95 per cent confident that only five times in a hundred (or 1 in 20) could these findings have arisen by chance. We can never be 100 per cent certain. There is always the possibility that our findings could be the result of some chance occurrence or the result of sampling error.

ETHICS

When planning *any* type of research we need to pay particular attention to ethical issues. Ethics should inform decisions made about every aspect of the research from start to finish. It is important to be aware of professional bodies providing guidance within our academic discipline(s), but also current legislation, for example, data protection and intellectual property law. It is also important to be aware of the European Union Directive (2004) which means that all research involving the NHS must be awarded ethical approval by an ethics committee. Moreover, these ethics committees are now answerable to strategic health authorities in England and to the Central Office of Research Ethics Committees (COREC). These are now enshrined in law. The application process has now been merged with the National Research Ethics Service (http://www.nres.npsa.nhs.uk). Similarly, the Research Governance Framework for health and social care defines the broad principles of good research governance and is key to ensuring that health and social care research is conducted to high scientific and ethical standards.

There is a vast literature on ethics and social research and debates exist between those who take a 'deontological' perspective (moral absolutism) and those who take a 'utilitarian' perspective (cost/benefit). Some argue against the use of 'ethics codes' (Douglas 1976) while others argue that 'codes' are too general to be practically helpful (Punch 2005). A useful overview is provided by Gomm (2008) which includes information about the ethicality of randomised controlled trials. Within the field of qualitative research, ethics has been written about in depth and takes on particular importance because of the length of time that researchers spend with participants. There are debates in particular about the nature of research with children and young people (Mishna *et al.* 2004; Alderson 2004). What ethical issues arise when conducting research with children and are they different? Much of the debate centres on the vulnerability of children and the differential power relations between adults and children. Mishna *et al.* (2004) argue this has particular importance when the research involves more qualitative techniques such as interviewing as opposed to a standard questionnaire.

There is also a need to pay particular attention to research that takes place online. A good introduction to qualitative research on the internet is by Mann and Stewart (2002). The question is asked to what extent computer mediated communication (CMC) engenders 'new' ethical principles. Is a 'new' set of ethics required or are the ethical considerations the same? In fact, the British Psychological Society has recently devised a separate set of guidelines for its members doing research online (http://www.bps.org.uk/the-society/code-of-conduct/code-of-conduct_home.cfm).

The ethical and legal context of online research is discussed in a recent edited collection by Fielding *et al.* (2008). It is worth noting that online research comes in many shapes and forms, from 'internet surveys' to 'virtual ethnography' (Hine 2000) and the analysis of archival data.

Gaiser and Schreiner (2009) offer guidance on designing, analysing and presenting online research. An issue that arises again and again is the blurring of the boundaries between the 'private' and the 'public' domain. Does textual data in a chat room or discussion group constitute publicly available or private data? Some argue that it depends upon the views of the participants (Mann and Stewart 2002). If textual data is obtained online and findings are published, will it be possible to trace the original postings using a search engine? Online research raises a number of new questions that have not yet been successfully tackled. It is important to weigh up all of the arguments for and against using online research and how you would approach this before embarking on a study. It is also important as a consumer of research to be aware of these debates for your own critical analyses.

It is important to be aware of research ethics that apply to both the online and offline world and also to be aware of the nature of research ethics as they impact upon both quantitative and qualitative research. The following is a brief overview of some of the key issues.

THE KEY PRINCIPLES

1   Informed consent (voluntary informed consent).
2   Right to privacy.
3   Anonymity and confidentiality.
4   Right to withdraw.
5   Covert research.
6   Protection from harm.
7   Obligations to sponsors/funders.

Have a look at the following ethical guidelines and explore these 'key principles':

- British Psychological Society
  http://www.bps.org.uk/the-society/code-of-conduct/code-of-conduct_home.cfm

- British Society of Criminology
  http://britsoccrim.org/ethical.htm

- British Sociological Association
  http://www.britsoc.co.uk/NR/rdonlyres/468F236C-FFD9-4791-A0BD-4DF73F10BA43/0/StatementofEthicalPractice.doc

- Medical Research Council
  http://www.mrc.ac.uk/Ourresearch/Ethicsresearchguidance/index.htm

- National Patient Safety Agency: National Research Ethics Service (NHS)
  http://www.nres.npsa.nhs.uk/

- Royal Statistical Society
  http://www.rss.org.uk/main.asp?page=1875

ETHICAL CONCERNS IN RELATION TO METHOD

Survey research

The main issues of survey research to consider are:

- Do participants have the right to withdraw?
- Are respondents given the chance to opt out of particular questions?
- How is debriefing provided?
- Is 'informed consent' truly informed?
- It is important to avoid coercion although inducements to take part are sometimes used.
- It is important not to breach anonymity and confidentiality. Do not make promises you cannot keep.
- How will data be stored? Will it be digital? Who will have access to it? Will pseudonyms be used to protect identities?
- These issues need to be addressed with online research and may reveal different solutions.

Experimental research

Will the aims and objectives of the research be explained to respondents before the research begins? This is essential to the process of obtaining 'informed consent'. Deception is most common in this type of research and sometimes 'informed consent' is sought later. However, this would need to be built into the application for ethical approval.

Interviews

- What consideration is given to respondents being harmed by the research?
- What support is offered? Are respondents aware that they can refuse to answer questions or can terminate the interview at any time?
- It is important not to take advantage of the respondents' generosity – do not assume you can overrun with the interview – agree a time and stick to it.
- Be respectful! Assuming that the research is taking place face to face, what are the safety issues for the respondent and the researcher to consider?

Fieldwork

Typically the researcher spends a long time with participants. In such instances, informed consent is not a once and for all event. Over time, people may come and go. It is important that consent is renegotiated as the research progresses, especially if the research changes direction. This is an important difference between quantitative and qualitative research. It is vital for both the sake of the research and the respondents that the researcher acts with integrity at all times and respects participants. If the researcher fails to do so, trust is broken and this can damage the quality of the data and also the reputation of the organisation to which you belong.

An important distinction is made between 'procedural ethics' and 'ethically important moments' in research (Guillemin and Gillam 2004). These are the difficult and unpredictable moments with ethical and legal implications that arise in the practice of doing research. It is a good idea when planning research to brainstorm and try to anticipate potential problems that could emerge.

RESEARCH IN A HEALTH AND SOCIAL CARE SETTING

Increasingly, health and social care workers are involved in practice based research (Hek and Moule 2006). Whether they are directly responsible for research, or not, they need to be aware of research ethics. Ethics are not simply a matter of 'filling in a form', getting it past an ethics committee and then forgetting all about it. Ethics are important to each and every stage of the research process, from choosing a topic, right through to analysis and reporting of research findings. It is not acceptable to conduct research that is poorly designed or shoddy, in the same way that it is not acceptable to publish research which is flawed. Doyal (2005) identified that the large volume of student research projects within the health care system was putting large numbers of patients under unnecessary pressure. The justification for this was questioned. In the majority of cases it was found that the research was designed to aid student understanding rather than contribute to the stock of knowledge. It was argued, therefore, that the principles underlying the Declaration of Helsinki (based upon prioritising the rights of the participants over and above the needs of the research) should apply equally to student projects as to professional researchers. This has made primary research by students increasingly difficult.

Furthermore, Oliver (2003) argues that research participants within a health and social care context are particularly vulnerable because of the circumstances of their lives:

> The essential ethical dilemma is whether it is morally acceptable to approach people who are ill or who are living in adverse circumstances, and ask them to help with a research programme.
>
> (Oliver 2003: 110–11)

Within a health and social care context, therefore, researchers need to be extremely sensitive to ethics and ensure that research is designed appropriately. Always think about the needs of your respondents over and above the needs of your research and try to brainstorm potential difficulties (Grbich 2003).

MOMENT FOR REFLECTION

Activity – Ethics

Explore the key ethical principles identified above and look at a set of ethical guidelines, for example, from the British Criminological Society. Next, find a published research paper within the same discipline and read this closely. How well are ethical issues explained? Are there any particular problems and how are they overcome?

NOTES

1 Experiments which took place at the Hawthorne Plant of factory workers found that productivity increased no matter what changes were made to the factory workers' conditions. This was explained by the fact that those observed reacted to employers' taking an interest in them.

2 Popper (1959) talked about black swans as examples of phenomenon which help to disprove a theory. A theory may hold true until we find such a negative instance. In terms of the nature of knowledge, truth can never be certain. All knowledge is provisional. If we believe that 'all swans are white' once we come across a black swan the theory no longer holds true.

REFERENCES

Alderson, P. (2004) 'Ethics', in Fraser, S. (Ed.) *Doing Research with Children and Young People*, London: Sage, pp. 97–112.

Ammenwerth, E., Iller, C. and Mansmann, U. (2003) Can Evaluation Studies Benefit from Triangulation? A Case Study, *International Journal of Medical Informatics*, 70 (2–3), 237–48 [online]. Available at: http://www.sciencedirect.com/science/journal/13865056 (Accessed 9 April 2009).

Applebaum, S. and Patton, E. (2003) The Case for Case Studies in Management Research, *Management Research News*, 26 (5), 60–71 [online]. Available at: http://www.emeraldinsight.com/10.1108/01409170310783484 (Accessed 10 April 2009).

Aveyard, H. (2008) *Doing a Literature Review in Health and Social Care*, Maidenhead: Open University Press.

Barker, E. (1984) *The Making of a Moonie: Choice or Brainwashing?*, Oxford: Blackwell.

Bateman, T. and Pitts, J. (2005) 'Conclusion: What the Evidence Tells Us', in Bateman, T. and Pitts, J. (Eds) *The RHP Companion to Youth Justice*, Lyme Regis: Russell House.

Beharrell, P. (1993) 'Aids and the British Press', in Eldridge, J. (Ed.) *Getting the Message: News, Truth and Power*, Glasgow University Media Group, London: Routledge, pp. 210–52.

Bell, J. (1997) *Doing Your Research Project: A Guide for First-Time Researchers in Education and Social Science*, Buckingham: Open University Press.

Benson, A. and Blackman, D. (2003) Can Research Methods ever be Interesting?, *Active Learning in Higher Education*, 4 (1), 39–55. DOI: 10.1177/1469787403004001004.

Booth, S., Booth, A. and Falzon, L. (2003) The Need for Information and Research Skills Training to Support Evidence-Based Social Care: A Literature Review and Survey, *Learning in Health and Social Care*, 2 (4), 191–201.

Borreani, C., Miccinesi, G., Brunelli, C. and Lina, M. (2004) An Increasing Number of Qualitative Research Papers in Oncology and Palliative Care: Does it Mean a Thorough Development of the Methodology of Research?, *Health and Quality of Life Outcomes*, 2 (1), 7. DOI: 10.1186/1477-7525-2-7.

Bowling, A. (2007) *Research Methods in Health: Investigating Health and Health Services*, 2nd edition, Berkshire: Open University Press.

Boynton, P. (2004) Selecting, Designing and Developing Your Questionnaire, *British Medical Journal*, 328 (7451), 1312–15. DOI: 10.1136/bmj.328.7451.1312.

Bradburn, N., Sudman, S. and Wansink, B. (2004) *Asking Questions: The Definitive Guide to Questionnaire Design, for Market Research, Political Polls, and Social and Health Questionnaires (research methods for the social sciences)*, Chichester: John Wiley.

British Psychological Society (2007) *Conducting Research on the Internet: Guidelines for Ethical Practice in Psychological Research Online* [online]. Available at: http://www.bps.org.uk/the-society/code-of-conduct/code-of-conduct_home.cfm (Accessed 15 March 2009).

Bryman, A. (2008) *Social Research Methods*, 3rd edition, New York: Oxford University Press.

Bryman, A. and Burgess, B. (1994) *Analyzing Qualitative Data*, London: Routledge.

Burger, J. (2009) Replicating Milgram: Would People Still Obey Today? *American Psychologist* 64 (1), 1–11. DOI: 10.1037/a0010932.

Burke Johnson, R. and Onwuegbuzie, A. (2004) Mixed Methods Research: A Research Paradigm Whose Time has Come, *Educational Researcher*, 33 (7), 14–26. DOI: 10.3102/0013189X033007014.

Burke Johnson, R., Onwuegbuzie, A. and Turner, L. (2007) Toward a Definition of Mixed Methods Research, *Journal of Mixed Methods Research*, (April 2007), 1 (2), 112–33. DOI: 10.1177/1558689806298224.

Burr (1988) Contextualizing Critical Care Family Needs through Triangulation: an Australian Study, *Intensive and Critical Care Nursing*, 14 (4), 161–9. DOI: 10.1016/S0964-3397(98)80473-4.

Caracelli, V. and Greene, J. (1993) Data Analysis Strategies for Mixed Methods Evaluation Designs, *Educational Evaluation and Policy Analysis*, (Summer 1993), 15, 195–207 [online]. Available at: http://www.jstor.org/stable/1164421 (Accessed 12 May 2009).

Charmaz, K. (2006) *Constructing Grounded Theory: a Practical Guide through Qualitative Analysis*, London: Sage.

Creswell, J. (2003) *Research Design: Qualitative, Quantitative, and Mixed Methods Approaches*, 2nd edition, London: Sage.

Creswell, J. (2007) *Qualitative Inquiry and Research Design: Choosing among Five Traditions*, 2nd edition, London: Sage.

Davies, H., Nutley, S. and Smith, P. (Eds) (2000) *What Works? Evidence-Based Policy and Practice in Public Services*, Bristol: The Policy Press.

Davies, M. (2007) *Doing a Successful Research Project: using Qualitative or Quantitative Methods*, Basingstoke: Palgrave Macmillan.

Denscombe, M. (2007) *The Good Research Guide for Small-Scale Social Research Projects*, 3rd edition, Maidenhead: Open University Press.

Denzin, N. (1989) *The Research Act: a Theoretical Introduction to Sociological Methods*, 3rd edition, London: Prentice Hall International.

Department of Health (2005) *Research Governance Framework for Health and Social Care*, 2nd edition, London: HMSO.

Department of Health (2001) *Research Governance Framework for Health and Social Care*, 2nd edition, London: HMSO.

Dick, B. (2004) Action Research Literature: Themes and trends, *Action Research*, 2 (4), 425–44. DOI: 10.1177/1476750304047985.

Douglas, J. (1976) *Investigative Social Research: Individual and Team Field Research*, Beverly Hills, CA: Sage Publications.

Doyal (2005) *The Ethical Governance and Regulation of Student Projects: A Proposal Working Group on Ethical Review of Student Research in the NHS* [online]. Available at: http://www.dh.gov.uk/prod_consum_dh/groups/dh_digitalassets/@dh/@en/documents/digitalasset/dh_4120898.pdf (Accessed 18 May 2009).

Edwards, A. and Talbot, R. (1999) *The Hard-Pressed Researcher*, 2nd edition, London: Longman.

Ferguson, H. (2003) Outline of a Critical Best Practice Perspective on Social Work and Social Care, *British Journal of Social Work*, 33, 1005–24.

Fetterman (1998) *Ethnography: Step by Step*, 2nd edition, London: Sage.

Fielding, N., Lee, R. and Blank, G. (Eds) (2008) *The Sage Handbook of Online Research Methods*, London: Sage.

Fink, A. (2006) *How to Conduct Surveys: A Step-by-Step Guide*, 3rd edition, Thousand Oaks, CA: Sage.

Fink, A. (2005) *Conducting Research Literature Reviews: from the Internet to Paper*, Thousand Oaks, CA: Sage.

Flyvbjerg, B. (2006) Five Misunderstandings about Case-Study Research, *Qualitative Inquiry*, 12 (2), 219–45. DOI: 10.1177/1077800405284363.

Gaiser, T. and Schreiner, T. (2009) *A Guide to Conducting Online Research*, London: Sage.

Gelsthorpe, L. and Morris, A. (1988) Feminism and Criminology in Britain, *British Journal of Criminology*, Spring 1988, 28 (2), 93–110.

Glaser, B. (1992) *Basics of Grounded Theory Analysis: Emergence vs Forcing*, Mill Valley, CA: Sociology Press.

Glaser, B. and Strauss, A. (1967) *Discovery of Grounded Theory: Strategies for Qualitative Research*, New York: Aldine Publishing.

Glasziou, P., Irwig, L., Bain, C. and Colditz, G. (2001) *Systematic Reviews in Health Care: A Practical Guide*, Cambridge: Cambridge University Press.

Gleeson, R., Forde, E., Bates, E., Powell, S., Eadon-Jones, E. and Draper, H. (2008) Medical Students' Attitudes Towards Abortion: a UK Study, *Journal of Medical Ethics*, 34, 783–7. DOI:10.1136/jme.2007.023416.

Gomm, R. (2008) *Social Research Methodology: A Critical Introduction*, 2nd edition, Basingstoke: Palgrave Macmillan.

Gomm, R., Hammersley, M., and Foster, P. (Eds) (2000a) *Case study method: key issues, key texts*, London: Sage.

Gomm, R., Needham, G., and Bullman, A. (Eds) (2000b) *Evaluating Research in Health and Social Care: A Reader*, London: Sage.

Gray, D. (2004) *Doing Research in the Real World*, London: Sage.

Gray, M. and Mcdonald, C. (2006) Pursuing Good Practice? The Limits of Evidence-based Practice, *Journal of Social Work*, 6 (1), 7–20.

Grady, K. and Wallston, B. (1988) *Research in Health Care Settings*, London: Sage.

Greene, J., (2008) Is Mixed Methods Social Inquiry a Distinctive Methodology?, *Journal of Mixed Methods Research*, January 2008, 2 (7), 7–22. DOI: 10.1177/1558689807309969.

Grbich, C. (2003) *Qualitative Research in Health: An Introduction*, London: Sage.

Guillemin, M. and Gillam, L. (2004) Ethics, Reflexivity, and 'Ethically Important Moments' in Research, *Qualitative Inquiry*, April 2004, 10 (2), 261–80. DOI: 10.1177/1077800403262360.

Hammersley, M. and Atkinson, P. (2007) *Ethnography: Principles in Practice*, 3rd edition, New York: Routledge.

Hansen, E. (2006) *Successful Qualitative Health Research: A Practical Introduction*, McGraw Hill: Open University Press.

Hek, G. and Moule, P. (2006) *Making Sense of Research: An Introduction for Health and Social Care Practitioners*, 3rd edition, London: Sage.

Hine, C. (2000) *Virtual Ethnography*, London: Sage.

Hockley, J. and Froggatt, K. (2006) The Development of Palliative Care Knowledge in Care Homes for Older People, *Palliative Medicine*, 20 (8), 835–43. DOI: 10.1177/0269216306073111.

Homan, R. (1991) *The Ethics of Social Research*, London: Longman.

Hopkins-Burke, R. (2008) *Young People, Crime and Justice*, Devon: Willan.

Hughes, D. (1989) Paper and people: the work of the casualty reception clerk, *Sociology of Health and Illness*, 11 (4), 382–408.

Humphreys (1970) *Tearoom trade: A Study of Homosexual Encounters in Public Places*, London: Duckworth.

Kelle, U. and Erzberger, C. (2004) 'Qualitative and Quantitative Methods: Not in Opposition', in Flick, U., Von Kardoff, E. and Steinke, I. (Eds) *A Companion to Qualitative Research*, London: Sage, pp. 172–7.

Kember, D. (2000) *Action Learning and Action Research: Improving the Quality of Teaching and Learning*, London: Kogan Page.

Kimchi, J., Polivka, B. and Stevenson, J. (1991) Triangulation: Operational Definitions, *Nursing Research*, 40 (6), 364–66.

Lambert, H. and McKevitt, C. (2002) Anthropology in Health Research: From Qualitative Methods to Multidisciplinarity, *British Medical Journal*, July 2002, 325, 210–13. DOI: 10.1136/bmj.325.7357.210.

Lawton, J. (2001) Gaining and Maintaining Consent: Ethical Concerns Raised in a Study of Dying Patients, *Qualitative Health Research*, September 2001, 11 (5): 693–705. DOI: 10.1177/104973201129119389.

Leininger, M. and McFarlane, M. (2002) *Transcultural Nursing: Concepts, Theories, Research and Practice,* 3rd edition, New York: McGraw Hill.

Lincoln, Y. and Guba, E. (1985) *Naturalistic Enquiry*, Newbury Park, CA: Sage.

Lofland, J. and Lofland, L. (1984) *Analyzing Social Settings: A Guide to Qualitative Observation and Analysis*, 2nd edition, Belmont: Wadsworth Publishing.

Luthy, C., Cedraschi, C., Pautex, S., Piguet, V. and Allaz, A. (2009) Difficulties of Residents in Training in End-of-Life Care: A Qualitative Study, *Palliative Medicine*, January 2009, 23 (1), 59–65.

Mann, C. and Stewart, F. (2002) *Internet Communication and Qualitative Research: A Handbook for Researching Online*, Sage: London.

Milgram, S. (1974) *Obedience to Authority: An Experimental View*, London: Tavistock.

Mishna, F., Antle, B. and Regehr, C. (2004) Tapping the Perspectives of Children: Emerging Ethical Issues in Qualitative Research, *Qualitative Social Work*, 3 (4), 449–68.

Moser, C. and Kalton, G. (2001) *Survey Methods in Social Investigation*, Aldershot: Ashgate.

Moule (2005) *E-learning for Healthcare Students: Developing the Communities of Practice Framework*. EdD thesis, Bristol: University of the West of England.

Nicolson, P., Burr, J. and Powell, J. (2005) Becoming an Advanced Practitioner in Neonatal Nursing: A Psycho-Social Study of the Relationship Between Education Preparation and Role Development, *Journal of Clinical Nursing*, July 2005, 14 (6), 727–38. DOI: 10.1111/j.1365-2702.2005.01137.x.

Oliver, P. (2003) *The Student's Guide to Research Ethics*, Berkshire: Open University Press.

Onwuegbuzie, A. and Leech, N. (2004) *On Becoming a Pragmatic Researcher: The Importance of Combining Quantitative and Qualitative Research Methodologies*, Manuscript submitted for publication.

Oppenheim, A.N. (2001) *Questionaire Design and Attitude Measurement*. London: Continuum.

Pastrana, T., Jünger, S., Ostgathe, C., Elsner, F. and Radbruch, L. (2008) A Matter of Definition – Key Elements Identified in a Discourse Analysis of Definitions of Palliative Care, *Palliative Medicine*, April 2008), 22 (3), 222–32.

Patton, M. (1990) *Qualitative Evaluation and Research Methods*, London: Sage.

Pawson, R. and Tilley, N. (1997) *Realistic Evaluation*, London: Sage.

Pawson, R. and Tilley, N. (1994) What Works in Evaluation Research?, *British Journal of Criminology*, Summer 1994, 34 (3), 291–306.

Plummer, K. (2001) *Documents of Life 2: An Invitation to a Critical Humanism*, 2nd edition, London: Sage.

Popper, K. (1959) *The Logic of Scientific Discovery*, London: Hutchinson.

Procter (1994) Analyzing Survey Data in Gilbert (Ed.) *Researching Social Life*, London: Sage.

Punch, K. (2006) *Developing Effective Research Proposals*, 2nd edition, London: Sage.

Punch, K. (2005) *Introduction to Social Research: Quantitative and Qualitative Approaches*, London: Sage.

Ragin, C. and Becker, H. (Eds) (1992) *What is a Case? Exploring the Foundations of Social Inquiry*, Cambridge: Cambridge University Press.

Rapport, F. (Ed.) (2004) *New Qualitative Methodologies in Health and Social Care Research*, London: Routledge.

Rosen, A., Proctor, E. and Staudt, M. (1999) Social Work Research and the Quest for Effective Practice, *Social Work Research*, 23 (1), 4–14.

Rugg, (2007) *Using Statistics: A Gentle Introduction*, McGraw Hill: Open University Press.

Saks, M. and Allsop, J. (2007) *Researching Health: Qualitative, Quantitative and Mixed Methods,* London: Sage.

Seale, C. (1999) Quality in Qualitative Research, *Qualitative Inquiry*, December 1999, 5 (4), 465–78. DOI: 10.1177/107780049900500402.

Shaw, I. (2000) Research in Social Work, in Davies, M. (Ed.) *Blackwell Encyclopaedia of Social Work*, Oxford: Oxford University Press.

Sheldon, B. (2000) Cognitive Behavioural Methods in Social Care: A Look at the Evidence, in Stepney, P. and Ford, D. (Eds) *Social Work Models, Methods and Theories*, Lyme Regis: Russell House, pp. 65–83.

Sibbald, B. and Roland, M. (1998) Why are Randomised Controlled Trials Important?, *British Medical Journal*, 17 January 1998, 316 (7126), p. 201 [online]. Available online: http://www.bmj.com/cgi/content/full/316/7126/201 (Accessed 21 February 2009).

Sidell, M. (1995) *Health in Old Age*, Buckingham: Open University Press.

Silverman, D. (2006) *Interpreting Qualitative Data: Methods for Analyzing Talk, Text and Interaction*, 3rd edition, London: Sage.

Smart, C. (1977) *Women, Crime and Criminology*, London: Routledge and Kegan Paul.

Stake, R. (1995), *The Art of Case Study Research*, London: Sage.

Strauss, A. (1987) *Qualitative Analysis for Social Scientists*, Cambridge: Cambridge University Press.

Strauss, A. and Corbin, J. (2008) *Basics of Qualitative Research: Techniques and Procedures for Developing Grounded Theory*, 3rd edition, London: Sage.

Tashakkori, A. and Creswell, J. (2007) Editorial: The New Era of Mixed Methods, *Journal of Mixed Methods Research*, January 2007, 1 (1), 3–7. DOI: 10.1177/2345678906293042.

Tashakkori, A. and Teddlie, C. (Eds.) (2003) *Handbook of Mixed Methods in the Social and Behavioural Sciences*, Thousand Oaks, CA: Sage.

Trevithick, P. (2005) *Social Work Skills: A Practice Handbook* (2nd edition), Berkshire: Open University Press.

Trinder, L. (2000a) Introduction: The Context of Evidence-based Practice, in Trinder, L. and Edwards, S. (Eds) *Evidence-based Practice: A Critical Appraisal*, Oxford: Blackwell Science, pp. 1–16.

Trinder, L. (2000b) Evidence-based Practice in Social Work and Probation, in Trinder, L. and Edwards, S. (Eds) *Evidence-based Practice: A Critical Appraisal*, Oxford: Blackwell Science, pp. 138–62.

Trinder, L. and Reynolds, S. (Eds) (2000) *Evidence-Based Practice: A Critical Appraisal*, Oxford: Blackwell Science.

Van der Velde, J., Williamson, D. and Ogilvie, L. (2009) Participatory Action Research: Practical Strategies for Actively Engaging and Maintaining, *Health Research*, 19 (9), 1293–302, DOI: 10.1177/1049732309344207.

Walker, W. (2005) The Strengths and Weaknesses of Research Designs Involving Quantitative Measures, *Journal of Research in Nursing*, 10 (5), 571–82. DOI: 10.1177/13614 0960501000505.

Webb, S. (2001) Some Considerations on the Validity of Evidence-based Practice in Social Work, *British Journal of Social Work*, 31 (1), 57–79.

Williams, D. and Garner, A. (2002) The Case Against 'the Evidence': A Different Perspective on Evidence Based Medicine, *British Journal of Psychiatry*, 180 (1), 8–12 [online]. Available at: http://bjp.rcpsych.org/cgi/content/full/180/1/8 (Accessed 17 April 2009).

Yin, R. (2003) *Case Study Research: Design and Methods*, 3rd edition, London: Sage.

Yin, R. (1994) *Case Study Research: Design and Methods*, 2nd edition, London: Sage.

CHAPTER 11

INTRODUCTION TO THE CRIMINAL JUSTICE SYSTEM

PHILIP HODGSON

OBJECTIVES

After reading this chapter you should be able to:

▪ Identify the origins of and current debates concerning the police, the national offender management service [the prison and probation services] and other relevant organisations dealing with crime.

▪ Introduce a range of contemporary issues influencing policy and practice in dealing with specific groups of offender and specific types of offence.

▪ Understand the origins of the modern police, prison and probation services and the climate and contexts in which they currently operate.

After reading this chapter you will know the meaning of the following terms:
The police, prosecution, courts, probation, prison, multi-agency working, victims.

INTRODUCTION

Before a person enters the criminal justice system they will have committed or be suspected of committing a criminal offence. Whilst common sense suggests that we all know what constitutes a crime, like many other common sense assumptions, this is not entirely true (Hodgson and Webb 2005), as actually defining what is a crime can present a host of dilemmas. Definitions of crime can be socially constructed, politically motivated, ever changing and differ from country to country. Consequently an act itself is not a crime until it has been defined as being so. For example, prior to 31 January 1983 it was acceptable to ride in the front seat of a car in England or Wales without wearing a seat belt. Since that date it has been an offence to do so.

Whilst there are a number of issues to consider when attempting to define crime, an oft cited legalistic definition suggests that an act is a crime when it, 'is capable of being followed by criminal proceedings, having one of the types of outcome (for example, punishment), known to follow these proceedings' (Williams 1955: 123). Thus, hitting an opponent and breaking their rib during a boxing match would not be considered a crime as it is not capable of being followed by criminal proceedings. Conversely, punching an individual in a nightclub which leaves the victim with a broken rib would be considered a crime as criminal proceedings could follow resulting in the perpetrator being punished.

Having established that it is not a straightforward task to define what a crime actually is, it is equally difficult to assess levels of crime not least because a large percentage of crimes are not reported to the police. As official crime statistics rely on police recorded crime data, such statistics therefore only offer a limited overview of actual crime levels. Since 2005, in response to the limitations of official data and to assess the 'Hidden figure of crime' (that is crime that goes unreported), official publications such as *Crime in England and Wales* now offer both police recorded statistics and data derived from the British Crime Survey (BCS) (which is an annual victimisation survey reporting on people's experiences of crime the previous year). The difference between police recorded statistics and British Crime Survey data can be dramatic. For example, in 1981, when the first British Crime Survey of England and Wales was conducted less than three million crimes had been recorded by the police whereas through their victimisation survey the BCS estimated that during the same period 11 million crimes had been committed. Whilst there are a number of reasons for this under-reporting (for example the victim considers the matter too trivial or believes that the police will be uninterested/unable to do anything), when studying criminology and reviewing crime statistics it is worthwhile comparing and contrasting both data sources to assess levels of crime.[1]

The remainder of this chapter will focus upon the agencies that comprise the criminal justice system. However, a point to note prior to discussing the criminal justice system is that the 'system' is actually a collective of autonomous and semi-autonomous agencies operating within an interconnected process and each of the individual agencies that comprise the system have their own principles and core responsibilities. As such, Ashworth and Redmayne (2005: 67) suggest that it is impossible to formulate one meaningful aim that would be relevant to each stage of the criminal justice system but that it is possible to offer a cluster of aims which are relevant to all agencies, such as preventing crime, treating suspects fairly, having respect for victims and supporting the efficient and effective delivery of justice. Responsibility for the criminal justice system falls across three main government departments – those of the Ministry of Justice, the Home Office and the Attorney General's Office.[2]

THE POLICE

Most people's first encounter with the criminal justice system will be with the 'gatekeepers', the police, who are the most visible agency of the criminal justice system. Indeed, it is estimated that around 40 per cent of the adult population have some kind of contact with the police each year (Allen 2006).

Whilst the history of the police is well documented (*see* for example Reiner 2000, Rawlings 2001, Gitchley 1978), the idea of a state organised specialist policing organisation is a fairly modern concept with a formalised police service not appearing in England and Wales until the nineteenth century as a result of the 1829 Metropolitan Police Act. The police are of significant importance in the criminal justice system as representatives of the service are empowered by the state to enforce the law and to ensure public and social order through the legitimised use of force which is not generally available to others.

Currently there are approximately 140,000 police officers operating in England and Wales and they work within one of the 43 separate police forces that are responsible for policing local areas. Whilst most studies on policing tend to focus on the police, there are many aspects of policing which are undertaken via a plurality of agencies such as private security firms, Custom and Excise officers, special constables, community support officers, neighbourhood and street wardens (Crawford 2008). As such, police and policing are two different concepts and as Bowling and Phillips (2002: 980) comment:

> Police refers to a particular kind of social institution, while policing implies a set of processes with specific social functions. Police are not found in every society; however, policing is arguably a necessity in any social order.

Consequently, the police are one of a number of agencies that actually perform a 'policing function'. Whilst traditionally the police have been regarded as the agency for responsibility for crime reduction, since the Crime and Disorder Act 1998 this responsibility has shifted beyond the police and responsibility now lies within the collaborative and partnership working arrangements that exist in the locality. However, despite the move towards collaborative work the police service still remain the lead agency in crime reduction partnerships (Crawford 1998) and ultimately the police still have, through their application (or in indeed non-application) of the law, a major input into which sections of the community enter the criminal justice system.

Policing in the UK experienced its mythical 'golden age' during the 1950s when police legitimacy was at its highest point and the police enjoyed the confidence of the general public. In part, this golden age has been attributed to the cohesive community relations that existed within this era together with the population's blind faith in authority and general ignorance of what the police were actually doing! (Downes and Morgan 1994). However, public confidence began to wane as a result of a number of high profile scandals involving the police, increasing crime rates and concerns about youth culture and public order policing (Reiner 2000). As a response, a Royal Commission in Policing (1962) was established leading to the Police Act 1964 which reformed police governance. The Act remains a milestone in policing history, and provided the foundation of the modern police service by introducing the tripartite system of police governance. Each police force in England and Wales is managed through a structure of governance comprising of the Home Secretary, the Chief Constable and the local Police Authority. Whilst the roles and responsibilities of each of these stakeholders have not remained static, essentially the Chief Constable is responsible for day-to-day operational management of the service and the Police Authority act as a 'critical friend' to ensure the quality of local policing is maximised and is carried out effectively and efficiently and provides 'best value'. The Home Secretary has overall responsibility for ensuring the delivery of an efficient and effective police service in England and Wales.[3]

Historically, the police may have enjoyed support from significant sections of the population; Newburn (2008) nevertheless suggests that the last twenty years have witnessed a substantial decline in public satisfaction with the police and that contemporary policing faces a number of challenges. Key debates centre upon issues such as occupational culture, accountability, performance and effectiveness, terrorism, methods of policing and policing in a diverse society (for an overview of the key issues, see Newburn 2008) Central to the latter issue is the relationship between the police and minority ethnic communities and incidents such as the Brixton Riots in 1981 and the murder of Stephen Lawrence in 1993, that led to public enquiries and subsequent publication of reports (Scarman (1982) and Macpherson (1999)), which have highlighted the need for change in policing practice. One of the key findings contained in the latter report was the suggestion that the police service was 'institutionally racist' and over 70 recommendations were outlined, designed to increase trust and confidence in policing amongst black and minority ethnic groups. One of the recommendations was the need to increase the numbers of police officers from black and minority ethnic (BME) groups, which almost ten years after the publication of the report still remains relatively low (4.1 per cent[4])and does not reflect the ethnic composition of the population of England and Wales.

As mentioned earlier the police are 'gatekeepers' to the criminal justice system and through the application of their various powers of stop, search, arrest and detention they essentially have discretion as to who will enter the criminal justice system. This discretionary element has been called into question by Sanders and Young (2007: 123) who suggest that the police overuse their powers on certain groups, with Reiner describing some low status and powerless groups being viewed by officers as 'police property'. Despite the Scarman and Macpherson recommendations, statistics suggest that some BME groups continue to be 'over policed', for example black people are nearly eight times more likely to be stopped and searched per head of population than white people.[4]

Each year around 1.5 million persons are arrested for notifiable offences[5] in England and Wales of whom approximately 80 per cent are males (Povey *et al.* 2009). The term 'arrest' as it is currently used generally refers to the beginning of the investigative process with the power of arrest falling under S.24 Police and Criminal Evidence Act 1984 (PACE)[6], and a lawful arrest requires first that a person is involved or suspected of involvement or attempted involvement in the commission of a criminal offence and there are reasonable grounds for believing that the person's arrest is necessary. Once arrested the suspect's detention and treatment by the police is governed by the Codes of Practice that accompanied PACE and the suspect can be detained for up to 36 hours during which time regular reviews are made by a custody sergeant (or by a more senior officer). When 36 hours have elapsed an application to a magistrates court can·be made to extend the period of detention to 60 hours, otherwise the suspect has to be released or charged or given an out of court disposal.[7][8] It is worthwhile noting that there are separate systems for 10–17 year olds and for adult offenders.

PROSECUTION

Historically the prosecution of an offence was the responsibility of the victim but with the development of a formal police service in the nineteenth century the responsibility of prosecution shifted towards the police who soon became the main prosecution authority in England and Wales.

In 1962 a Royal Commission indicated that it was not acceptable for the police to use the same officers to investigate and prosecute cases and recommended that all police forces should have their own prosecuting solicitor's departments. Whilst some police forces took on board these recommendations, concerns over the role of the police in the prosecution process continued and resulted in the Royal Commission on Criminal Justice Procedure 1981. This was followed by the Prosecution of Offenders Act 1985 which established the Crown Prosecution Service (CPS), who since 1986 have been responsible for prosecuting offenders in England and Wales (Customs and Excise and the Inland Revenue can mount their own prosecution).

The relationship between the police and the CPS has at times been strained with questions centring upon issues such as independence, accountability and competence often being the source of conflict between the two agencies. After the initial problems working relations have improved and the Glidewell Review (1998) established the foundations for greater inter-agency collaboration and increased the number of CPS geographical areas from 14 to 42 making them coterminous with existing police force areas (apart from CPS London which covers the forces of the City of London Police and the Metropolitan Police).

More recently, the Criminal Justice Act 2003 expanded the role of the CPS through the introduction of 'statutory charging' and the majority of charging decisions are now taken by the CPS. This expanded role allows the CPS to advise the police at the investigatory stage and in some instances it is responsible for framing the charge and ensuring that relevant and sufficient evidence is obtained to charge the suspect and that they are charged with the appropriate offence. Finally, the CPS reviews the case and decides whether to proceed with or discontinue the case. This decision to prosecute is based upon the criteria listed in the Code for Crown Prosecutors (CPS 2000) and centres upon two basic issues. First, is there sufficient evidence to secure a conviction?; and second, is a prosecution in the public interest? The CPS then prepares the case for court and presents the case at court.

THE COURTS

Within England and Wales a two tier court system operates (magistrates' and Crown courts), for adults aged 18 years or over[9]. The lower criminal court (magistrates' court) is used for summary cases that include most motoring offences and other relatively minor matters such as drunkenness, common assault and prostitution, and those 'triable either way' which are not referred or directed to Crown courts. Most cases (approximately 95 per cent) are heard in magistrates' courts, with the more serious crimes (indictable offences, such as homicide, rape and robbery) being heard in Crown court. Offences triable either way, such as theft and burglary, arson and criminal damage, can be heard in either magistrates' court or Crown court.

Cases in magistrates' courts are usually heard by a panel of three magistrates (Justices of the Peace). They are not paid and do not usually have any legal qualifications but are supported by a legally qualified court clerk who advises them on the law. In addition, there are also about 130 district judges (formerly known as stipendiary magistrates), who sit in magistrates' courts and are required to have at least seven years' experience as a barrister or solicitor and two years' experience as a deputy district judge. They sit alone and deal with more complex or sensitive cases. Punishments ordered by magistrates cannot exceed six months' imprisonment (or 12 months for consecutive sentences), or fines exceeding £5000[10]. If a case is triable either way the offender may be committed by the magistrates to the Crown court for sentencing if it is thought that a more severe sentence is warranted. During the court hearing, the court will, if the case is adjourned (postponed to a later date), have to make a decision as to whether the defendant is released on bail or remanded in custody. Whilst there is a presumption that the defendant will be granted unconditional bail, the court may impose conditions on the bail such as drug testing, residency or an exclusion order.

Crown courts deal with more serious cases, that is, those that are based on an indictment (a formal document containing the alleged offences). Cases are heard by a single 'professional' judge (who will be a lawyer or solicitor of at least ten years' experience), and a 12 person jury selected randomly from the electoral register.

If convicted and when deciding a sentence, courts refer to the statutory sentencing framework contained in the Criminal Justice Act 2003, as to the appropriate sentence to impose. For the Crown court judge, the maximum penalty will be specified in the statute creating the offence. Possible punishments include discharges, financial penalties (fines), a community order or imprisonment. Once the type of penalty has been decided the court must then decide the sentence tariff (for example, length of prison sentence or content of Community Order).[11] The Criminal Justice Act 2003 also sets out in statute for the first time the purpose of sentencing adults; namely – punishment, crime reduction, reform and rehabilitation, public protection and reparation.

As there are a number of sentencing options available to the court in order to determine the suitability of a sentence and prior to imposing a custodial or community sentence, the court will request a pre-sentence report (PSR) which is compiled by the Probation Service. This report comments on the suitability of particular sentences and assesses the details and circumstances of the offence(s). In addition, the report will contain an assessment of the consequences of the offence(s) including the impact on the victim, the risks of further offending by the individual and any personal circumstances which may be relevant to the offence(s).

THE PROBATION SERVICE

Whilst the probation service through completion of a PSR has involvement with offenders at the pre-sentence stage, the bulk of work takes place following sentence. The main aims of the service are to protect the public, reduce reoffending, punish offenders within the community, ensure that the offender has an awareness of the effects of their crime on their victim(s) and rehabilitate the offender.

The probation service originated from informal court practices of the nineteenth century, whereby local courts sought information on young offenders to ascertain their suitability for discharge or bind over to an individual (often an employer), who would be willing to supervise them. From around 1876, the Church of England Temperance Society started to offer a presence in some city police courts in order to offer 'salvation' to suitable offenders who were willing to pledge abstinence, and such informal court practices provided the origins of the modern day probation service (McWilliams 1983).

The 1907 Probation of Offenders Act placed probation work on a statutory footing and empowered courts to appoint officers who were to advise, assist and befriend those placed on probation orders by the court. Whilst this philosophy remained influential for sometime, the organisation has undergone numerous changes since its formation (*see*, for example, Stratham and Whitehead). Whilst reducing reoffending and the rehabilitation of the offender remain, the service now has a much wider remit which includes a 'public protection' and risk management function as well as a role in ensuring that the offender is properly punished. Since 1991 the probation service has additionally been required to work with victims of crime and make sure that the offender is aware of the effects of their crime on their victims and the community.

While the probation service provides just under 250,000 pre-sentence reports to the courts each year, the majority of the work undertaken by probation is to supervise adult offenders who have been sentenced by the court to a community sentence and those who have been released from prison on licence, for example; it is estimated that they supervise around eight million hours of unpaid work per year. Since the Criminal Justice Act 2003, only one community sentence, the Community Order, is now available to the court. However, through the imposition of requirements that can be attached to the order (such as curfews, drug treatment, unpaid work), the Order can essentially be tailored to meet the offender's need and meet the court's sentencing aims.

Recent concerns over the weaknesses of the case management of offenders and the lack of connectivity between the courts, probation and prison resulted in the publication of the Carter Report (2003), which recommended the establishment of a National Offender Management Service (NOMS) with the aim of reducing re-offending through consistent and effective offender management. NOMS was established in June 2004 as an executive agency of the Ministry of Justice and is structured to link up prison and probation services and is responsible for the commissioning and delivery of adult offender management services for England and Wales.

PRISON

Prison historically existed as a holding institution for those awaiting sentences such as execution or transportation and for debtors. From the late eighteenth century the concept of prison changed as a result of prison reformers such as Elizabeth Fry and John Howard and philosophers such as Jeremy Bentham, and prisons became places where it was thought that individuals' attitudes and behaviours could be altered. Prison regimes, whilst harsh, moved away from the use of punishments such as the tread wheel and crank, and the nineteenth century saw the introduction of new systems such as the 'silent and separate systems', which were used either to keep a regime of silence or to keep prisoners in solitary confinement in order that prisoners could not 'infect' one another with criminal ways and to ensure that they had time for personal reflection.

The Prison Act 1898 asserted reformation as the main role of prison regimes and led to a dilution of the separate system, the abolition of hard labour, and a shift towards the idea that prison work was to be productive and beneficial to the prisoner. The question of whether prisons should seek to reform and rehabilitate those who have broken the law or just serve as institutions which sanction and separate offenders from society continues to fuel contemporary debate. The current objectives of Her Majesty's Prison Service are to protect the public through holding prisoners securely and reducing the risk of prisoners re-offending on release.[12]

Since the abolition of capital punishment a custodial sentence is the toughest penalty a court can impose upon an individual and therefore should only be used if the offence is so serious that there is no appropriate alternative. However, the use of prison has risen dramatically over the last twenty years and the prison population of England and Wales has steadily risen from less than 50,000 in 1990 to over 83,000 in 2009.[13] Current projections suggest that the prison population could continue to rise by up to an additional 15 per cent by 2015 (Ministry of Justice 2008). The Carter Report (2003) suggested that the reason for the increase in the prison population was not attributable to an increase in numbers being caught or convicted or to an increase in the seriousness of crimes being committed but to the increasing severity of sentences being imposed by the court. These high rates of imprisonment make England and Wales one of the highest incarcerators in Western Europe with a rate of 142 people per 100,000 of the population (Walmsley 2005). Not surprisingly, the increase in the prison population has led to issues of overcrowding, which in turn limits the prison's ability to provide little more than secure accommodation. Another problem within prisons is that a substantial number of prisoners have mental health problems and it is questionable whether prisons are the most suitable places to treat individuals who have mental health disorders.[14]

When a prison sentence is imposed by a court the length of sentence specified by the court is the maximum length of sentence that is to be served by the offender. Offenders are eligible for parole (early release), at specified points in their sentence, with individuals sentenced to less than four years being automatically released from prison at the half way point of their sentence and offenders who are sentenced to four or more years being considered for parole halfway through their sentence. If they are refused parole they are automatically released when they have served two thirds of their sentence. Additionally, prisoners who are serving sentences of between three months and under four years can be released early under the Home Detention Curfew (HDC) scheme for between two weeks and four and a half months before their automatic release date, depending on the length of the sentence. If an individual is released on HDC they are required to submit to a curfew and wear an electronic monitoring tag for the duration of the scheme. On release, all prisoners who are given a custodial sentence of 12 months or more are released with licence conditions, which places them under supervision by the probation service for the duration of their original sentence. The licence can contain conditions such as residency, curfew, supervision and drug testing requirements and if the offender fails to comply with their licence conditions they can be recalled to prison to serve the remainder of their sentence.

MULTI-AGENCY WORKING

In line with other public service provision the last decade has required organisations operating within the criminal justice arena to fundamentally change their method of service delivery. As a result of the Crime and Disorder Act 1998, the police service and local authorities were mandated to act as the 'responsible authorities' for their local area and as such were required to bring together an array of other agencies to form a partnership (Crime and Disorder Reduction Partnership (CDRP)), in order to generate strategies to tackle crime and disorder in their local area. The move to collaborative and partnership working has signalled the demise of traditional individual agency responsibility within the criminal justice system and further legislation has widened the range of agencies that are 'responsible authorities'. The push towards partnership working has been driven by the notion that resource sharing and common agendas across agencies will not only lead to efficiencies but will allow problem focused solutions to be formulated which transgress traditional organisational boundaries and will lead to a shift away from the previously prevailing 'silo' mentality. There are numerous examples of collaborative working arrangements in the Criminal Justice System, for example the Multi-Agency Public Protection Arrangements (MAPPA) were introduced in 2001 to support the assessment and management of serious sexual and violent offenders. MAPPA brings together the police, probation and prison services into what is known as the MAPPA Responsible Authority (other agencies have a duty to cooperate). MAPPA identifies offenders to be supervised, ensures information is shared about offenders and that risks posed by offenders are assessed and managed. Prior to MAPPA it was not uncommon for agencies supervising or working with offenders to work in isolation and to be completely unaware of the involvement of other agencies with the same individual.

Responsibility for crime has also been extended to individuals and communities under what Garland (1996) terms a 'responsibilisation strategy', which has shifted the responsibility of governing the 'crime problem' from being solely a state function to one of shared responsibility amongst individuals such as property owners, residents, town planners, employers, parents and individuals. The emphasis on engaging communities in tackling crime has been re-emphasised in Casey's (2008) aptly named report 'Engaging Communities in Fighting Crime' and public involvement is considered to be the solution to reinvigorating public confidence with the criminal justice system.

One concluding comment regarding collaboration and partnership working is that despite the commitment by policy makers to collaborative working arrangements, reports of success of such arrangements are not often reported in practice (Gray *et al.* 2003; Joyce 2000: 184).

VICTIMS

Victims were often the forgotten party in discussions about the criminal justice system. However, they have become key players in both policy and academic research and as Zedner (2004: 1207) suggests:

> Studying victims has become one of the growth industries of criminology. Since 1980 there has been an extraordinarily rapid increase in national and local victim surveys and in studies of the impact of crime, of victim needs and services.

Agencies working across the criminal justice system are now required to note victims' interests as well as those of the community and the offender. The rise in interest in victims has been attributed in part to penal reformers, high profile cases which drew the attention of the media, a recognition of the existence of vulnerable groups and increased knowledge through victimisation surveys (Dignan 2005). Victim surveys have indicated that certain groups are more likely to be victims than others, for example the Home Office research estimates that a small percentage of the population suffers a significant amount of all crime and even suggest that previous victimisation is the single best predictor of future victimisation. However, there are a lot of misconceptions regarding the likelihood of being victimised which are perhaps fuelled by alarmist tabloid headlines, and, for example, old aged pensioners are not the group most at risk from assault and children are more likely to be sexually assaulted by family members than a stranger.

In 1990 the Home Office published the Victims' Charter which set out the rights of victims and the standards of service that they could expect to receive from agencies working across the criminal justice system. This was replaced in 2006 by the Victims' Code of Practice which gives victims of crime statutory rights. Whilst increasing emphasis on victims is welcome there is still, for some, insufficient attention paid to victims' needs.

SUMMARY OF MAIN POINTS

You should be able to:

- Demonstrate a critical appreciation of a range of issues influencing policy and practice within the criminal justice system.
- Understand the origins of the criminal justice system and apply this to contemporary practice.
- Identify the major explanations of crime, criminality and punishment.
- Demonstrate an appreciation of the origins of and current issues affecting the institutions of criminal justice.

NOTES

1 Current crime statistics for England and Wales can be found at: http://www. crimereduction.homeoffice.gov.uk/sta_index.htm#Crime

2 The Ministry of Justice is responsible for criminal law and sentencing, for reducing reoffending and for prisons and probation. The Home Office is responsible for crime and crime reduction, policing, security and counter-terrorism, borders and immigration, passports and identity. The Office of the Attorney General oversees the Crown Prosecution Service, the Serious Fraud Office and the Revenue and Customs Prosecutions Office.

3 The Home Secretary also publishes an annual policing plan and monitors the quality of policing through the Inspectorate of Constabulary and the Police Standards Unit and can intervene in 'failing forces'.

4 *Statistics on Race and the Criminal Justice System 2007/8* A Ministry of Justice publication under Section 95 of the Criminal Justice Act 1991 (April 2009).

5 Notifiable offences cover a wide spectrum of crimes, from homicide to minor thefts.

6 Since 1 January 2006, all offences will carry the power of arrest (Serious Organised Crime and Police Act 2005).

7 Time limits for terrorist cases fall outside PACE and are covered by the Terrorism Act 2000, 2006.

8 See Home Office (2007) *Out of Court Disposals for Adults: A guide to alternatives to prosecution*, London: Office for Criminal Justice.

9 The Criminal Justice Act 1991 established the Youth Court (replacing the Juvenile Court), to deal with offences of children (aged 10 to under 14) and young people (aged 14-17).

10 The Criminal Justice Act 2003 increased the length of imprisonment a magistrate could impose to 12 months but this has not been implemented.

11 For further reading on sentencing *see* Ashworth, A. (2005) *Sentencing and Criminal Justice*, Cambridge: CUP.

12 http://www.hmprisonservice.gov.uk/abouttheservice/statementofpurpose/

13 Female prisoners comprise just under six per cent of the total prison population and 27 per cent of prisoners identify themselves as being from BME groups (Home Office Statistics on Race and the Criminal Justice System 2007/08).

14 For a detailed discussion of prison issues *see* Cavadino, M. and Dignan, J. (2007) *The Penal System*, (4th edition), London: Sage.

REFERENCES

Allen, J. (2006) *Policing and the criminal justice system – public confidence and perceptions: findings from the 2004/05 British Crime Survey*, Home Office Online report, July 2006.

Ashworth, A. and Redmayne, M. (2005) *The Criminal Process* (3rd edition), Oxford: Oxford University Press.

Bowling, B. and Phillips, C. (2002) *Racism, Crime and Justice*, Harlow: Longman.

Casey, L. (2008) *Engaging Communities in Fighting Crime*, London: Home Office.

Cavadino, M. and Dignan, J. (2007) *The Penal System. An Introduction*, London: Sage.

Crawford, A. (2008). Plural policing in the UK: policing beyond the police, in Newbury, T. *A Handbook of Policing*, Cullompton: Willan.

Crawford, A. (1998). *Crime prevention and community safety: Politics, policies and practices*, London: Longman.

Critchey, T. A. (1978) *A History of the Police in England and Wales*, London: Constable.

Dignan, J. (2005) *Understanding Victims and Restorative Justice*, Buckingham: Open University Press.

Downes, D. and Morgan, R. (1994) Hostages to Fortune? The Politics of Law and Order in Post-War Britain, in M. Maguire *et al.* (Eds) *The Oxford Handbook of Criminology*, Oxford: Oxford University Press.

Garland, D. (1996) The limits of the sovereign state, *British Journal of Criminology*, 36, 451–71.

Gray, A., Jenkins, B. and Leeuw, F. (2003) Collaborative Government and Evaluation: The Implications of a New Policy Instrument, in Gray, A., Jenkins, B., Leeuw, F. and Mayne, J. (Eds) *The Challenge for Evaluation: Collaboration in Public Service*, London: Transaction Publishers.

Hodgson, P. and Webb, D. (2005) Young People, Crime and School Exclusion: A Case of Some Surprises, *Howard Journal of Criminal Justice*, 44 (1), 12–28.

Joyce, P. (2000) *Strategy in the Public Sector: A Guide to Effective Change Management*, Chichester: Wiley.

McWilliams, B. (1983) The mission to the English Police Courts 1876–1936, *Howard Journal of Criminal Justice*, 22, 129–47, Oxford: Blackwell Publishing.

Ministry of Justice (2008) *Prison Population Projections 2008–2015 Ministry of Justice Statistics Bulletin*, London: Home Office.

Newburn, T. (2008) *A Handbook of Policing*, Cullompton: Willan

Povey, D., Smith, K., Hand, T. and Dodd, L. (2009) *Police Powers and Procedures England and Wales 2007/08*, London: Home Office.

Rawlings, P. (2001) *Policing: A short history*, Cullompton: Willan.

Reiner, R. (2000) *The Politics of the Police* (3rd edition), Oxford: Oxford University Press.

Sanders, A. and Young, R. (2007) *Criminal Justice* (3rd edition), Oxford: Oxford University Press.

Stratham, R. and Whitehead, P. *The History of Probation: Politics, Power and Cultural Change 1876–2005*, London: Shaw and Sons.

Walmsley, R. (2005) *World Prison Population List* (6th edition), Kings College London: International Center for Prison Studies, pp. 1–6.

Williams, G. (1955) The Definition of Crime, *Current Legal Problems*, 107.

Zedner, L. (2004) *Criminal Justice*, Oxford: Oxford University Press.

FURTHER READING

Whist this chapter only offers a brief 'taster' of issues in the criminal justice system, a number of good general textbooks exist and the following are recommended:

Crowther, C. (2007) *An Introduction to Criminology and Criminal Justice*, Basingstoke: Palgrave.

Hayward , K. J., Hale, C., Wahidin, A. and Wincup, E. (Eds) (2009) *Criminology*, Oxford: Oxford University Press.

Maguire, M., Morgan, R. and Reiner, R. (Eds) (2007) *The Oxford Handbook of Criminology*, Oxford: Clarendon Press.

Newburn, T. (2007) *Criminology*, Cullompton: Willan.

CHAPTER 12

THEORIES OF COUNSELLING

MARTYN HARLING AND GRAHAM WHITEHEAD

O B J E C T I V E S

After reading this chapter you should be able to:

▓ Define the term counselling.

▓ Chart the factors that have contributed to the historical development of counselling activity in Britain.

▓ Differentiate between the main theoretical paradigms of counselling theory.

▓ Comprehend the significance of multicultural counselling practice in Britain.

After reading this chapter you will know the meaning of the following terms: Psychodynamic, cognitive behavioural, humanistic, multicultural.

There is a Moment of Reflection at the end of the chapter.

INTRODUCTION

This chapter provides a broad introduction to the body of theory that underpins counselling activity in contemporary Britain. It starts by exploring definitions of counselling and discusses how counselling activity fits within contemporary health and social care provision in Britain. The discussion identifies the theoretical foundations of the major approaches to counselling theory, and charts their development into a historical context. It then identifies key theorists and describes the basic assumptions and explanations which underpin each of the major counselling traditions. Consideration is given as to how these explanations engender differing models of helping. The chapter also provides a case study to enable the reader to consider how theoretical perspectives might be applied in practice and directs the reader to reference material with suggestions for further study.

DEFINITIONS OF COUNSELLING

Before engaging in discussions around the theoretical assumptions underpinning counselling theory, it is important to develop a shared understanding of what we mean by the term 'counselling'. Each text book will present a slightly different definition of counselling, its role within society and the processes involved in the professional activity. Workers in health and social care often say that they are 'counselling' a patient, client or service user when they are simply engaged in a private conversation. In order to clarify such misconceptions, the British Association for Counselling and Psychotherapy (BACP), the professional body representing counselling and psychotherapy in the United Kingdom (*see* www.bacp.co.uk), offers the following definition:

> Counselling takes place when a counsellor sees a client in a private and confidential setting to explore a difficulty the client is having, distress they may be experiencing or perhaps their dissatisfaction with life, or loss of a sense of direction and purpose.
>
> (BACP 2009)

This definition, whilst providing an indication of the depth of relationship between a counsellor and their client and the purpose of such a relationship, does not indicate how the process of counselling is actually carried out. BACP (2009) goes on to state that:

> By listening attentively and patiently the counsellor can begin to perceive the difficulties from the client's point of view and can help them to see things more clearly, possibly from a different perspective. Counselling is a way of enabling choice or change or of reducing confusion. It does not involve giving advice or directing a client to take a particular course of action. Counsellors do not judge or exploit their clients in any way.
>
> (BACP 2009)

This additional information goes some way to define counselling as an activity, but allows a certain amount of flexibility in connection with what a counsellor actually does. This flexibility is important as there are many different theoretical approaches to counselling. Even individual practitioners using the same theoretical approach differ in the way they work with their clients and may focus on different issues.

In very general terms, counselling occurs where a trained practitioner works with a client to address issues relating to the client's psychological health and well-being. This activity is an agreed relationship between both parties with explicit clarification required about the boundaries, constraints and focus of the activity. (Further discussion about the definition of counselling can be found in Chapter 19, The Practice of Counselling.)

Students often find it difficult to distinguish between the terms 'counselling' and 'psychotherapy'. There is considerable debate within the profession about the overlap between the role of a counsellor and that of a psychotherapist, and this distinction is one reason why the forthcoming regulatory framework is aiming to clarify a greater distinction between these activities (*see* Home Office 2007 and BACP website in resource list). There is also considerable debate about whether a distinction is necessary. In general terms, one distinction to bear in mind is that a psychotherapeutic intervention is normally carried out over a much longer period of time than a counselling intervention and usually deals with clients presenting issues in more depth and detail. In this chapter, we have used the term 'intervention' and 'practitioner' to introduce theoretical variations although other terms used widely in the profession include 'therapy' and 'therapist'.

HISTORY OF COUNSELLING

Counselling evolved during the twentieth century as a means of addressing the problems faced by individuals in their daily lives. The history of counselling is often presented as a chronological list of the key theorists and their theories, but as Pilgrim (1996) points out, it is important to consider the contributions of key theorists alongside more general social factors such as politics, economics, significant historic events and importantly society's changing view on mental health.

The origins of counselling can be traced back to the Victorian era, a time when great developments occurred in medicine, science, engineering and the structure of Western societies. Prior to this point in history, psychological problems were mainly treated from a religious perspective, dealt with by the clergy within the local community (McLeod 2009). Europeans generally lived in small rural communities and were employed in farming. Individuals with mental health problems or learning difficulties could remain within their community, accepted or tolerated by those living around them. As early as the sixteenth century, houses of correction had been established for 'the punishment of vagabonds and the relief of the poor' (Foucault 1967/2001: 40). Such institutions were often established alongside prisons, allowing the detainment of individuals who fell outside the expected moral standards of the time. These institutions later evolved into the workhouse system and asylums of the Victorian era (Foucault 1967/2001).

The industrial revolution meant that a large number of the population began to migrate into the cities from small rural communities. The rise of capitalism as the dominant economic and political force resulted in a shift in moral values as the development of the work ethic led to a decline in religious and spiritual values (McLeod 2009). Individuals, who were less productive, such as the old, disabled or mentally ill, were increasingly seen as a burden, locked up in workhouses or asylums. Initially the control of such institutions was viewed as a moral undertaking, instigated by individuals or groups in society who considered it a social obligation to become involved in such work.

During the nineteenth century the power of the medical professions grew and through intense lobbying was allowed to gain control of asylums and thus of mental health issues (Pilgrim 1996). Whilst asylums still fulfilled a role in incarcerating those who could be problematic in society, medical and biological explanations for insanity began to be developed (McLeod 2009). Residents of the asylums were often viewed as objects of study (and at times experimentation) and kept in appalling conditions. This was particularly true for women. Foucault (1967/2001) describes the care of female residents at Bethlem Hospital stating:

violent madwomen were chained by their ankles to the wall of a long gallery; their only garment was a homespun dress.

(Foucault 1967/2001: 67)

Towards the end of the Victorian era an Austrian physician, Sigmund Freud (1856–1939), developed a model to explain how the mind consists of conscious and subconscious areas and theorised about how emotional disorders could develop in individuals. Freud's ideas were instrumental in developing approaches aimed at helping individuals in emotional distress and were the foundations for developing counselling as a helping profession.

Freud suggested that individuals develop toward adulthood, progressing through a series of stages. When an individual has problems or becomes fixated in one of these stages this can result in psychological problems in later life. The approach to counselling, which evolved from Freud's work, is often referred to as 'psychodynamic'. During Freud's lifetime and after his death many other theorists (such as Freud's daughter Anna, Melanie Klein and Carl Jung) adapted and added to his original ideas.

Much of Freud's work was considered controversial in the society in which it was first described. Many ideas were based on sexual drives and the possibility of abuse which were taboo subjects in Victorian society. During Freud's lifetime significant events such as the First World War (1914–18) and the persecution of the Jews under the Nazis were significant in adding to his ideas, suggesting destructive as well as sexual drives as significant factors in driving human behaviour.

The First World War has been credited as ending the Victorian focus on biological and moral deviancy as explanations for insanity. The large number of returning troops with 'shell shock' led to the fact that:

[it] was out of the question to tolerate the unpatriotic notion that these men were in any sense degenerate.

(Pilgrim 1996: 4)

Psychological distress caused by the First World War, within large sections of the population who were considered to have made an unprecedented sacrifice to society, was instrumental in establishing Freudian ideas alongside medicine as a way of dealing with psychological disturbances (Pilgrim 1996).

Around the time of the First World War a second approach to explaining human actions started to be developed. An American, J. B. Watson (1878–1958) is often credited as founding the 'behavioural approach' where the experimentally observable behaviour of animals, described by theorists such as Ivan Pavlov (1878–1936), is linked to human behaviour. Behaviourists consider that behaviour is learnt and can therefore be unlearnt, given the correct reinforcement and circumstances. Behaviourist approaches paid little attention to internal processes in the psyche (as described by Freud), focusing on the observable actions of the individual. This approach to therapy grew in popularity after the First World War, particularly in the USA (McLeod 2009).

Experience gained from dealing with the psychological consequences of the First World War enabled theorists to predict the possibility of problems emerging in the Second World War (1939–45). Some theorists were encouraged to develop approaches to counselling which were more focused on the current emotional needs of the individuals seeking support. Such 'humanistic' approaches were based on an optimistic view of the human psyche, suggesting that there is an ultimate drive toward self-actualisation where an individual strives to reach their full potential (as described by Abraham Maslow 1908–70). Approaches within the humanistic tradition (such as 'gestalt' and the person-centred approach) vary in how they approach counselling and their view on the role of a counsellor, but share a positive view on the individual's potential for emotional growth and development.

Since the Second World War many Western societies, such as Britain, have developed consumer based societies with an increasing acknowledgement of the role behaviour can play on an individual's health and well-being. Cognitive behavioural therapy (CBT) has emerged as an important approach in the UK, with the government increasing access to counselling through the NHS, through initiatives such as IAPT (Improving Access to Psychological Therapies). In addition to the improved access to CBT, Britain is an increasingly multicultural nation requiring a more considered approach to counselling application. Traditional approaches to counselling (psychodynamic, behavioural, humanistic and cognitive) have been criticised for their focus on the needs of 'Western (mainly American) industrial society' (McLeod 2009: 288). Multicultural counselling theory and practice has developed considerably over recent decades to respond to the demands of delivering counselling provision in a multicultural and multiracial society.

There is considerable research evidence that clients from non-Caucasian backgrounds are less likely to make use of counselling services and there are many reasons why this appears to be true (for further discussion *see* Littlewood and Lipsedge 1982). The major paradigms of counselling theory have tended to replicate the predominant philosophical and psychological concepts popular within Western society. As a multicultural society develops, there is a need to develop multicultural training and practice for counsellors so that the profession is equipped to respond more appropriately to a widening cultural and racial demographic. D'Ardenne and Mahtani (1989) suggest that counsellors should aim to become culturally sensitive, enabling the profession to provide a more effective transcultural service to clients, patients or service users.

MAJOR TRADITIONS OF COUNSELLING

Psychodynamic

The psychodynamic approach has its origins in the ideas of Sigmund Freud (1856–1939) although current theory and practice has gone beyond Freud's initial formulation with developments and adaptations by individuals such as Carl Jung (1875–1961) and Melanie Klein (1882–1960).

One of the most important and at the time unique contributions made by Freud was to present a model of the mind based on thought processes rather than biological ideas. Freud's model consisted of three elements:

- The id – which is present from birth, containing the instincts and biological drives which demand immediate gratification.
- The ego – which develops from the id, at about two years of age, as a result of contact with the outside world. It can be linked to reason and common sense, allowing an individual to function in a socially acceptable way.

- The superego – contains the conscience and moral principles, which the individual starts to assimilate at around five years of age. The superego develops from contact with significant others (such as parents) and is the cause of self criticism.

These elements form the conscious (the area we are aware of) and subconscious (the area we are unaware of) mind. A tension exists between the demands of each element, and they are often in conflict with one another. States of conflict may lead to the unpleasant sensation of anxiety developing, which people deal with in different ways.

One way of dealing with such conflict is to use ego defence mechanisms, which are coping strategies, allowing id impulses to be expressed in ways acceptable to the ego, thus reducing anxiety. These defence mechanisms are quite effective, in the short term, but may lead to psychological problems if used over extended periods of time. Freud described several mental defence mechanisms which were later elaborated on and added to by his daughter Anna. They include:

- Repression (motivated forgetting) – the instant removal from awareness of any threatening impulse, idea or memory.
- Denial (motivated negation) – blocking of external events and information from awareness.
- Projection (displacement outwards) – attributing to another person one's own unacceptable desires or thoughts.
- Displacement (redirection of impulses) – channelling impulses (typically aggressive ones) on to a different target.
- Reaction formation (asserting the opposite) – defending against unacceptable impulses by turning them into the opposite.
- Sublimation (finding an acceptable substitute) – transforming an impulse into a more acceptable form of behaviour.
- Regression (developmental retreat) – responding to internal feelings triggered by an external threat by reverting to 'childlike' behaviour from an earlier stage of development (McLeod 2009: 87).

In addition to dividing the mind into three areas, Freud proposed that humans progress through five stages of development during their early life consisting of:

1 The oral stage (first year) where the main source of comfort is from sucking.
2 The anal stage (roughly two to three years of age) where the main source of pleasure is from withholding and passing faeces.
3 The phallic stage (roughly four to six years of age) where the focus 'for both boys and girls in conventional Freudian thinking is the penis (this is very controversial and raises questions about how Freud viewed the sexes)' (Beckett 2002: 36). This stage is also marked by the Oedipus complex (for boys) and Electra complex (for girls) where 'both boys and girls desire to have an exclusive sexual relationship towards their opposite-sex parent, and become murderously jealous of their same-sex parent' (Beckett 2002: 37). It is easy to understand how such theoretical views are criticised heavily today in the light of a greater acceptance of same-sex relationships.

4   The latency stage (from seven years of age to adolescence) is a quieter period where the child has resolved the Oedipus or Electra conflict prior to adolescence.

5   The final genital stage (adolescence onwards) is where the individual seeks a more permanent resolution of the earlier conflicts by seeking a partner in place of the parent.

Adults may become fixated in an earlier stage of development if they fail to receive the appropriate amount of stimulation (that is, overindulgence or deprivation) at the appropriate age.

See Beckett (2002: 35–8) for a more comprehensive discussion of these stages.

Focus of the counselling intervention

In psychodynamic counselling, the intervention focuses on the unconscious mind. Childhood experiences and instinctual drives are considered to have a direct influence on adult personality. The counsellor uses what happens in the immediate, unfolding relationship with their client to explore and understand the root causes of the client's presenting problems. The counsellor focuses on the client's history, their maternal and paternal relationship and considers the client's use of defence mechanisms. This information is used to explain the client's current issues, problems or maladaptive behaviour.

The role of the practitioner

Traditionally, Freud used a couch where his clients would lie facing away from him during therapy. More recently counsellors, using the psychodynamic approach, have tended to sit facing their clients in the same way as counsellors working in other orientations. The role of the therapist is to uncover the unconscious mind to the client. Transference, where the client relates to the therapist as if they are a key individual in their present or past life, is encouraged in order to expose problems in past relationships. Techniques such as 'free association' where the client links a series of words together quickly as a 'stream of consciousness' and dream analysis may be used to raise issues buried in the subconscious mind.

Practical implications

The intervention does not tend to concentrate on a specific, presenting issue. Whilst recent debate has focused on brief psychodynamic therapy, historically individuals engage in psychodynamic therapy over extended time frames.

COGNITIVE BEHAVIOURAL THERAPY

Cognitive behavioural therapy (CBT) can be seen as a fusion between behavioural and cognitive approaches to counselling. Theorists and researchers in both areas realised that there was a 'natural affinity between the two perspectives' (McLeod 2009: 143).

J. B. Watson (1878–1958) is often considered to be the founder of behavioural approaches, with later contributions by individuals such as B. F. Skinner (1904–90).

Behavioural therapy is based on the assumptions that all behaviour is learnt, universal laws can predict behaviour and such assumptions may be applied to individuals seeking therapeutic support. A great deal of experimental research has been conducted to verify the ideas and theories underpinning the behavioural approach. However, it is unusual for a counsellor to adopt a purely behavioural stance in therapy. Simply focusing on the factors, which can stimulate a particular behaviour, tends to ignore the cognitive thought processes which can also influence an individual's behaviour. This aspect of psychology has been considered by cognitive psychology. Theorists such as Aaron T. Beck (1921) and Albert Ellis (1913–2007) have emphasised the role of thought processes in influencing or modifying a particular course of action or behaviour.

CBT counsellors consider the cognitive thought processes around a particular behaviour as well as the actual behaviour. In support of cognitive approaches Ellis suggested an A-B-C model where an individual's actions are connected by an 'activating' event. This raises 'beliefs' about the event, which in turn can lead to a set of 'consequences'. A does not necessarily lead to C as B is significant to the outcome. Beck described a set of cognitive distortions:

- Arbitrary inference – drawing conclusions with no supporting evidence.
- Selective abstraction – interpreting events out of context.
- Over-generalisation – drawing conclusions on limited experience.
- Magnification and minimisation – wrongly evaluating the significance of events.
- Personalisation – blaming self for an outcome when there is no logical reason.
- Placing all experiences at polar extremes – viewing one's actions as either a saint or sinner (Nelson-Jones 2006).

Considering the impact of thought processes on subsequent behaviour adds the cognitive element to the CBT approach.

CBT counsellors employ a wide range of therapeutic techniques aimed at helping an individual to change their actions or performance in social situations. These techniques can be rehearsed in the therapeutic environment or practised in the real world through the use of structured exercises and interventions.

Focus of the counselling intervention

The focus of the counselling intervention is on the thought processes (cognitions) which control behaviours and how to adapt the problematic behaviour into a more acceptable form. Often therapy is focused on a particular presenting behaviour such as smoking tobacco or eating disorders, which the therapist attempts to address in a relatively tight time-frame. This solution focused, brief approach to therapy fits in well with modern consumerist Western societies and often appeals to funding agencies due to its focus on measurable changes in behaviour.

The role of the practitioner

The practitioner in CBT acts as a 'trainer' assisting the client to alter patterns of maladaptive behaviour. A rapport needs to be established between counsellor and client in order to facilitate engagement and discussions around cognitive aspects, however the developing relationship between the counsellor and client is not seen as a therapeutic tool as it is in other approaches to counselling. The counsellor seeks to diminish a presenting problem identified by the client rather than suggest an overall improvement in their psychological well-being.

There are many different techniques used in CBT. These are agreed with the client at the onset of therapy and are dependent upon the nature of the individual's presenting problem or issue. The overall focus is to concentrate on the specific goals set out at the start of therapy. Approaches can vary from challenging irrational beliefs to assisted exposure to a fear evoking stimulus.

Challenging irrational beliefs, attached to the presenting problem, is often achieved through 'Socratic' dialogue. Named after the Greek philosopher Socrates (470–399BC) this process requires the therapist to employ carefully considered questions in order to challenge the client's irrational beliefs (Westbrook *et al.* 2007). Relaxation techniques can also be taught to the client in order to enable them to consider their reactions, in a given situation, from a calmer perspective.

Behavioural aspects of therapy can include experiments either within the real world or in the therapeutic environment. Clients may be asked to expose themselves to a fear evoking situation, on a gradual basis, in order to desensitise themselves to the stimulus. Clients are often set 'homework' tasks to achieve between sessions or given self-help literature linked to relaxation techniques (Westbrook *et al.* 2007).

Practical implications

CBT focuses on a presenting issue and is aimed at working toward solving a set problem within a relatively tight time-frame. There is a considerable amount of research evidence to support this approach, especially using the research method of random controlled trials (RCTs), and this has led to the popularity of this approach with funding bodies such as the NHS. Clients also see the logic of focusing on a particular problem and developing solutions in a relatively short period of time. Whether underlying issues can be usefully addressed in a short time-frame has been questioned by many authors such as Stiles *et al.* (2006, 2007).

HUMANISTIC

Humanistic approaches to counselling are based on phenomenological philosophy. Phenomenology attempts to challenge the idea that universal laws and theories govern our existence. Such a viewpoint considers that each individual will experience and perceive reality differently. It is therefore important to work with the individual rather than trying to explain their problems or modify their behaviour. Humanistic approaches to counselling present an optimistic view that, given the right environment, the human capacity of creativity, growth and choice will enable individuals to reach their own solutions to life's problems or challenges.

There are many variations in counselling approaches, developed by different theorists, which can be described as 'humanistic'. These include gestalt therapy (Fritz Perls 1893–1970), transactional analysis (Eric Berne 1910–70), person-centred approach (PCA) (Carl Rogers 1902–87) and existentialist counselling (for example, logo therapy, Victor Frankl 1905–97).

Whilst the humanists share the view that their clients construct their own reality, there are major differences in their approaches to therapy and the underlying assumptions made. Since it is not possible to consider all of these approaches in this brief chapter, the most commonly used approach within the humanistic tradition, the PCA first described by Carl Rogers (1902–87), will be used as a focus for discussion.

The view of the individual

Carl Rogers shared Abraham Maslow's (1908–70) view that individuals have a motivational drive toward self-actualisation or fulfilling their potential.

The PCA, whilst focusing on the significance of the 'here and now', within the therapeutic setting, is based on a developmental model of personality. Early childhood experiences relating to how an individual receives love and affection from significant others such as their parents are considered to be influential in developing an individual's self-concept. An individual's self-concept or 'conceptual construction of him-self' (or her-self) (Mearns and Thorne 2007: 10) is a crucial factor in the way they interpret life's experiences.

A person with a high self-concept will accurately perceive experiences, whereas an individual with a low self-concept will distort experiences according to their internal value structure. For example, a student with a high self-concept will attribute a good grade to their level of subject knowledge, whereas a student with a low self-concept could attribute the same result to the marker missing their mistakes (Nelson-Jones 2006). Such an internal frame of values is referred to as the individual's 'conditions of worth' and is a major focus of the PCA to therapy (for a more detailed discussion *see* Mearns and Thorne 2007).

Focus of the counselling intervention

The focus of the counselling intervention in humanistic counselling is to allow time for the client, patient or service user to express his/her concerns in a supportive and developmental manner. The 'client' is seen as being the expert about his/her issues and the practitioner will aim to focus on the interpersonal dynamics of the therapeutic relationship. There is considerable debate amongst humanistic practitioners about whether an initial assessment of a client presenting issues is seen as helpful, or conversely whether it could be seen as stigmatising the client and medicalises his/her presenting concerns. There is, however, consensus that the general aim of working with the client is to move toward self-actualisation.

The role of the practitioner

The role of the counsellor is to create an environment and relationship in which self-actualisation can occur. In the PCA the three elements of empathy, congruence and unconditional positive regard are central to this process. Mearns and Thorne (2007) define these as:

> Empathy is a continuing process whereby the counsellor lays aside her own way of experiencing and perceiving reality, preferring to sense and respond to the

experiencing and perceptions of her clients. This sensing may be intense and enduring with the counsellor actually experiencing her client's thoughts and feelings as powerfully as if they had originated in her (p. 67).

Congruence is the state of being of the counsellor when her outward responses to her client consistently match her inner experiencing of her client (p. 121).

Unconditional positive regard is the label given to the fundamental attitude of the person-centred counsellor towards her client. The counsellor who holds this attitude deeply values the humanity of her client and is not deflected in that valuing by any particular client behaviours. The attitude manifests itself in the counsellor's consistent acceptance of and enduring warmth towards her client (p. 95).

Continually showing empathy to the client, being congruent and demonstrating the attitude of unconditional positive regard is considered central to the success of the person-centred approach.

Practical implications

The PCA does not seek to expose the reasons for a client's presenting issues, as with psychodynamic approaches, or focus on one presenting issue or problem, as with CBT. The PCA attempts to facilitate the client's inbuilt drive toward self-actualisation. It is this positive view of humanity which characterises PCA and other humanistic approaches of counselling.

The counselling process may last for some time and it may prove difficult to ascertain when the process has reached its conclusion. The PCA is very dependent upon the counsellor's interpersonal skills and their ability and experience around demonstrating the core conditions in the counselling interaction. Clients may be unused to the level of attention given by the counsellor and hence resistant to the counselling process. This is particularly true of clients with poor social skills and low self-confidence levels.

MULTICULTURAL COUNSELLING

A broad definition of the term 'multiculturalism' embraces a wide range of variables or differences. This may include factors such as gender, disability, social class, religion, age, sexual orientation, racial and ethnic origin. Pederson (1991) proposed a broad definition of multicultural counselling which includes:

ethnographic variables such as ethnicity, nationality, religion and language; demographic variables such as age, gender and place of residence; status variables such as social, educational and economic; and affiliations including both formal affiliations to family or organisations and informal affiliations to ideas and a lifestyle.

(Pederson 1991: 229)

This definition indicates how a person might construct their cultural and racial identity and is a starting point for working with a client. Pedersen argues that multiculturalism emphasises both the way a person perceives him/herself as different from and similar to other people. It challenges those who have presumed that differences do not matter as well as those who have overemphasised differences which are frequently referred to as stereotyping.

Ivey *et al.* (1997: 134) describe multicultural counselling as a 'metatheoretical approach that recognises that all helping methods ultimately exist within a cultural context'. This definition of multiculturalism emphasises awareness of difference, the significance of cultural factors that shape the way a person may view the world and is in essence a challenge to those training in counselling to consider the relevance and efficacy of counselling within a multicultural context.

Bimrose (1996) traces the origins of multicultural counselling to the American civil rights movement in the mid 1970s. Around this time, questions were asked about the groups of people who never requested counselling, or, if they came along for a first session, did not return. A clear pattern emerged. Clients from minority ethnic groups were the least likely to request and/or continue with counselling.

The most widely accepted explanation is that counselling practice is an ethnocentric activity. Many authors (Lago and Thompson 1996; Sue *et al.* 1996; Sue and Sue 1999) have argued that mainstream approaches are white, middle class activities that operate with many distinctive values and assumptions. For example, that clients will be future and action orientated. Such approaches are ethnocentric or 'culturally encapsulated' (Wrenn 1985), holding at their centre a notion of normality derived from white culture, which is irrelevant to many clients and has the potential for alienating them.

Focus of counselling intervention

The focus of multicultural counselling is to support the client in exploring their self-perception and to consider how these perceptions influence their approach to life and the challenges they face.

The role of the practitioner

The role of the counsellor requires understanding and consideration of the challenges that multicultural counselling poses and to provide a therapeutic response that is relevant and sensitive to presenting cultural and racial concerns. D'Ardenne and Mahtani (1989: 12) challenge counsellors to acknowledge their own ethnocentricity, and this is viewed as being particularly pertinent for non-Caucasian practitioners.

Practical implications

The issue that non-Caucasian clients can find mainstream counselling unhelpful has equal relevance to other client variables such as gender, sexual orientation and disability. The counsellor is required to consider such needs when applying mainstream approaches to diverse groups of clients and to consider fully the requirements of such groups in practice delivery.

CONCLUSION

This chapter has provided the reader with a broad introduction to the key approaches to counselling. The following case study can be used as an exercise to apply the broad principles and approaches described to a practical scenario. This will give the reader the opportunity to differentiate between the main theoretical paradigms. However, it is important to acknowledge that becoming an effective counsellor requires a clear knowledge of their chosen approach and that the necessary interpersonal skills develop with professional training over time. In order to pursue counselling as a career, it is important to develop a theoretical knowledge base through an accredited training course and develop effective counselling skills via supervised practice. The British Association for Counselling and Psychotherapy provides further information about this on their website (www.bacp.co.uk) along with information about their nationally recognised professional accreditation procedure and an ethical code of conduct.

As the profession moves towards a regulatory framework, future professional training and continuing professional development requirements will be determined by the regulatory body, the Health Professional Council (HPC). This position was set out by a government White Paper outlining the intent to regulate counselling and psychotherapy (Home Office 2007). It is highly likely that this process will clarify the distinct professional roles in counselling and psychotherapy service delivery and develop appropriate professional codes of conduct for professional practice.

MOMENT OF REFLECTION

Case study: Irene

Irene is 66 years of age and has been referred for counselling by her doctor. She has been married twice and has two grown up children, a son aged 27 and daughter 31. As a child she had extended periods of illness necessitating long stays in hospital. She comes from a large family. Her father worked long hours in the local factory but died soon after his retirement, and her mother, still alive, struggled with raising her seven brothers and sisters. She says that she has always had problems developing close relationships with people and this has been the case with both her former and current husband, and with both her children. She has a very difficult relationship with her daughter and only speaks occasionally with her mother. She feels isolated from her husband at present and considers the relationship to be deteriorating. She tells her doctor she has been very low for some time and just cannot open up to people. She does not relish the thought of discussing her feelings with a counsellor but does wonder what counselling involves.

1   How might a counsellor, using the three main approaches to counselling discussed in this chapter explain Irene's presenting issue?
2   How might the counsellor plan to work with Irene according to his/her theoretical approach?

Discussion points

What can Irene expect from counselling?

How might the counselling outcomes be affected by the theoretical approach used by the counsellor?

Assuming the counsellor is of a different ethnic background to Irene, what transcultural themes might emerge during the initial sessions (if any)?

SUMMARY OF MAIN POINTS

You should be able to:

- Describe how the counselling profession has developed to meet the needs of service users seeking emotional and psychological support.
- Outline the main counselling paradigms and apply them to a real life scenario.
- Appreciate the need to develop multicultural competencies in counselling interventions.
- Understand the complexity of counselling as an activity and the need for professional regulation.

REFERENCES

Beckett, C. (2002) *Human Growth and Development,* London: Sage.

Bimrose, J. (1996) Multiculturalism, in Bayne, R., Horton, I. and Bimrose, J. (Eds) *New Directions in Counselling*, London: Routledge.

British Association for Counselling and Psychotherapy (BACP) (2009). What is Counselling? [online]. Available at: http://www.bacp.co.uk/information/education/whatiscounselling.php

D'Ardenne, P. and Mahtani, A. (1989) *Transcultural Counselling in Action,* London: Sage.

Foucault, M. (2001 [1967]) *Madness and Civilisation,* (Howard, R., Trans.), Abingdon: Routledge Classics.

Home Office (2007) *Trust, Assurance and Safety: The Regulation of Health Professions in the 21st century,* London: The Stationary Office.

Ivey, A. E., Ivey, M. B. and Simek-Morgan, L. (1997) *Counselling and Psychotherapy: a Multicultural Perspective* (4th edition), Boston: Allyn & Bacon.

Lago, C. and Thompson, J. (1996) *Race, Culture and Counselling,* Buckingham: Open University Press.

Littlewood, R. and Lipsedge, M. (1982) *Aliens and Alienists: Ethnic Minorities and Psychiatry*, Harmondsworth: Penguin.

McLeod, J. (2009) (4th edition) *An Introduction to Counselling,* Buckingham: Open University Press.

Mearns, D. and Thorne, B. (2007) *Person Centred Counselling in Action* (3rd edition), London: Sage.

Nelson-Jones, R. (2006) *Theory and Practice of Counselling and Therapy* (4th edition), London: Sage.

Pedersen, P. B. (1991) Multiculturalism as a generic framework, *Journal of Counselling and Development,* 70 (1), 6–12.

Pilgrim, D. (1996) British Psychotherapy in Context, in Dryden, W. (Ed.) *Handbook of Individual Therapy,* London: Sage.

Stiles, W. B., Barkham, M., Mellor-Clark, J. and Connell, J. (2007) Effectiveness of cognitive-behavioural, person-centred, and psychodynamic therapies as practised in UK primary care routine practice: replication in a larger sample, *Psychological Medicine*, published online 10 September 2007, doi:10.1017/S0033291707001511.

Stiles, W. B., Barkham, M., Twigg, E., Mellor-Clark, J. and Cooper, M. (2006) Effectiveness of cognitive-behavioural, person-centred and psychodynamic therapies as practised in UK National Health Service settings, *Psychological Medicine, 36,* 555–56.

Sue, D. W. and Sue, D. (1999) *Counselling the Culturally Different: Theory and Practice* (3rd edition), New York: Wiley.

Sue, D. W., Ivey, A. I. and Pederson, P. B. (1996) *A Theory of Multicultural Counseling and Therapy,* Pacific Grove: Brooks/Cole.

Westbrook, D., Kennerley, H. and Kirk, J. (2007) *An Introduction to Cognitive Behaviour Therapy: Skills and Applications,* London: Sage.

Wrenn, C. G. (1985) The culturally encapsulated counsellor revisited, in Pedersen, P. (Ed.) *Handbook of cross-cultural counselling and therapy*, Westport, CT: Greenwood.

USEFUL WEBSITES

British Association for Counselling and Psychotherapy (BACP):
www.bacp.co.uk

The British Psychological Society (BPS):
www.bps.org.uk

United Kingdom Council for Psychotherapy (UKCP):
www.psychotherapy.org.uk

Counselling and Psychotherapy in Scotland (COSCA):
www.cosca.org.uk

Irish Association for Counselling & Psychotherapy (IACP):
www.irish-counselling.ie

MIND Mental Health Charity:
www.mind.org.uk

Health Professions Council (regulatory body):
www.hpc-uk.org

CHAPTER 13

PLACE, NEIGHBOURHOOD AND HEALTH

JAMES HUNTER

OBJECTIVES

After reading this chapter you should be able to:

■ Discuss the concept of place and its relationship with socio-economic forms of deprivation and exclusion.

■ Understand neighbourhood-based explanations of health inequalities, including: Individual characteristics, physical environment, location of communities vis-à-vis each other, community cohesion, lack of access to services, quality of local services, resource allocation and local politics.

■ Identify and measure neighbourhood effects involving the issues in, and contemporary approaches to, the quantitative measurement of local health and social care environments.

■ Identify and measure local service provision.

■ Understand contemporary approaches to the measurement and evaluation of the quantity and quality of local public services.

After reading this chapter you will know the meaning of the following terms: Neighbourhood function, spill-over effects, the physical and built environment, social capital, community engagement, access to services, resource allocation and local politics.

There are two Moments of Reflection for you to work on at the end of the chapter.

INTRODUCTION

Does where you live shape your life chances and opportunities in respect of suffering from poor health and lack of access to quality health care? Does a lack of geographical mobility condemn certain individuals to endure a higher prevalence of health problems because of the neighbourhood they reside in? A growing body of evidence in the UK indicates a distinctive geographical pattern to the distribution of social problems including poor health (*see* for example, McCormick and Philo 1995; Shelton *et al.* 2006; Dorling *et al.* 2007; Thomas and Dorling 2007; Shaw *et al.* 2009). Furthermore, once factors concerning individual characteristics, circumstances and life choices are taken into account, geographical variations in health outcomes cannot be entirely explained by simply examining the type of individuals living within different localities (*see* for example, Congdon *et al.* 1997; Curtis *et al.* 2004; Dibben *et al.* 2006). This is not to say that current policy initiatives designed to tackle 'problematic' individual behaviour (for example, smoking, alcohol, drugs and obesity), along with strategies that seek to address the link between household income, poverty and health deprivation (for example, minimum wage and working family tax credits) are not important. However, this present situation both highlights the extent to which 'people' based diagnoses still predominantly feature in policy initiatives designed to tackle health inequalities – and supports the argument by Powell *et al.* (2001) that there has been an over-emphasis upon people poverty conceptions of social problems at the expense of placed based factors.

Why does place matter? Our own direct experience of living within specific neighbourhoods tells us that place matters in terms of the positive and negative attributes of localities. In deciding where to live, we make decisions based upon (often highly subjective) judgements about the merits of areas that are as much shaped by our view of the place as it is by our opinion concerning the individuals who live there. The extent to which place, and the complex set of circumstances, processes and interactions that operate within and around the communities we live in, really impacts upon our circumstances and life opportunities is, however, open to considerable conjecture and debate. In part this stems from arguments concerning the type of methodological approach and evidence required to demonstrate that place exerts a significant and independent impact upon our lives (*see* for example McCulloch 2001; Dietz 2002; Sampson *et al.* 2002; Diez Roux 2004). More importantly, however, disputes concerning the link between place and social problems are crucially centred around whether place or 'area effects' really exist at all – and if so, what aspects of place exert a causal influence on our lives? Do poor neighbourhoods make their residents poorer (Friedrichs 1998), or is it the presence of poor residents that renders neighbourhoods poorer places in which to live? Should our attempts to tackle health inequalities centre on 'people poverty' orientated solutions, or should we equally be concerned with addressing the structural, interpersonal, institutional context of health and health care that is embodied within the neighbourhoods in which we reside?

The aim of this chapter is to explore the concepts of place, and neighbourhood effects, as a mechanism for understanding the presence of health inequalities within certain communities. The chapter seeks to develop a more holistic conception of *place poverty* as a theoretical framework for evaluating health inequalities, one that takes us beyond narrow conceptions of poverty that predominantly focus the attention of governments and health care organisations upon deprived individuals living within deprived communities. Having examined the concept of place poverty, the discussion moves on to identify different types of neighbourhood effect that need to be considered in evaluating the health environment operating within specific localities, and finally introduces an analytical approach that enables the evaluation of place and health in relation to both the scale of health problems and the quality of health care operating within different areas.

PLACE POVERTY AND NEIGHBOURHOOD EFFECTS: MOVING BEYOND THE CONCEPTION OF POVERTY AS THE PRESERVE OF DEPRIVED INDIVIDUALS LIVING IN DEPRIVED PLACES

The concept of place poverty

The geography of social problems has become characterised in the UK by the use of terms such as 'the North–South divide' and the 'postcode lottery'. An examination of the contemporary evidence on the spatial distribution of a wide range of social problems in the UK quickly reveals, however, that both the concept of a North–South divide, and the notion that urban areas are uniformly poor whilst rural areas are prosperous, is both overly simplistic and misleading. For example, according to the English Indices of Multiple Deprivation 2007 (Noble *et al.* 2008), 30 different counties or metropolitan areas are represented in the top 100 most deprived local authority areas in England – with only 12 of these located in the North of England[1]. Furthermore, ten per cent of the top 100 most deprived local authorities in England also fall into the two most rural categories of the local authority urban/rural classification developed by DEFRA[2].

This failure to understand properly the relationship between place and the nature/distribution of social problems, however, is not simply a problem that stems from perpetuating place-based stereotypes in spite of the available empirical evidence. It is equally the product of the conceptual straightjacket that we tend to fall into when we are charged with considering the concepts of poverty, deprivation and exclusion. Our natural inclination in this situation, which is mirrored to an unfortunate extent within policy and academic circles, is to conceive of these terms in the form of deprived *individuals*. Even if our immediate focus shifts away from people towards place, our gaze naturally falls upon deprived neighbourhoods rather than considering the nature of all localities. It is akin to the problem of having difficulty in stepping outside the confines of needs based welfare systems to recognise that any criteria deemed acceptable by society can form the basis of a just distribution of resources or services – and when the distribution of resources does not match the distribution of need, that is not automatically grounds for demanding an end to this apparent form of 'injustice'.

The problem we face here is that the very concept of poverty itself is imbued within an entrenched conception of deprivation that is both material and urban in nature. The limitation of considering income based definitions and measures of deprivation is highlighted by Townsend (1979), who asserts that these represent a limiting demand side conception of poverty that fails to take account of variations in the supply of public services and initiatives designed to address the impact of deprivation. Whilst in the context of rural deprivation, Cloke *et al.* (1995) argue that the policy failure of official agencies to recognise the scale and nature of rural deprivation is one of the main forms of deprivation that rural communities experience. So what do we mean by place poverty? What circumstances does the concept seek to encapsulate, and how does this shape which localities are defined as being 'poor'? Whilst few would disagree with Atkinson and Kintrea (2003: 437) that 'it is worse to be poor in a poor area than one that is socially mixed', and that 'residence in a neighbourhood of concentrated poverty has an independent negative effect on both the quality of life and the life chances of poorer individuals and households' (Fitzpatrick 2008: 9), the criteria by which we judge an area inevitably shapes our identification of neighbourhoods that can be deemed 'problematic'. Alternative conceptions of poverty, social exclusion and cohesion, and the distribution of resources and public expenditure are just some of the legitimate alternative criteria for judging neighbourhoods that produce very different maps of the distribution of social problems within and across administrative areas.

The attachment of the 'place' moniker to the concept of poverty clearly implies that we are concerned here with 'the way in which poverty is distributed unevenly across space' (Cotter 2002: 537). The spatial focus of place poverty therefore requires us to clearly distinguish conceptually between the dimensions of poverty that relate to people and those that relate to place. According to Smith (1977: 112), people poverty occurs 'where low-income people occupy certain parts of a city by virtue of their low income, but their money incomes are not low because of where they live', whereas place poverty 'emerges when other benefits or penalties compound the advantages or disadvantages of particular groups by virtue of where they live'. Traditional approaches to explaining the presence of health inequalities within specific neighbourhoods that focus upon individual characteristics (for example, age, gender and social class), circumstances (for example, unemployment and homelessness) or life choices (for example, smoking and binge drinking) can therefore be equated with people based conceptions of poverty. Conversely, perspectives that concentrate upon aspects of neighbourhoods (for example, the function of and relationship between communities, the physical and built environment, pollution, etc.) are underpinned by a place based conception of poverty. Place poverty shifts our attention away from people towards place. This in itself, however, is not sufficient to move us beyond 'economic' or resource based conceptions of poverty that inevitably take us once more towards the downtrodden and marginalised neighbourhoods that constitute the 'usual suspects' in terms of providing the subject matter for studies of health-related forms of social deprivation and exclusion. For us to escape the clutches of narrow conceptions of poverty, and hence place poverty, it is necessary to understand the nature of neighbourhood and the aspects of neighbourhood that shape how poverty manifests itself within the context of communities and localities.

The concepts of neighbourhood and neighbourhood effects

The concepts of neighbourhood and neighbourhood effects are intrinsically linked – and many of the conceptual and methodological problems surrounding the assessment of the impact of neighbourhood relate to this dynamic interrelationship (Buck

2001; Atkinson and Kintrea 2001). If we wish to understand what it is about the neighbourhoods in which we live that provides us with advantages/disadvantages, then we need to understand what we mean by neighbourhood, and how individuals relate to the local communities in which they live. The concept of neighbourhood enjoys many different definitions within the academic literature. According to Davies and Herbert (1993) these include proximity to other neighbourhoods, physical and territorially defined boundaries, socially defined boundaries, a focal point for social interaction and networks, community cohesion and common identity, opportunity, history and sentiment. Whilst some definitions focus on the physical and geographical dimensions of neighbourhood, for example 'place and people, with common sense limit as the area one can easily walk over' (Morris and Hess 1975: 6), or 'a physical or geographical entity with specific (subjective) boundaries' (Golab 1982: 72), others have emphasised the interaction between the physical and social dynamics of neighbourhood, for example 'A neighbourhood is a distinct territorial group, distinct by virtue of the specific physical characteristics of the area and the specific social characteristics of the inhabitants' (Glass 1948: 18), 'a place with physical and symbolic boundaries' (Keller 1968: 89), 'Geographic units within which certain social relationships exist' (Downs 1981: 15), or 'a limited territory within a large urban area, where people inhabit dwellings and interact socially' (Hallman 1984: 13). Other definitions have focused on the presence of key local institutions, for example 'Common named boundaries, more than one institution identified with the area, and more than one tie of shared public space or social network' (Schoenberg 1979: 69), or 'A set of sub-areas of the city each of which could be regarded as having a history of its own community, a name, an awareness on the part of its inhabitants of community interests, and a set of local businesses and organisations orientated to the local community' (Kitagawa and Taeubeur 1963: 13). The dynamic nature of the processes located within neighbourhoods is emphasised by Wilkenson (1989: 339), 'Community is not a place, but it is a place orientated process. It is not the sum of social relationships in a population but it contributes to the wholeness of social life. A community is a process of interrelated actions through which residents express their shared interest in the local society'. For Healey (1998: 69), neighbourhood is about the opportunities and social interactions which shape a sense of community identity, 'A key living space through which people get access to material and social resources, across which they pass to reach other opportunities and which symbolises aspects of the identity of those living there, to themselves and to outsiders'.

The problem of defining and understanding the nature of neighbourhood is that the development of a meaningful definition of neighbourhood is complicated by two factors. First, there is the need to incorporate a wide range of factors, processes and interactions that inhabit localities and communities. How people relate to their neighbourhood is important in understanding how neighbourhoods operate and shape the lives of their residents. Davies and Herbert (1993) identify a range of ways in which the sentiment of individuals towards their neighbourhood are expressed: attachment, satisfaction or dissatisfaction with their locality; security and safety; empowerment, physical environment and aesthetics; symbolism; latent participation; common values; and empathy or a sense of belonging. Different people react to different circumstances in different ways at different points of time. This brings us to the second problem in defining and understanding the concept of neighbourhood. The problem of measuring and classifying neighbourhood is, as Keller (1968: 87) points out, made more problematic by the varying presence and unique interaction of the dimensions of neighbourhood identified above within specific localities:

> The term neighbourhood ... refers to distinctive areas into which large spatial units may be subdivided. The distinctiveness of these areas stems from different sources whose independent contributions are difficult to assess: geographical boundaries, ethnic or cultural characteristics of the inhabitants, psychological unity among people who feel they belong together, or concentrated use of an area's facilities for shopping, leisure and learning ... Neighbourhoods containing all four elements are very rare in modern cities ... geographical and personal boundaries do not always coincide.
>
> (Keller 1968: 87)

Thus, in exploring the nature of neighbourhood we need to recognise that there are a range of factors that we need to take into account, all or some of which will be operational to varying degrees at different points in time. This is important in the context of official attempts to classify similar types of neighbourhood in a generic sense (for example, ONS Area Classification 2001[3]) or in relation to a specific policy issue (for example, Home Office Crime Families in relation to Crime and Disorder Reduction Partnership areas or Basic Command Units which enjoy a similar propensity for crime to occur within them[4]) for the purposes of administering common policy initiatives to solve common policy problems. Neighbourhoods that to all intents and purposes appear to be highly similar to one another (for example, deprived inner city estates) may actually exhibit unique, and often subtle, differences that render them quite different from the other localities that they have been grouped with.

Neighbourhoods are multifaceted and dynamic entities – but in what forms do they impact upon the lives and opportunities of their residents? What do we actually mean by a 'neighbourhood effect', and how do they relate to the presence of health problems within specific localities? Unsurprisingly, there is an extensive literature that has sought to define and develop typologies/classifications of neighbourhood effects (*see* for example, Jencks and Mayer 1990; Atkinson and Kintrea 2001; Buck 2001; Galster 2001; Friedrichs *et al.* 2003; Lupton 2003). Drawing on both the specific literature on neighbourhood, and the wider discourses concerning aspects of place, space, design, human/social/economic and political geography, it is possible to identify a series of distinctive types of neighbourhood effect that can be deployed to explain the presence of health inequalities (or the factors that give rise to them) within specific communities:

1   *Function of, and relationship between, neighbourhoods*: Life within neighbourhoods is shaped substantially by the function (for example, residential, industrial, commercial, leisure) or mix of functions assigned to cities, towns and villages and the sub-divided areas within them. Area or neighbourhood function shapes the presence of the type of individuals, facilities, institutions, organisations and activities within localities. Crucially, these in turn also shape the presence of both social problems and opportunity within neighbourhoods. The relationship between places, localities and neighbourhoods is an equally important aspect to consider. Within cities and towns, the concept of identifiable zones of transition and stability has been employed to explain both the distribution of deprivation

and wealth, and patterns of growth and development within urban environments (*see* Park *et al.* 1925; Hoyt 1939). The ability, or lack of ability, to move between the different function-based zones of cities and towns in order to secure resources, employment, accommodation, leisure, etc. becomes a crucial factor in shaping the lives of individuals. The concept of urban hierarchies (*see* for example Hall *et al.* 2001) which seeks to understand the relative fortunes over time of localities, based upon core economic and institutional characteristics, points to the importance of understanding places within the context of other localities that are around them. Echoing the underlying principles developed by von Thünen (1826), Christaller (1933) and Losch (1938), the spatial distribution of places in terms of their optimum theoretical, and actual, distance from one another can play a crucial role in shaping the sustainability of communities, and the degree of social and geographical mobility enjoyed by their respective populations.

2   *Spillover effects*: Social problems are dynamic elements that do not respect our attempts to bring order to places in the form of political, administrative, organisational or policy initiative boundaries. The contagious nature of deprivation and exclusion means that the ills of one specific neighbourhood (be it the symptoms or causes of social problems) can quickly spread to other surrounding communities (Jencks and Mayer 1990). Spillover effects, however, also materialise in a positive format. The location of new employment opportunities, a new school, or a new health centre within a specific neighbourhood may prove beneficial to a much wider group of individuals and communities than simply those living within immediate proximity to the new facilities. On a larger spatial scale, the concept of positive spillover effects, in terms of employment and prosperity transforming the quality of life within the surrounding hinterlands of major cities, was very much present within the policy emphasis on the significance of regions and core cities as key economic and social drivers placed by the last Labour government (*see* for example DCLG 2006).

3   *Physical infrastructure, physical spaces and the built environment*: There is a clear link between the physical conditions of our accommodation and our health (*see* for example, Martin *et al.* 1987). There is also substantial evidence linking the infrastructure of neighbourhoods in terms of road networks and streetscape to health problems such as higher levels of pollution and increases in the incidence of childhood asthma (*see* for example, Ferguson *et al.* 2004), or to variations in mortality in road traffic accidents (*see* for example, Jones *et al.* 2008), or to the drastically higher incidence of road fatalities amongst children from lower social classes (*see* for example, Roberts and Power 1996). The link between the design of the physical environment and the presence of crime has been long recognised (*see* for example, Poyner and Webb 1991; Schneider and Kitchen 2002), and has given rise to the concept of crime prevention through environmental design (CPTED). However, out of environmental criminology and the wider social sciences has emerged an important body of literature that has recognised the importance of exploring the link between the physical environment and social problems, how individuals relate to the physical spaces which they inhabit and utilise (*see* for example, Jacobs 1961; Wood 1961; Newman 1973; Hillier 1984) – and has sought to question the perceived suitability of 'utopian' urban housing design (Coleman 1985). The 'broken window' thesis (Wilson and Kelling 1982) which argues that poorly maintained physical environments will attract social

problems, will enhance the negative stigma associated with localities that are deprived in appearance, and discourage local residents from taking pride in their communities, is a good example of a perspective that makes the link between the physical environment, social problems and social interactions.

4   *Social networks and interrelationships*: The importance of community interaction, networks and collective efficacy as a mechanism for achieving neighbourhood cohesion (*see* for example, Forrest and Kearns 2001; Bridge 2002; Bridge *et al.* 2004) has come to the fore with the emergence of both social exclusion and social capital onto the policy agenda. The growing recognition of the importance of lacking connection or engagement with fellow neighbours and citizens as a form of poverty can be attributed directly to shifts in policy discourses away from deprivation towards exclusion. Physical regeneration that is not accompanied by social regeneration can often result in the construction of new or reconstituted residential areas that do not work as living, organic and sustainable communities, because the quality of the physical environment cannot mask the lack of soul possessed by places, or the sense of ownership or belonging displayed by the indigenous population to their new surroundings. This can particularly be the case where physical regeneration results in the relocation of the materially poor, but community rich, existing population in favour of supposedly more desirable or 'essential' populations (*see* for example, Palen and London 1984). It is, however, important to recognise that lower levels of community spirit and deprived neighbourhoods do not automatically go hand in hand. Whilst the 'broken windows' thesis makes the link between physical decay, social deprivation and lack of community ownership of physical spaces, there are plenty of deprived neighbourhoods that exhibit markedly high levels of social capital and community engagement. This can be placed in direct contrast to the leafy middle and upper class suburbs in many cities and towns which are often materially rich, but poor in respect of social interaction.

5   *Political networks and participation*: Connected in part to the social interaction/community spirit form of neighbourhood effect, is the extent to which localities possess the mechanism to generate change from within, through participation in the local democratic process and the deployment of political contacts and networks. Under the last Labour government there was a strong policy emphasis upon a direct engagement by local public service organisations with local communities in terms of transforming their surroundings, which involved both participation and consultation of local residents (for example, New Deal for Communities). However, the ability to engage, interact with and utilise local, regional and national policy-making systems via representation and direct action varies across communities. Affluent neighbourhoods can employ the policy relevant knowledge of the 'system' and professional connections of their residents to much greater effect than deprived communities when it comes to either campaigning for the provision of a service/facility, or in order to prevent an undesirable physical or policy development (for example, new bypass, wind turbines, or closure of a local school).

6   *Public services and institutions*: The presence of schools, hospitals, GP surgeries, pharmacies, police stations, etc. within nearby proximity is vital not only in responding to, and preventing, health and wider social problems, but also in terms of maintaining the existence of communities. The devastating impact of the loss of local food shops or pubs within rural communities is evidence of the need for the preservation of core community institutions (Commission for Rural Communities

2008). The type and quality of services provided to residents within neighbourhoods, as well as levels of access to service centres, also clearly have an impact upon the quality of life experienced by local residents. This is not only in respect of the direct services that are provided to the local community, but also in relation to the public service infrastructure required to create individual opportunity and to increase social/geographical mobility. In an increasingly fragmented policy environment, the need for the local public to successfully work in partnership with one another is equally crucial in shaping local circumstances and opportunities. Furthermore, in the current performance assessment culture within which public service organisations operate, the increasing link between quality of performance, partnership working and the ability to secure additional funding/policy initiatives is creating a new form of place poverty. Afflicted by deprivation, with possibly poor access to services, the exposure of local populations to poor performing schools, hospitals, police forces, etc. can potentially have a longer-term impact as previous levels of success, efficiency, commitment to partnership working amongst local public service agencies are increasingly being deployed by central and regional government as criteria for distributing public resources.

7   *Ownership, attachment and stigma*: The final type of neighbourhood effect concerns our emotional relationship with places and communities, and the stigma attached to certain types of locality (Ellaway *et al.* 2001; Watkins and Jacoby 2007). What outsiders might see as an irrational sense of belonging and attachment to places can result in individuals choosing to continue living within deprived and excluded neighbourhoods. Equally, the lack of connection with neighbourhoods and the desire to get out of the area as soon as possible on the part of substantial elements of the local population can frustrate the best intentions of policy initiatives and public service organisations in terms of physically and economically regenerating localities, investing in the local institutional infrastructure, and seeking to turn round failing public service institutions (for example, schools). The stigma, often unfairly acquired by specific neighbourhoods, that operates as a barrier to employment and other forms of opportunity can often explain the low level of attachment felt by individuals to specific localities. The importance of social stigma attached to postcodes in relation to accessing education, employment, housing and the relationship between residents of 'sink' estates and public servants (for example, the police) is a widely recognised problem in analyses of barriers to social inclusion (Fitzpatrick 2004).

Buck (2001: 2254) couches the neighbourhood effects identified above in terms of alternative models of neighbourhood:

- Epidemic – the potential for peer pressure to transform negative individual and group behaviour into a contagious entity.
- Collective socialisation – the potential for positive peer group and role models to mould individual and group behaviour into positive neighbourhood attributes.
- Institutional model – the ability of public service agencies to recruit high quality professionals and to utilise resources effectively in order to generate quality public services.
- Relative deprivation – the apparent relative adverse situation of individuals in relation to their neighbours results in adverse behaviour, for example, the higher

drop-out rate amongst poor children occupying classes containing affluent high performing pupils.

- Competition – the competition between neighbourhoods for scarce public and private resources.
- Network – the presence of links within the community to more affluent and socially integrated networks within and beyond the confines of the neighbourhood.
- Expectations – the impact of varying degrees of expected success in ventures – the 'he's done very well for a boy from a council estate' phenomenon.
- Insecurity – modified forms of behaviour arising from crime, social disorder and fear of victimisation.
- Physical isolation – the lack of proximity of communities to centres of employment, resources, opportunities and influence.
- Barriers to opportunity – the lack of access to services, opportunities and social well-being because of the infrastructure, mobility and public service distribution profile of the neighbourhood.

In some respect these models of neighbourhood (effect) work more effectively in terms of encapsulating the circumstances, developments and processes that are operating both within and outside neighbourhoods. The jury is still very much out on the extent to which these neighbourhood effects operate in isolation or in combination to advantage or disadvantage local populations within different localities (*see* for example Kleinman 2000; Lupton 2003; Lupton and Power 2004). The same jury is still waiting to pass verdict on the relative merits of people-poverty versus place-poverty based explanations of spatial variations in health inequalities and wider social problems. Yet conceptually, few of us would disagree with the potential for utilising these different types of neighbourhood effect as a heuristic device for exploring questions concerning the nature of place and neighbourhood, and why some localities 'work' whilst others do not in terms of sustainability and the quality of life that they afford their residents.

EVALUATING THE HEALTH ENVIRONMENT WITHIN DIFFERENT LOCALITIES IN ENGLAND[5]

The previous section identified a range of neighbourhood effects that can impact upon the health outcomes of people living within different localities. For the purposes of illustrating a methodological approach to the mapping of local health environments, our focus now will concentrate upon one specific neighbourhood effect: the quality of local public services. Faced with individual circumstances and forms of neighbourhood deprivation that are likely to result in lower employment prospects, lower income levels, poorer housing conditions and greater health problems, excluded communities are vitally dependent upon: (a) the provision of quality services that will positively impact upon the immediate consequences of deprivation and exclusion; and (b) the ability of local public service agencies to engender strategic change and development, secure scarce resources from regional/central government, and implement policy initiatives effectively. There is a significant body of literature that has pointed to the presence of a strong relationship between deprived areas and poor public services (*see* for example, Harvey 1973; Galbraith 1992; Jargowsky 1997; Shaw *et al.* 1999; Andrews *et al.* 2005). Unfortunately, the conclusions drawn from such research have

manifested themselves into a universalism that deprived places always equal poor services. This not only creates a false perception of neighbourhoods but has, arguably, also
resulted in the narrow socio-demographic and economic focus of attempts to develop
empirical classifications of localities. Crucially, it also fails to recognise that lack of
access to quality public services (including health care) is a form of place poverty that
is not automatically restricted to urban, deprived neighbourhoods. Users of health
care services from within affluent or rural localities who experience problems accessing treatment in terms of long waiting times, who are denied access to specific drugs
simply by the virtue of which primary care trust's jurisdiction they fall under, or who
endure poor quality services once they arrive at their local GP or hospital, equally suffer a form of postcode lottery in relation to health.

A persistent problem in the assessment of the health environments operating within different localities is the failure to utilise and integrate the available data
in a manner that develops a picture that reflects both the scale of health problems
and the quality of health care being provided within specific localities. For example, the Community Health Profiles developed by the Association of Public Health
Observatories[6] concentrate purely on measuring the scale of health inequalities and
associated lifestyle factors displayed by individuals living within specific localities
without exploring issues relating to access or the quality of local health care. Equally,
the performance assessment framework utilised by the Healthcare Commission in rating service provision by the different types of NHS trust operating within each area
is done without reference to the prevailing health conditions within the locality in
question. The Health Poverty Index does produce a spider chart representation of the
relative conditions within individual local areas of England and incorporates aspects
of health outcomes, contextual factors, and access to/quality of health care provision.
Closer inspection, however, reveals that quality of health care is measured by indicators relating to aspects of health care that are either too generic or which concern
very specific niche forms of health services – whilst access to health care services is
measured in terms of available resources of staffing and places rather than the spatial
proximity of services to local populations.

What we require, therefore, is an analytical approach that enables us to assess
the dimensions of health related forms of place poverty operating within different local
areas that reflects both the scale of health problems and the quality of health care provision. As we have argued above, many places which appear to be ideal localities within
which to live in respect of high life expectancy and lower rates of death from cancer,
smoking, heart disease, etc. cannot be treated as such if the quality of public health care,
when it is required, is of a poorer standard than that available within other areas. The
approach adopted here is to construct a matrix that maps the relative 'performance' of
health environments within different localities in respect of both health problems and
the quality of health care (see Figure 13.1). The relative position of individual localities
within this matrix can be plotted in respect of their relative score on different aspects
of health inequality (for example, life expectancy, infant mortality, deaths from cancer)
against the performance of local health care organisations that are responsible for providing the services which are designed to respond to/prevent the specific health issue
under consideration (for example, primary care, acute, mental health and ambulance
trusts). The score for each local area is plotted on the horizontal and vertical lines relative to the minimum and maximum health problem/quality of services scores attained
across the range of localities under consideration.

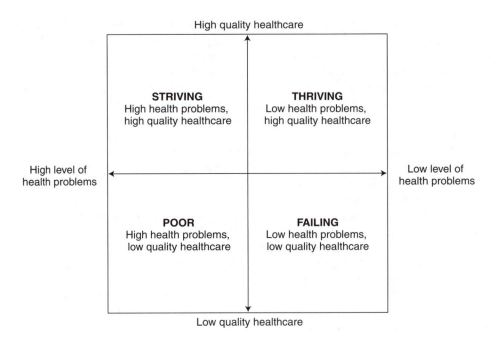

Figure 13.1 Local health environment matrix

Each locality plotted within the matrix can then be assigned to one of four categories (thriving, striving, failing and poor) depending upon which cell of the matrix they are located in. Ideally we would like as many localities as possible to end up in the thriving category since this would indicate a situation in which poor health was less likely, and when treatment was required, the quality of health care was of a high standard. Equally, we would wish as few localities as possible to be located in the poor category since this would suggest a double disadvantage suffered by residents living within these areas – a higher disposition to experiencing poor health which is then compounded by access to poorer quality health care services. Areas ending up in the striving category have the prospect of high quality local health care services operating as compensation for the greater prevalence of health problems within these localities, whilst areas located in the failing category experience place poverty in the form of poorer quality health care. However, it is important to recognise that in employing such a matrix to evaluate health-related aspects of place poverty, we are not assuming a causal relationship between the scale of health problems and the quality of local health care. To achieve this situation we would have to allow for a sufficient period of time to pass in order for the quality of local health care services at a specific point in time to result in a reduction in health problems occurring at a later point in time. More importantly, we would have to allow for all of the external factors that operate outside of the control or remit of local health care organisations, which are likely to result in high levels of health problems, in order to discover the independent impact of the quality of health care provision upon the prevalence of a specific health problem within different local areas.

Figures 13.2 and 13.3 represent the application of the methodology to the mapping of local health environments in respect of female life expectancy/deaths from cancer against quality of local health care in England in 2007/8. For the purposes of this exercise, the quality of local health care has been measured on the basis of the combined quality of overall service scores (graded in terms of excellent, good, fair and weak) attained by primary care, acute and ambulance trusts in England, operating within each locality, on the basis of the performance assessment framework implemented by the Healthcare Commission (2008). Each diamond plotted in the matrix represents a local authority area in England. If the theory that poorer areas will suffer poorer quality public services is valid, then we would expect to see the majority of localities with low female life expectancy/high rates of death from cancer located within the 'poor' category of the matrix. Conversely, if local health care agencies operating in localities with high female life expectancy/low rates of death from cancer find it easier to deliver high quality services, then this should result in these areas appearing within the 'thriving' category of the matrix.

In Figure 13.2, an examination of the distribution of localities in relation to female life expectancy reveals that the above propositions concerning the relationship between the incidence of poor health and quality of local health care are not entirely supported. The majority of local areas with lower female life expectancy do fall within the 'poor' category (that is, lower levels of female life expectancy accompanied by lower quality health care provision). However, there are a significant number of localities with lower female life expectancy that appear to enjoy higher quality health care (that is, they fall into the 'striving' category). Equally, when we shift to localities with higher levels of female life expectancy we can see that a majority of these represent areas with poorer quality health care. In Figure 13.3, the overall pattern for the data relating to deaths from cancer has shifted both upwards and to the right within the matrix, that is, there are more areas that are doing better in terms of the incidence of cancer related mortality, and more areas are delivering higher quality health care services. Crucially, however, there now appears to be a situation in which there are more problem localities, in terms of high rates of death from cancer, that are delivering high quality health care, than there are areas delivering lower quality health care. Conversely, areas with lower rates of deaths from cancer appear to be dominated by localities in which the quality of health care is also lower. It is important to emphasise that in employing the chosen methodology, we are not seeking to imply a causal link between the incidence of health problems and the quality of health care (that is, we are not seeking to make a direct link between poorer quality health care and an increased risk of death from cancer or a lower level of female life expectancy). We are merely utilising the approach to illustrate that in terms of place poverty there are (a) deprived areas which are also afflicted by poorer quality public services; (b) deprived areas whose population has the compensation of higher quality health care services; and (c) that many supposedly good places to live, in the context of lower incidence of health problems, can turn out to be problematic areas within which to reside when the local population has to call upon health care services that are performing at a poorer standard compared to other places in England.

The evidence in Figures 13.2 and 13.3 does, however, enable us to make some important comments both in relation to the link between place and health, and in respect of the concept of place poverty. First, an enshrined principle both within the concept of a 'national health service', and the policy statement of intent by New Labour that within 10–20 years no one should be seriously disadvantaged by where they live (Social Exclusion Unit 2001), implies the goal of a uniform quality of local health care for all. The evidence presented above appears to indicate in relation to quality of local health care we have a long way to go before a situation of spatial justice is arrived at. Second, the

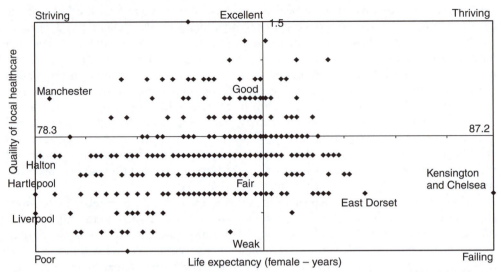

Figure 13.2 Local health environment matrix – life expectancy (female) against quality of local health care in England 2007–8

Source of data: Community Health Profiles/Healthcare Commission

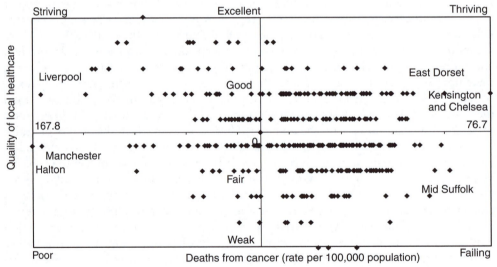
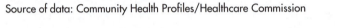

Figure 13.3 Local health environment matrix – deaths from cancer against quality of local health care in England 2007–8

Source of data: Community Health Profiles/Healthcare Commission

argument that poorer areas endure poorer quality public services is not borne out by the evidence in relation to local health care services. Third, in utilising the concept of place poverty, we need to move away from the notion of 'poverty' as being the sole preserve of urban and deprived neighbourhoods. A geography of health constructed on the basis of spatial variations in quality of local health care reveals a postcode lottery in which the traditional delineators of urban/rural, and North/South, are no longer appropriate.

CONCLUSION

In this chapter we have explored the concept of place poverty and neighbourhood effects. We have examined the different types of area effect that can operate within specific localities, and have seen how these can directly influence the pattern of health operating within different neighbourhoods. We have also advanced a methodological approach that makes the link between the prevalence of social problems and quality of local public services. This has enabled us to think about both the importance of public services in terms of addressing social problems within different areas and shaping the quality of life and opportunity for residents living within different neighbourhoods. It has also enabled us to reveal that the geography of health and health care is more complex and diverse than the conventional North/South and urban/rural conceptions of the postcode lottery might initially suggest. The test of whether the ideas explored within this chapter have helped the reader to understand a wider range of factors that underpin the presence of health inequalities within certain localities lies in the application of these concepts to real neighbourhoods and communities (*see* the exercise below). If the reader has either become awakened to the possibility of using place as a mechanism for analysing and evaluating social problems, or has developed a more nuanced understanding of the concept of place and neighbourhood, then the seeds will have been sown for unpicking the conventional mindset of focusing solely upon deprived individuals living in deprived neighbourhoods.

SUMMARY OF MAIN POINTS

You should be able to:

*   Understand the geographical nature of social deprivation and exclusion.
*   Appreciate the concept of place poverty, and neighbourhood-based explanations of social problems and regional inequalities in health and social care problems and outcomes.
*   Evaluate approaches to the quantitative measurement of social problems and the quantity and quality of local services/policy responses.
*   Undertake a quality of life assessment within a specific locality.

MOMENT OF REFLECTION

Activity One

1   What do you understand by the terms 'place' and 'neighbourhood'?

2   Choose a particular type of health issue (for example, teenage pregnancy or obesity). How can you utilise the concepts of place and neighbourhood to explain the prevalence of your chosen health issue within specific localities?

MOMENT OF REFLECTION

Activity Two: Evaluating your own place or neighbourhood

Think of a place that is familiar to you. It can be somewhere you grew up, somewhere that you live permanently now, somewhere that you live when you are studying. Think of this place in terms of the immediate area that surrounds the house/flat that you live in (that is, a particular neighbourhood rather than a whole city or town). Think about how you would rate this neighbourhood in terms of the quality of life and opportunities that it provides you. Now think about whether this would be true for other types of household (for example, families with children, households with disabled members, the elderly). What conclusions have you reached? Does your chosen place have the same impact on all of its residents? Now think about the localities that surround your chosen neighbourhood. To what extent is the quality of life and level of opportunities in your chosen neighbourhood shaped by the areas around it? Do these surrounding areas have a positive or negative impact on your chosen locality? Finally, think about the characteristics of your chosen neighbour-hood that might impact upon its residents. How do you think the function, physical and built environment, levels of community spirit and political engagement, access to key services and facilities, the quality of local public services, and the sense of attachment and ownership shape the neighbourhood that you live in?

NOTES

1 North of England defined as including the regions of the North East, North West and Yorkshire and Humberside.
2 These categories are Rural-50 (at least 50 per cent but under 80 per cent of the local population located in rural settlements and larger market towns); Rural-80 (80 per cent or over of the local population located in rural settlements and larger market towns). DEFRA (2005) *Rural and Urban Area Classification 2004* [online]. Available at: available at www.defra.gov.uk.
3 Office for National Statistics, Area Classification of local authorities, wards, health authorities, super output areas 2001 (Available at: www.statistics.gov.uk).
4 *See* for example, G. Harper *et al.* (2002) *Family Origins: Developing Groups of Crime and Disorder Reduction Partnerships and Police Basic Command Units for comparative purposes*, Home Office RDS website (Available at: www.homeoffice.gov.uk/rds).
5 This conceptual approach can be applied to the health context operating within any country or region subject to the data being available. The discussion presented here in relation to England is simply for illustrative purposes.
6 Community Health Profiles available at: www.apho.org.uk.
7 Health Poverty Index available at: www.hpi.org.uk.

REFERENCES

Andrews, R., Boyne, G.A., Law, J. and Walker, R.M. (2005) External Constraints on Local Service Standards: The Case of the Comprehensive Performance Assessment in English Local Government, *Public Administration*, 83 (3), 639–56.

Atkinson, R. and Kintrea, K. (2001) Disentangling Area Effects: Evidence from Deprived and Non-Deprived Neighbourhoods, *Urban Studies*, 38 (12), 2277–98.

Atkinson, R. and Kintrea, K. (2003) 'Opportunities and Despair, it's all in there': Fractioned Experiences and Explanations of Area Effects and Life Chances, *Sociology*, 38 (3), 147–66.

Bridge, G. (2002) *The Neighbourhood and Social Networks*, Bristol/Glasgow: ESRC Centre for Neighbourhood Research, CNR Paper No. 4.

Bridge, G., Forrest, R. and Holland, E. (2004) *Neighbouring: A Review of the Evidence*, Bristol/Glasgow: ESRC Centre for Neighbourhood Research, CNR Paper No. 24.

Buck, N. (2001) Identifying Neighbourhood Effects on Social Exclusion, *Urban Studies*, 38 (12), 2251–75.

Christaller, W. (1933/1966) *Die Zentralen Orte in Suddeutschland*, Jena: Gustav Fischer, Translated (in part) by C. W. Baskin (1966) *Central Places in Southern Germany*, London: Prentice Hall.

Cloke, P., Goodwin, M., Milbourne, P. and Thomas, C. (1995) Deprivation, Poverty and Marginalisation in Rural Lifestyles, *Journal of Rural Studies*, 11 (4), 351–65.

Coleman, A. (1985) *Utopia on Trial: Vision and Reality in Planned Housing*, London: Hilary Shipman.

Commission for Rural Communities (2008) *State of the Countryside Report*, Cheltenham: Commission for Rural Communities.

Congdon, P., Shouls, S. and Curtis, S. (1997) A Multi-level Perspective on Small-Area Health and Mortality: A Case Study of England and Wales, *International Journal of Population Geography*, 3, 243–62.

Cotter, D. (2002) Poor People in Poor Places: Local Opportunity Structures and Household Poverty, *Rural Sociology*, 67 (4), 534–55.

Curtis, S., Southall, H., Congdon, P. and Dodgeon, B. (2004) Area Effects on Health Variation over the Life-course: Analysis of the Longitudinal Study Sample in England using New Data on Area of Residence in Childhood, *Social Science and Medicine*, 58, 57–74.

Davies, W. and Herbert, D. (1993) *Communities within Cities: An Urban Social Geography*, London: Belhaven Press.

Department for Communities and Local Government (2006) *Strong and Prosperous Communities: The Local Government White Paper*, London: The Stationery Office.

Dibben, C., Sigala, M. and Macfarlane, A. (2006) Area Deprivation, Individual Factors and Low Birthweight in England: is there Evidence of an 'Area Effect'?, *Journal of Epidemiology and Community Health*, 60, 1053–9.

Dietz, R. (2002) The Estimation of Neighbourhood Effects in the Social Sciences: An Interdisciplinary Approach, *Social Science Research*, 31, 5399–75.

Diez Roux, A. (2004) Estimating Neighbourhood Health Effects: The Challenges of Causal Inference in a Complex World, *Social Science and Medicine*, 58, 1953–60.

Dorling, D., Rigby, J., Wheeler, B., Ballas, D., Thomas, B., Fahmy, E., Gordon, D. and Lupton, R. (2007) *Poverty, Wealth and Place in Britain 1968 to 2005*, Bristol: Policy Press.

Downs, A. (1981) *Neighbourhoods and Urban Development*, Washington DC: Brookings Institution.

Ellaway, A., Macintyre, S. and Kearns, A. (2001) Perceptions of Place and Health in Socially Contrasting Neighbourhoods, *Urban Studies*, 38 (12), 2299–316.

Ferguson, E., Maheswaran, R. and Daly, M. (2004) Road-traffic Pollution and Asthma – Using Modelled Exposure Assessment for Routine Public Health Surveillance, *International Journal of Health Geographics*, 3, 24–31.

Fitzpatrick, T. (2008) *Applied Ethics and Social Problems: Moral questions of birth, society and death*, Bristol: Policy Press.

Forrest, R. and Kearns, A. (2001) Social Cohesion, Social Capital and the Neighbourhood, *Urban Studies*, 38 (12), 2125–43.

Friedrichs, J. (1998) Do Poor Neighbourhoods make their Residents Poorer? Contextual Effects of Poverty Neighbourhoods on Residents, in H-J. Andress (Ed.) *Empirical Poverty Research in Comparative Perspective*, Aldershot: Ashgate.

Friedrichs, J., Galster, G. and Musterd, S. (2003) Neighbourhood Effects on Social Opportunities: The European and American Research and Policy Context, *Housing Studies*, 18 (6), 797–806.

Galbraith, J. (1992) *The Culture of Contentment*, London: Sinclair-Stevenson.

Galster, G. (2001) On the Nature of Neighbourhood, *Urban Studies*, 38 (12), 2111–24.

Glass, R. (1948) *The Social Background to a Plan: The Study of Middlesbrough*, London: Routledge and Kegan Paul.

Golab, C. (1982) The Geography of the Neighbourhood, in R. Bayer (Ed.) *Neighbourhoods in Urban America*, Port Washington: Kennikat.

Hall, P., Marshall, S. and Lowe, M. (2001) The Changing Urban Hierarchy in England and Wales 1913–38, *Urban Studies*, 35 (9), 775–807.

Hallman, H. (1984) *Neighbourhoods: Their Place in Urban Life*, Beverley Hills, CA: Sage Publications.

Harvey, D. (1973) *Social Justice and the City*, London: Edward Arnold.

Healey, P. (1998) Institutional Theory, Social Exclusion and Governance, in A. Madanipour *et al.* (Eds) *Social Exclusion in Cities*, London: Jessica Kingsley Publishers.

Healthcare Commission (2008) *Annual Health Check 2007/2008*, London: Healthcare Commission.

Hillier, B. (1984) *The Social Logic of Space*, Cambridge: Cambridge University Press.

Hoyt, H. (1939) *The Structure and Growth of Residential Neighbourhoods in American Cities*, Washington DC: US Government Printing Office.

Jacobs, J. (1961) *The Death and Life of Great American Cities*, New York: Vintage Books.

Jargowsky, P. (1997) *Poverty and Place: Ghettos, Barrios and the American City*, New York: Russell Sage Foundation.

Jencks, C. and Mayer, S. (1990) The Social Consequences of Growing Up in a Poor Neighbourhood, in L. Luynn and M. McGeary (Eds) *Inner City Poverty in the United States*, Washington DC: National Academy Press.

Jones, A., Haynes, R., Kennedy, V., Harvey, I. M., Jewell, T. and Lea, D. (2008) Geographical variations in mortality and morbidity from road traffic accidents in England and Wales, *Health and Place*, 14, 519–35.

Keller, S. (1968), *The Urban Neighbourhood: A Sociological Perspective*, New York: Random House.

Kitigawa, E. and Tauebeur, K. (1963) *The Chicago Local Community Fact Book*, Chicago, IL: Chicago University Press.

Kleinman, M. (2000) Include Me Out? The New Politics of Place and Poverty, *Policy Studies*, 21 (1), 49–61.

Losch, A. (1938) The Nature of Economic Regions, *Southern Economic Journal*, 5 (1), 71–8.

Lupton, R. (2003) 'Neighbourhood Effects': Can we Measure them and Does it Matter?, London: London School of Economics, Centre for Analysis of Social Exclusion, Paper No. 73.

Lupton, R. and Power, A. (2004) *What We Know About Neighbourhood Change: A Literature Review*, London: London School of Economics, CASE Report no. 27.

Martin, C., Platt, S. and Hunt, S. (1987) Housing Conditions and Ill Health, *British Medical Journal*, 294, 1125–7.

McCormick, J. and Philo, C. (1995) 'Where Is Poverty? The Hidden Geography of Poverty in the United Kingdom', in C. Philo (Ed.) *Off the Map: The Social Geography of Poverty in the UK*, London: Child Poverty Action Group.

McCulloch, A. (2001) Ward-Level Deprivation and Individual Social and Economic Outcomes in the British Household Panel Study, *Environment and Planning A*, 33 (4), 667–84.

Morris, D. and Hess, K. (1975) *Neighborhood Power*, Boston, MA: Beacon Press.

Newman, O. (1973) *Defensible Space: People and Design in the Violent City*, London: Architectural Press.

Noble, M., McLennan, D., Wilkinson, K., Whitworth, A. and Barnes, H. (2008) *The English Indices of Deprivation 2007*, London: Department for Communities and Local Government.

Palen, J. and London, B. (1984) *Gentrification, Displacement and Neighbourhood Revitalisation*, New York: SUNY Publications.

Park, R., Burgess, E. and McKenzie, R. (1925) *The City*, Chicago: University of Chicago Press.

Powell, M., Boyne, G. and Ashworth, R. (2001) Towards a Geography of People Poverty and Place Poverty, *Policy and Politics*, 29 (3), 243–58.

Poyner, B. and Webb, B. (1991) *Crime Free Housing*, Oxford: Butterworth Architecture.

Roberts, I. and Power, C. (1996) Does the Decline in Child Injury Mortality Vary by Social Class? A Comparison of Class Specific Mortality in 1981 and 1991, *British Medical Journal*, 313, 784–6.

Sampson, R.J., Morenoff, J.D. and Gannon-Rowley, T. (2002) Assessing 'Neighbourhood Effects': Social Processes and New Directions in Research, *Annual Review of Sociology*, 28, 443–78.

Schneider, R. and Kitchen, T. (2002) *Planning for Crime Prevention: A Transatlantic Perspective*, London: Routledge.

Schoenberg, S. (1979) Criteria for the Evaluation of Neighbourhood Viability in Working Class and Low Income Areas in Core Cities, *Social Problems*, 27, 69–85.

Shaw, M. *et al.* (1999) *The Widening Gap: Health Inequalities and Policy in Britain*, Bristol: Policy Press.

Shaw, M. *et al.* (2009) *The Grim Reaper's Road Map: an Atlas of Mortality in Britain*, Bristol: Policy Press.

Shelton, N., Birkin, M. and Dorling, D. (2006) Where not to Live: A Geo-demographic Classification of Mortality for England and Wales 1981–2000, *Health and Place*, 12, 557–69.

Smith, D. (1977) *Human Geography: A Welfare Approach*, London: Edward Arnold.

Thomas, B. and Dorling, D. (2007) *Identity in Britain: A Cradle-to-Grave Atlas*, Bristol: Policy Press.

Townsend, P. (1979) *Poverty in the UK*, Harmondsworth: Penguin.

von Thünen, J. H. (1826) *Der isolierte Staat (Isolated state)*, translated by C. M. Wartenberg, Oxford: Pergamon Press.

Watkins, F. and Jacoby, A. (2007) Is the Rural Idyll Bad for your Health? Stigma and exclusion in the English countryside, *Health and Place*, 13, 851–64.

Wilkenson, K. (1989) The Future for Community Development, in J. Christenson and J. Robinson (Eds) *Community Development in Perspective*, Ames, IA: Iowa State University Press.

Wilson, J. and Kelling, G. (1982) The Police and Neighbourhood Safety: Broken Windows, *Atlantic Monthly*, 3, 29–38.

Wood, E. (1961) *Housing Design: A Social Theory*, New York: CHPC.

CHAPTER 14

HEALTH, HOUSING AND REGENERATION

ANN MCCARTHY

OBJECTIVES

After reading this chapter you should be able to:

■ Discuss the link between housing and health and the role of housing standards and housing professionals in the amelioration of housing related health problems.

■ Evaluate the implications of an ageing housing stock to public health.

■ Consider current problems in housing that have the potential to affect public health and approaches to ameliorate them.

■ Consider key issues, impact on housing and sustainable development.

After reading this chapter you will know the meaning of the following terms: Healthy housing, poor housing, housing hazards, sustainable development, neighbourhood.

There is a Moment of Reflection for you to work on at the end of the chapter.

INTRODUCTION

This chapter examines the relationships between housing, health and well-being to inform an understanding of the most effective approaches to address potential health impacts associated with the built environments in which we live. To place housing in its proper public health context, the Chartered Institute of Environmental Health (CIEH 2008) provides an excellent comparison of statistics on the numbers of people killed or injured in the home, compared to on the road or at work. Eight times as many people in the UK are injured at home than are injured on the roads, and ten times as many people in the UK are killed at home than at work. Housing also compares strongly with the key lifestyle issues of the day. This chapter will outline evidence for the existence of neighbourhood-based housing related health disparities, to enable you to consider how theories of disease causation shape public health and health promotion strategies, and will explore specific research and intervention practices to generally address health disparities. Drawing from a range of frameworks, you should be able to begin to find ways to address health disparities in your research and practice. Clearly, more work will be necessary to explain whether particular interventions are effective in reducing health disparities.

HOUSING FOR HEALTH

The role of public health is to provide the circumstances under which people can be healthy. Housing can affect health in a number of relatively minor ways, which combine to form one of the key social determinants of health (Shaw 2004). Investment in housing can be more than just an investment in bricks and mortar, and can provide a foundation for the future health and well-being of residents (Shaw 2004). Increasingly in modern society and particularly in the UK, the focus for that investment is emphasised more and more as an individual responsibility rather than a collective, societal or governmental one. Housing is the conjunction of the dwelling, the home, the immediate environment and the community. Each of these four housing dimensions has the capacity to affect individual health status through physical, mental or social mechanisms, and they all interlink. It will become increasingly relevant to consider housing as a substantial element of public health and social welfare, and to integrate health aspects into strategies of sustainable housing construction and neighbourhood or urban planning (WHO 2004).

'Healthy housing' covers the provision of functional and adequate physical, social and mental conditions for health, safety, hygiene, comfort and privacy. A healthy home, therefore, is not a specially designed house; it is more a residential setting for a household. The Habitat Declaration, Istanbul (1996), defines the characteristics of an 'adequate shelter', which are very much in line with what healthy housing is:

> Adequate shelter means more than a roof over one's head. It also means adequate privacy; adequate space; physical accessibility; adequate security; security of tenure; structural stability and durability; adequate lighting, heating and ventilation; adequate basic infrastructure, such as water-supply, sanitation and waste-management facilities; suitable environmental quality and health-related factors; and adequate and accessible location with regard to work and basic facilities; all of which should be available at an affordable cost. Adequacy should be determined together with the people concerned, bearing in mind the prospect for gradual development. Adequacy often varies from country to country, since it depends on specific cultural, social, environmental and economic factors. Gender-specific and age-specific factors, such as the exposure of children and women to toxic substances, should be considered in this context.
>
> 2nd Habitat Conference in Istanbul, cited in WHO report (2004)

Housing is a key determinant of health, but identifying the independent effect of poor housing on health is difficult due to the complexity of potential causal pathways and confounding factors, which include the degree of individual and neighbourhood deprivation, the presence of multiple domestic hazards, and the amount of time spent in the home (Smith 1990). Work by Shaw (2004) distinguished the influences of housing on health into 'direct' and 'indirect', and then further broken down into 'hard/physical/material' and 'soft/social/meaningful' influences. This allows us to see how the various factors associated with housing can interact with a person's health. Shaw (2004) identified respiratory illness as the main health outcome related to housing, with the primary factors being cold and damp. With evidence of the health consequences that exist, it is important to understand the influences within housing that cause ill health effects.

Research highlights that persons of poor health are also those most likely to live in poor housing (Smith 1990), but it is difficult to measure the influence of housing on health in the face of other socio-economic and residential structures (Marsh *et al.* 2000; Smith 1990). Moreover, the impacts of poor housing on health can be indirect and often take years to manifest themselves (Marsh *et al.* 2000). Nevertheless, there are a number of studies that show a statistically significant association between poor housing conditions and poor health (Pevalin *et al.* 2008; Acheson 1998; Marsh *et al.* 2000; Miles and Jacobs 2008; Ineichen 1993; Lowry 1991). Marsh *et al.* (2000) concluded that housing deprivation, when controlling for other social factors, arises as a significant variable affecting health. A dose-response relationship exists, in which the longer the exposure to poor housing the greater the effect on a person's health is likely to be (BMA 2003: 25). Furthermore, effects can be seen in adults who experienced poor housing in earlier life much more than those who did not, where both adult groups now live in decent housing; it appears 'history matters' (Marsh *et al.* 1999, 2000; BMA 2003). It can thus be determined that by improving housing for children, not only is health improved directly at the time for the occupants, but that this action will also indirectly decrease the likelihood of those children experiencing poor health later in life.

Poor housing is often encountered alongside other indicators of social disadvantage (Marsh *et al.* 2000), and people who live in poor housing often suffer from many other deprivations that can lead to poor health in their own right (BMA 2003), for example, fuel poverty, whereby the effectiveness of insulation and/or heating provision to the dwelling, linked to the disposable income of the occupiers, is such that in excess of 10 per cent of income has to be spent on effectively heating the home. The joined-up relationship of housing with other environmental impacts can clearly be demonstrated. For example, residential location can be linked to access to health care, as well as environmental hazards such as noise, air pollution, radon, etc. (Smith 1990).

The link between poor health and housing can be dated back to Edwin Chadwick's *Report into the Sanitary Conditions of the Labouring Population of Great Britain* in 1842. This was supported by Friedrich Engels (1845) in *The Conditions of the Working Class in England*. The result of such reports was that health concerns were high on the agenda of all housing legislation towards the end of the nineteenth century (Smith 1990; Malpass and Murie 1999), and the link between housing and health became a recurrent topic for investigation throughout the twentieth century (Marsh *et al.* 2000). Black *et al.* (DHSS, 1980) produced what is now an infamous report on the inequalities that existed in health within the UK, and placed emphasis on decent housing as a prime requisite for health. Yet still, in 1997, it was noted that there had been surprisingly little scientific research carried out (Marsh *et al.* 2000). Towards the end of the twentieth century, the link between housing and health moved up the UK political agenda once more, due mostly to the *Acheson Independent Inquiry into Inequalities in Health* report in 1998 (Marsh *et al.* 2000). Acheson (1998) highlighted housing and the environment as key areas for future policy if inequalities in health were going to be tackled. At this time over 1.5 million properties were estimated not to meet fitness standards required under the Housing Act 1985, and for many already deprived communities, the only available housing was substandard (DETR 2000). The government White Paper *Saving Lives: Our healthier nation* (DoH 1999), identified housing as a key environmental factor affecting public health. The British Medical Association report *Housing and Health: Building for the Future* (BMA 2003) highlighted the true importance of housing in tackling health issues and ensured that health played a pivotal role in the development of all current housing policy (DoH 2005). The Housing Act 2004 identifies and addresses health issues directly related to the home. New enforcement powers for local government, through the Housing Health and Safety Rating System (HHSRS) tackle a range of health influences including: lighting, noise, crowding, heat, cold, damp and mould, and entry by intruders. Evidence from the WHO, described by CIEH (2008), suggests that the most significant housing hazards in the UK are as follows:

- damp
- cold
- falls
- entry by intruders
- crowding and space (particularly in the south of the country and areas with high migrant workforces)
- radon (some parts of the country only)
- fire.

The HHSRS identifies 29 factors that are hazardous to health. Although the first factor, thermal conditions, is largely addressed, with welcome proposals to continue to tackle fuel poverty and improve energy efficiency, the wider hazards to health (such as indoor pollution, space and overcrowding, security, light and noise, infection and accidents) appear to receive less attention, currently.

Although there is undoubtedly a need for more systematic research into which housing interventions have the greatest effects on health and health inequalities, a wide range of studies have now shown health (particularly mental health) improvements following housing improvements such as heating system improvements or installation or eradication of house dust mites.

Social factors

Health can also be affected by social behaviour in the home, for example you might consider smoking in the home a major indoor air pollutant. Influencing behaviour in the home is no easy task; however, it is necessary to consider the many initiatives that are being promoted across the country to encourage smoke-free homes. A focus on indoor pollution should also consider the potential of 'eco-homes' and regulations to reduce the health effects associated with a range of pollutants such as formaldehyde (in MDF, carpets, etc.), volatile organic compounds (in paints and varnishes), house dust mites and so on. Investment in green technologies has the potential to both improve health – by targeting the most vulnerable households – and tackle employment and skills, alongside the environment, by effectively training people to become skilled in using renewable technologies to retrofit existing properties to make them more energy efficient.

The BMA (2003) report identified a number of housing circumstances that impact upon health. These primarily focused on the homes' condition and described the importance of housing to health. They suggested that the health of homeless people – whilst extremely poor – is comparable to that of many tenants in the social and private rented sector, due to high levels of stress, poor diet and living conditions. It is vital to consider the needs of those on low incomes as a particularly vulnerable group in housing terms; other vulnerable groups include women at risk of domestic violence, people with drug/alcohol problems, migrants, asylum seekers and refugees, and people with mental health problems or learning disabilities. The 2005 NICE guidance on housing provides evidence on the potentially negative short-term effects on health of rehousing. This has implications for policy around housing, for example, supporting policies that promote 'lifetime homes', whereby occupants of all sectors are encouraged to remain in their homes as they age, via housing standards which account for mobility and adaptability. This is highly pertinent given the aging population.

Affordability

There are also wider issues linking housing and health which include affordability. A range of estimates have been proposed since the mid 1990s of the number of affordable new homes needed to be built annually in the UK to meet demand, and government policy since 2004 has emphasised increasing housing supply generally, and the level of affordable housing within that. As well as building affordable new homes, affordability can be addressed by schemes such as shared ownership and alliances between local authorities and mortgage lenders. The focus of efforts to achieve the decent homes target has concentrated on social housing until 2010, despite the fact that around 80 per cent of the population reside in the private sector. In 2007, 45 per cent of private rented housing was non-decent (English House Condition Survey). As a consequence, professional bodies active in the field have argued that 'Private sector housing is in danger of being lost in the Government's new agenda of social housing and new build' (CIEH 2008). According to the Department of Communities and Local Government (DCLG), 22 per cent of privately rented homes do not have central heating. Housing policy, the right to buy and the growth of owner occupation have meant that around a half of the poorest sections of society are living in this sector, with no access to the sorts of support that those in social housing receive. The traditional ways and means of characterising poverty via housing tenure have now changed, and we all need to reflect on the implications of this; a focus on health inequalities should not mean that owner occupiers are ignored.

The Green Paper (DCLG 2007) *Homes for the Future: more affordable, more sustainable* took forward recommendations from the Cave (2007) report, an independent review entitled *Every Tenant Matters: A review of social housing regulation* and recognised the need for more affordable housing, but also identified the need for more sustainable and mixed communities. This builds on the issues tackled by the HHSRS to look at the wider determinants of health within the housing community and not just the home itself. Through the Housing and Regeneration Act 2008, the Homes and Communities Agency (HCA) was formed, replacing the Housing Corporation, to provide more social and affordable housing, and to promote regeneration. The HCA is responsible for driving forward the requirements of the 2007 Green Paper, and is the primary regulator of housing associations. Minimising the adverse effects of poor housing is a key challenge for government both nationally and locally, and for all stakeholders (BMA 2003). The recent drive initiated by a focus on the Decent Homes Standard and the Housing Act 2004 has gone a long way in tackling the health issues associated with poor housing, arguably reconnecting public health and housing agendas, but issues of affordability and choice still remain.

THE HOLISTIC APPROACH

The interrelated social issues associated with housing mean that by tackling health issues, other problems such as crime, noise and air pollution, employment and climate change are also addressed. Homes themselves must be recognised as important, but the community in which they are situated is also vital and if housing issues are to be tackled, it is a holistic approach that is required. Corburn (2004: 541) has argued that in much of the developed world:

> public health and urban planning emerged with the common goal of preventing urban outbreaks of infectious disease, but in our lived environments, there appears to be little overlap between the fields today. The separation of the fields has contributed to uncoordinated efforts to address the health of urban populations and a general failure to recognise the links between, for example, the built environment and health disparities facing deprived communities.

Instead of searching for the one cause, we need to understand health disparities as the result of complex and overlapping interactions between, and differences among, population groups in relation to the social, economic and physical conditions in which they live and the resources they have to engage in health-promoting activities. As public health disparities are increasingly understood as a product of social, economic, political and physical inequalities in places – not just between people – the field of urban planning will need to play a more active role in understanding and addressing these health inequities. To paraphrase the words of Corburn (2005: 123), whether or not we can meet the challenges that urban (spatial) health disparities present for research and practice is yet to be determined, but the health of the least well off (and indeed a sustainable future for our modern societies and environments) hangs in the balance. This illustrates where our efforts can be best placed to reduce the burden of the health hazards we all face. The point to be made here is that to seriously address underlying inequalities in health, we need to address the root causes in terms of economic, environmental and social conditions; making individuals stronger to cope with the potential health hazards, whether it be by providing immunisations or additional welfare benefits, will not make the base problems go away. A balanced and equitable distribution of social, economic and environmental benefits will also deliver good health across the whole population. Sustainable development is the ultimate preventative agenda. Health and social care activities must increasingly be understood as the province of practitioners who strive to mitigate conflicts over power and values that arise at the community level.

By way of an example, one can explore how asthma disparities lend themselves to interventions in at least three traditional domains, which can reduce the spatial concentration of health disparities more generally. Corburn (2005) advocates that planning interventions aimed at addressing asthma might be effective public health remedies; approaches should include specific interventions targeted at individual homes, those directed at the entire neighbourhood through land-use planning and even across a region. Sub-standard housing contributes to asthma by concentrating allergens that trigger the disease (Hynes *et al.* 2000). In-home environmental interventions to reduce asthma triggers, such as integrated pest management, can improve asthma outcomes in the short term. One can advocate for physical housing improvements and more affordable housing in neighbourhoods hardest hit by asthma since unaffordable and/or unstable housing also triggers asthma by increasing stress and fear of displacement, homelessness and family safety (Krieger and Higgins 2002). Gentrification and resulting residential displacement can also contribute to asthma through diminished social networks. Planners have long recognised that housing quality, affordability and stability must be linked to changes in regional policy, such as eliminating residential segregation (Massey and Denton 1993) and improving land-use decisions beyond those impacting housing, aspects that might affect preferred transport methods for example. Environmental justice research is important here in revealing that toxic exposures from a range of pollution sources are more likely to be located in poor, minority, inner-city neighbourhoods. Particular premises, while separately only emitting small amounts of toxins, often combine to create cumulative environmental health risks, disproportionately burdening residents of already disadvantaged neighbourhoods. Research has also highlighted that deprived communities often have fewer desirable environmental assets that can promote health, such as parks, access to open space and street trees (Hurley 1995; Pellow 2002).

What might be termed 'walkable neighbourhoods' have a role in building community familiarity and thereby enhancing mental well-being (and also leading to greater potential reliance on the local neighbourhood and increased reduction of travel outside it). A disassociation between home and work can both disrupt an individual's sense of place, as well as contributing to chronic transport problems. Distribution of services (both in type and quality) helps to determine how the built environment supports those who live there in ways that are integral to health. Spatial planning and provision of services interacts with the smaller scale built environment – for example, location of work in relation to housing. Pollution experts tend to see air pollution as merely a problem caused by transport; current evidence from the UK's Local Air Quality Management process shows that whilst transport is the main cause of air pollution, the key determinant of whether people are exposed to harmful levels of pollution is likely to be controlled by buildings – for example, how narrow streets are, as this determines how well the pollution is able to disperse. There is important scope for looking at how health concerns about planning issues can be used to influence very micro-scale planning decisions about the design of individual buildings – such as the set-back distance of the facade from the roadside, accessibility, aesthetics and character, usability of space, noise insulation, etc.

It is particularly important to look at what it is about urban areas that leads to much higher incidences of problems with mental health. Numerous studies have demonstrated the significant impact this can have on physical health – how should mental and physical health impacts and outcomes be weighed against each other? As the built environment contains so many factors involving health, it is vital that we begin to determine ways of valuing and assessing different actions and impacts.

A decent home is one which is wind and weather tight, has modern facilities and can be readily warmed. There has been a change in how the fourth test will be measured. Property now has to have effective insulation and efficient heating to meet this criterion. Anyone who needs to spend more than 10 per cent of their disposable income to achieve the minimum heating standard deemed necessary for a healthy environment (18°C for living rooms, 16°C elsewhere) is fuel poor. There are thought to be around 40,000 extra deaths every winter than would be expected (premature deaths). Of greater concern is the incidence of cold-related illness. The Home Office also says that as well as having a decent home, people need to feel safe and secure in their communities and the Home Office are working jointly with them to coordinate a national drive against anti-social behaviour. The Department of Health says that providing decent housing contributes to their target to narrow the health gap between socio-economic groups and between the most deprived areas and the rest of the country. You need to contrast the rhetoric with the reality. Consultants to the Centre for Regional Economic and Social Research (CRESR) at Sheffield Hallam University used the principles of the HHSRS to estimate the health gains from housing improvement work undertaken by Sheffield Homes Ltd as part of their Decent Homes programme[1]. A similar project was undertaken in Ealing, London.

TOWARDS A MULTIDISCIPLINARY APPROACH

The aim of this chapter was to encourage you to analyse urban and rural living to understand the impact of current national and local policies and to evaluate strategies for the management of the built environment. The overall objective was to promote exploration of the knowledge and skills necessary for effective professional activity in the public health, housing and regeneration fields. A second challenge in reconnecting the fields is developing a coordinated, multidisciplinary approach toward eliminating health disparities. Much recent evidence suggests that disparities in health have not narrowed over time, are getting worse, and are increasingly linked to the physical and social environments that fall under the traditional domain of planning, such as housing, transportation, streetscapes, and community or social capital.

Public health, city planning, and civil engineering evolved together in much of the developed world. At the core of land use planning models was the idea of dividing up functions within the economy (for example, zoning), isolating those functions deemed unhealthy (for example, industry), and placing strict regulations on the kind of contact occurring between people and land use functions. This was aimed at 'immunising' urban populations from the undesirable externalities of the economy, such as industrial pollution. Professionals increasingly implemented public health measures in the mid to latter half of the twentieth century, and the field shifted toward addressing the 'hosts' (for example, individuals) of disease, because the 'environment' (for example, the world outside of micro-organisms) was harder to influence (Tesh 1990). During this era, public health largely ignored the social dimensions of disease and emphasised modifying individual 'risk factors' reflected in one's lifestyle, such as diet, exercise, and smoking (Susser and Susser 1996). Recent efforts have turned to promoting economic development through large infrastructure and transportation projects (Weir 2000). Planning shifted from attempting to restrain harmful 'spillovers' from private market activities in urban areas to promoting suburban economic development (Eishman 2000). Models of economic efficiency have been used in planning new towns, regional approaches were established to provide inexpensive and reliable resources to these areas, and an era of urban divestment and residential segregation took hold. By the latter half of the twentieth century, the biomedical model of disease (which attributes morbidity and mortality to molecular-level pathogens brought about by individual lifestyles, behaviours, hereditary biology, or genetics) was firmly entrenched as the dominant paradigm in epidemiology. Surprisingly, the biomedical model was oriented toward explaining molecular-level pathogenesis rather than explaining the distribution of disease among populations or disease incidence or distribution at a societal level. By the late twentieth century, the fields of planning and public health had moved apart both from their shared original mission of social betterment and from working collaboratively to address the health of urban populations. Urban planning underwent an analogous shift in its orientation toward environmental health by adopting the environmental impact assessment (EIA) process (Duhl *et al.* 2002).

The first challenge facing the recoupling of planning and public health is how to pay increased attention to the public health effects of land use, and places often referred to as the built environment, while simultaneously expanding our definition of planning to include the political processes that produce these outcomes. For example, the fields must develop new methods to understand the effects of the physical and social environment on human health by challenging the 'geographic neutrality' assumptions of most environmental laws. While reconnecting planning and public health will require increased attention to the health effects of plans in geographic places, it will also demand that the field recognise its democratic engagement role in the politics of 'place making'. In August 2008 the WHO Commission on the Social Determinants of Health concluded its work with the publication of a report entitled, *Closing the gap in a generation: Health equity through action on the social determinants of health*. While the Social Inclusion task group of the review acknowledges the need to reduce power inequalities, the reality is that '... holders of such power may relinquish it with reluctance' (Marmot 2009: 110). In relation to housing, the need for a partnership approach to delivering and sustaining healthy housing markets is now acknowledged by most local housing authorities within their local housing strategies. Consequently, what is needed now is political analysis and action. Intersectional scholarship, which analyses the intersections between and the common root causes of class, gender, racial and other inequalities, is the type of analysis required. Among other things it demonstrates that power inequalities need to be addressed by considering the nature of power itself – as opposed to the policies and practices through which it is manifested – in order to achieve lasting impact. This implies consideration of different types of power, their determinants and their distribution within housing systems.

CHAPTER SUMMARY

The overall objective of this chapter was to promote exploration of the knowledge and skills necessary for effective professional activity in the public health, housing and regeneration fields, as a health and social care professional with an appreciation of housing issues. The chapter has argued that it will become increasingly relevant to consider housing as a substantial element of public health and social welfare, and to integrate health aspects into strategies of sustainable housing construction and neighbourhood or urban planning. It has examined the relationship between health, housing and well-being to enable you to understand how potential health impacts associated with the built environment can be addressed, through a range of spatial levels and a consideration of a range of physical, social and economic stressors within the built environment that have the potential to impact upon the health of the public, and how to manage the risks they might pose. From here the focus was expanded to consider the influence and operation of the housing systems and housing policy in enabling society to meet the basic need for shelter within a decent, affordable home for the maximum number of citizens. You should now begin to understand the impact of a complex housing system, including the ability of key players to interact to achieve healthful housing. It is now necessary to explore the potential to deliver better health and well-being through considering the wider health issues associated with place making, and delivering sustainable communities. The intention was to enable you to begin to appreciate the kind of problems faced in practice and to understand the technical issues health and social care professionals might experience when faced with the real world of delivering healthy housing opportunities to communities.

SUMMARY OF MAIN POINTS

You should be able to:

- Discuss the link between housing and health and the role of housing standards and housing professionals in the amelioration of housing related health problems.
- Evaluate the implications of an ageing housing stock to public health.
- Consider current problems in housing that have the potential to affect public health and approaches to ameliorate them.
- Consider key issues, impact on housing and sustainable development.

MOMENT OF REFLECTION

Discussion points

1 Health and housing links are more societal than individual.

   Your discussion should consider both arguments *for* and *against* the statement.

   Current information on the statistical evidence of housing conditions is available from the Department of Communities and Local Government via their website. In April 2008, the English House Condition Survey (EHCS) was integrated with the Survey of English Housing (SEH) resulting in a new survey known as the English Housing Survey (EHS). Like the previous EHCS, it has three component surveys: a household interview, followed by a physical inspection and a market value survey of a subsample of the properties.

2 Consider the need for and role of evidence-based practice in the field of housing, health and social care.

   Good summaries of the impact of housing on physical and mental health are provided in BMA 2003 and Taske *et al.* 2005 (available on the NICE website at: www.publichealth.nice.org.uk).

3   In relation to the pivotal role played by housing in delivering effective public health, and in the light of political and market forces, obtain the housing strategy for an area in which you live or work and evaluate its commitment to promoting health and tackling health inequalities through policies concerned with housing, regeneration and sustainable development at the local level.

NOTE

1   *See* http://www2.warwick.ac.uk/fac/soc/law/research/centres/shhru/sdh_hia_report.pdf Decent Homes

REFERENCES

Acheson, D. (1998) *Independent Inquiry into Inequalities in Health,* London: The Stationery Office.

BMA (2003) *Housing and Health: Building for the Future* [online]. Available at: http://www. bma.org.uk/images/Housinghealth_tcm41–146809.pdf (Accessed 5 April 2009).

Cave, M. (2007) *Every Tenant Matters,* London: HMSO.

CIEH (2008) *Good Housing Leads to Good Health: A toolkit for environmental health practitioners.* London: CIEH.

Corburn, J. (2004) Confronting the challenges in reconnecting urban planning and public health, *American Journal of Public Health,* 94, 541–6.

Corburn, Jason (2005) Urban planning and health disparities: Implications for research and practice, *Planning Practice and Research,* 20 (2), 111–26.

DCLG (2007) *Homes for the future: more affordable, more sustainable,* London: The Stationery Office.

DETR (2000) *English House Conditions Survey,* Department of the Environment, Transport and the Regions, London: HMSO.

DHSS (1980) *Report of the Working Group on Inequalities in Health* (The Black Report), London: DHSS.

DoH (Department of Health) (1999) *Saving Lives: Our healthier nation White Paper* [online]. Cm. 4386. Department of Health, London: The Stationery Office. Available at: http:// www.webarchive.org.uk/wayback/archive/20071016205404/http://www.archive.official-documents.co.uk/document/cm43/4386/4386.htm (Accessed 19 March 2009).

DoH (2005) *Choosing Health: Making healthy choices easier* [online]. Cm. 6374. Available at: http://www.dh.gov.uk/en/Publicationsandstatistics/Publications/PublicationsPolicyAndGuidance/ Browsable/DH_4097491 (Accessed 19 March 2009).

Duhl, L. J. and Sanchez, A. K. (2002) *Healthy cities and the city planning process* [online]. Available at: http://www.who.dk/document/e67843.pdf (Accessed 4 December 2009).

Eishman, R. (2000) (Ed.) *The American Planning Tradition: Culture and Policy,* Washington, DC: Woodrow Wilson Center Press.

Fagan, J. and Davies, G. (2004) The natural history of neighborhood violence, *Journal of Contemporary Criminal Justice,* 20 (2), 127–47.

Fullilove, M. (2003) Neighborhoods and infectious disease, in Kawachi, I. and Berkman, L. F. (Eds) *Neighborhoods and Health,* New York: Oxford University Press, 211–23.

Greenberg, M. and Schneider, D. (1994) Violence in American cities: young Black males is the answer, but what was the question?, *Social Science and Medicine,* 39 (2), 179–87.

Hurley, A. (1995) *Environmental Inequalities: Class, Race, and Industrial Pollution in Gary, Indiana 1945–1980,* Charlotte, NC: University of North Carolina Press.

Hynes, H. P., Brugge, D., Watts, J. and Lally, J. (2000) Public health and the physical environment in Boston public housing: a community-based survey and action agenda, *Planning Practice and Research*, 15 (1/2), 31–49.

Ineichen, B. (1993) *Homes and Health: how homes and health interact*, London: E. & F.N. Spon.

Krieger, J. and Higgins, D. L. (2002) Housing and health: time again for public health action, *American Journal of Public Health*, 92, 758–68.

Lowry, S. (1991) *Housing and Health*, London: British Medical Journal.

Malpass, P. and Murie, A. (1999) *Housing Policy and Practice* (5th edition), Basingstoke: Macmillan.

Marmot, M. (2009) *Social Determinates of Health*, London: HMSO.

Marsh, A., Gordon, D., Heslop, P. and Pantazis, C. (1999) *Home sweet home? The impact of poor housing on health*, Bristol: The Policy Press.

Marsh, A., Gordon, D., Heslop, P. and Pantazis, C. (2000) Housing deprivation and health: a longitudinal analysis, *Housing Studies*, 15, 411–28.

Massey, D. S. and Denton, N. A. (1993) *American Apartheid: Segregation and the Making of the Underclass*, Cambridge, MA: Harvard University Press.

Miles, R. and Jacobs, D.E. (2008) Future Directions in Housing and Public Health: Findings from Europe with Broader Implications for Planners, *Journal of the American Planning Association*, 74 (1), 77–89.

Pellow, D. (2002) *Garbage Wars: The Struggle for Environmental Justice in Chicago*, Cambridge, MA: MIT Press.

Pevalin, D. J., Taylor, M. P. and Todd, J. (2008) The Dynamics of Unhealthy Housing in the UK: A Panel Data Analysis, *Housing Studies*, 23 (5), 679–95.

Shaw, M. (2004) Housing and public health, *Annual Review of Public Health* [online], 25, 397–418. Available at: http://web.ebscohost.com/ehost/pdf?vid=2&hid=4&sid=91defdbf-c50e-4348-ab94-8fca64930b0f%40SRCSM2 (Accessed 1 April 2009).

Smith, S. J. (1990) Health Status and the Housing System, *Social Science and Medicine*, 31, 753–62.

Susser, S. and Susser, E. (1996) Choosing a future for epidemiology: I. Eras and paradigms. *American Journal of Public Health*, 86, 668–73.

Taske, N., Taylor, L., Mulvihill, C. and Doyle, N. (2005) *Housing and public health: a review of reviews of interventions for improving health – Evidence briefing*, London: Health Development Agency.

Tesh, S. (1990) *Hidden Arguments: Political Ideology and Disease Prevention Policy*, New Brunswick, NJ: Rutgers University Press.

Wallace, D. and Wallace, R. (1998) *A Plague on Your Houses: How New York Was Burned Down and National Public Health Crumbled*, New York: Verso.

Weir, M. (2000) Planning, environmentalism and urban poverty, in Fishman, R. (Ed.) *The American Planning Tradition: Culture and Policy*, Washington, DC: Woodrow Wilson Center Press, pp. 193–215.

World Health Organization (2004) *Review of evidence on housing and health*, background document EUR/04/5046267/BD/1, 28 April 2004, presented at the Fourth Ministerial Conference on Environment and Health, Budapest, Hungary 23–5 June 2004.

FURTHER READING

Blackman, T. (2006) *Placing Health: Neighbourhood renewal, health improvement and complexity*, Bristol: The Policy Press.

Lupton, R. (2003) *Poverty Street. The dynamics of neighbourhood decline and renewal*, Bristol: The Policy Press.

Power, A. and Houghton, J. (2007) *Jigsaw Cities: Big Places, Small Spaces*, Bristol: The Policy Press.

USEFUL WEBSITES

Academy for Sustainable Communities:
  http://www.ascskills.org.uk/

Commission for Architecture and the Built Environment:
  http://www.cabe.org.uk/

Department for Communities and Local Government:
  http://www.communities.gov.uk/

Institute for Community Cohesion:
  http://www.cohesioninstitute.org.uk/

Institute for Public Policy Research:
  http://ippr.org.uk/

New Economics Foundation:
  http://www.neweconomics.org/gen/

The Joseph Rowntree Foundation is an important funder of research in this area of social science and their website contains excellent reports and summary findings:
  http://www.jrf.org.uk/

PART 3

CHAPTER 15

GLOBALIZATION AND HEALTH AND SOCIAL CARE

ADAM BARNARD

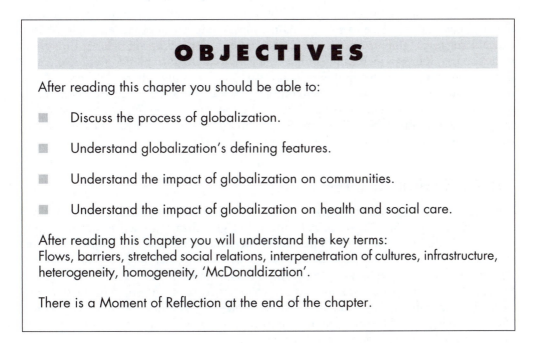

OBJECTIVES

After reading this chapter you should be able to:

- Discuss the process of globalization.

- Understand globalization's defining features.

- Understand the impact of globalization on communities.

- Understand the impact of globalization on health and social care.

After reading this chapter you will understand the key terms:
Flows, barriers, stretched social relations, interpenetration of cultures, infrastructure, heterogeneity, homogeneity, 'McDonaldization'.

There is a Moment of Reflection at the end of the chapter.

INTRODUCTION

This chapter aims to provide some contextual discussion on areas of health and social care practice. The current situation in the modern industrialized world is strongly built upon the processes that have become known as globalization. The following discussion looks at the dimensions of globalization and the processes associated with it, and the impact this has had on health and social care theory and practice. Globalization is framed in the context of current international policy and market pressures for trade and investment liberalization in health and social care services (UNRIGD 2007).

GLOBALIZATION

Children as young as two recognize the golden arches of McDonalds. Starbucks, Disney, Nike and Adidas have become global brands that are instantly recognizable and have permeated every high street and home. The Nike 'swooshstika' is reportedly the most requested tattoo in North America (Klein 2004). Political events from around the world are reported immediately, for example, 9/11 or the Asian tsunami. We mostly use Microsoft products on computers and most of us have shopped in a Wal-Mart store. The argument is that a process of globalization has led to distinct changes in our everyday life. Drugs, crime, sex, war, protest, terrorism, disease, people, ideas, images, news, information, entertainment, pollution, goods and money all travel the globe (Held 2004). Consequently, health and social care theory and practice have increasingly needed to become aware of, and respond to, the challenges of globalization.

In terms of culture (Hopper 2007), society (Barnett *et al.* 2005), politics (Bayart 2007) and economics (Held and Kaya 2006; Kaplinsky 2005) – rapid and dramatic changes have taken place due to globalization. Wikipedia, a good example of this process suggests 'globalization' (or 'globalisation', depending on which globalized term you use) refers to increasing global connectivity, integration and interdependence in the economic, social, technological, cultural, political and ecological spheres. What does this suggest to us about the contemporary world? How are we to understand this process? What impact does this have on health and social care? What does this mean for globalized communities? What challenges and opportunities does it raise for social care and helping professions in the twenty-first century?

WHAT'S GOING ON?

There is no question that the world is currently undergoing significant and profound acceleration in the process of globalization, but globalization itself is not new. For example, trade has existed for millennia between areas such as the Roman Empire, Arabia and China. The movement of peoples has a long, rich and troubled history. Knowledge, science, technology and culture have always been global throughout history. New forms of communication have emerged from the spoken, written and printed word, numerical systems or new technologies of communication such as the Victorian telegraph. However, many commentators would suggest we are now witnessing a qualitatively different set of processes.

Globalization although not new, has achieved unprecedented heights in the last half of the twentieth century and has accelerated further in the early twenty-first century. That dramatic growth has led to much work in many different fields on the topic of globalization and there have been many efforts to define it. Held (2004) suggests globalization involves four dimensions. The first dimension is social relations so stretched that cultural, economic and political networks are connected across the world. For example, different and dispersed communities are part of global 'diasporas' of peoples stretched beyond any nation or locality. Communities are constituted across territorial boundaries. Families can keep touch with relatives in Pakistan, India, China, Australia and Africa. Gilroy explores black people's experience in the 'black Atlantic' (Gilroy 1992) and the Jewish diaspora suggests that this aspect of globalization is nothing new. Health and social care theory and practice increasingly needs to recognize the significance of stretched social relations. For example, family members involved in receiving health and social care services may be in different countries, with different expectations and cultural understandings of health and social care. Diverse and heterogeneous cultural needs must be addressed by health and social care services. European enlargement has meant that health services are seeing increased use by migrant populations. Social care services are benefiting from older relatives moving to the UK to care for a new generation of children born to migrant communities.

The second dimension of globalization is an intensification of flows of interaction so that instant communication is available to many (if you have access to the mass media, TV, internet or telephone). Trade and commerce, entertainment, news and media, sport, art and culture are all experienced rapidly and in a far greater volume than before. Information on health and social care is communicated instantly so far flung, localized events take on a global significance, for example, the 'swine flu' epidemic of 2009. The relative success of web-based National Health Service information has been well received by most users.

The third dimension is the increasing interpenetration of distant cultures and events as societies come face to face with each other. For example, Bollywood films, the diversity of food available, the global recognition of brands such as Coke, Disney, Microsoft and McDonalds, suggests this interpenetration of culture. Events such as 9/11 show how we are influenced and affected by geographically distant and remote events. Health and social care services, theory and practice have needed to respond positively to transcultural understanding and action in the design and delivery of services.

Finally, the fourth dimension is the emergence of global infrastructures to support and drive these changes. The internet is often identified as a key emerging infrastructure that supports stretched social relations, intensified communication and brings people and places closer together, although in an uneven and divided way (Drori 2006). The emergence of 'health tourism' where people travel to, and access, health and social care services from global providers has been a recent development. So how might we summarize these changes and these processes?

TOWARDS A DEFINITION

Ritzer defines globalization as 'an accelerating set of processes involving flows that encompass ever greater numbers of the world's spaces and that lead to increasing integration and interconnectivity among those spaces' (Ritzer 2004). Giddens (2002) refers to these processes as a 'runaway world' and McLuhan and Powers (1989) speak of the 'global village'. Woodward (2003: 171) suggests globalization is:

> a social, cultural, political and economic phenomenon, which is subject to many different interpretations, ranging from those who see its impact as minimal and nothing new, to globalists or globalizers who argue that it is a recent and very significant phenomenon which has transformed life across the world. Some read this as a positive experience whilst others see it as having disastrous effects on local communities and those outside the western, especially US, mainstream. Most commentators agree that it has had some transforming impact.

Globalization transforms our everyday lives, from minor considerations of what to have for dinner to major world changing events. It involves social, economic, political, cultural and environmental processes and is characterized by conflict (such as terrorism and war) as well as consensus (such as communication and entertainment). It is also characterized by a weakening of boundaries of nation states (Woodward 2003: 137). Events in one country are no longer isolated, such as the fall of the Berlin Wall, pollution or natural disasters. All have far reaching effects that are transnational and global. Health and social care is not immune from these transformations and a globalized system of services and service users has emerged in response to these processes.

Another area that demands attention with globalization is the fact that it is divided between winners and losers. 'Positive globalizers' see everyone benefiting from the expansion of globalization, whilst 'negative globalizers' see losers missing out on the benefits and suffering increased exploitation. Global networks and flows operate differently for different groups of people and communities. Debates around class, 'race', gender, age, sexuality and disability, so often central to health and social care have been subsumed or marginalized in the mainstream of globalization (Adam 2002). For example, Saskia Sassen (2002) argues that in global cities (such as London, Tokyo and New York) most of the daily servicing jobs are carried out by women, immigrants and people from minority ethnic groups (often the same person). Health and social care provision is often delivered by a similar person.

Globalization allegedly presents opportunities of greater democracy and participation such as through the internet but this technology remains dominated by the wealthy areas of the world. There is rapid transmission of information, easy access for individuals and communities and new opportunities for ideas, markets, democracy and choice. However, speed is of more importance to rich nations and it is this very speed that leads us into a rapid and manic sense of consciousness where we often fail to reflect on the consequences of the impulse of the immediate or consequences of our actions. Health and social care is caught in trying to respond positively and appropriately to these impulses. Ideas can be censured, choice is restricted to global brands and products, and democracy can be blocked, stifled or monitored. Globalization has allowed easier movement of people across the globe but migration is often blocked for many refugees and migrants – migration is often economically driven and exploitation remains and deepens. Health and social care services have been reconstituted in terms of who accesses services and who provides these services. Any economic benefits of globalization need to be extended across all countries to challenge the health divides between rich and poor nations, economic benefits need to be translated into health benefits, adverse effects of globalization on population-level health influences (for example, on tobacco marketing and cross-border transmission of infectious disease) must be minimized, and globalization's change of infrastructures needs to recognize health provision (Woodward et al. 2001). Changes and reduction in health and social care services have often been motivated by a perceived need to reduce social provision, with a view to becoming more competitive within the global economy (Deacon 2000).

GLOBALIZATION AND COMMUNITIES

Let us consider just a few examples of money, communication, 'sameness' (homogeneity) and consumption with special emphasis on their impact on community (the discussion that follows draws heavily on the work of Appadurai (1996) and his sense of global 'scapes'). Vast sums of money circulate around the world through government treasuries, banks, brokerage houses and so on. However, most of this flow of money is largely invisible to us, although it can have a profound effect on us. The focus throughout this chapter is the impact of globalization on health and social care and communities, so how do global flows of money affect them? In many ways, of course, but one of the most important effects occurs when global traders in money decide that the currency of a given nation is overvalued. The result is a decline in the value of that currency with devastating effects on whole societies (for example, several East Asian countries in 1997; Argentina in 2002), as well as most communities within them. Buying power declines as local currencies are devalued. Jobs are lost and increasing numbers find themselves out of work and short of money. The community suffers in various ways without any control over the process. Globally, the poor are at risk from globalization.

Let us also consider communication. Some commentators have suggested the world has become 'flat' (Friedman 2005) due to the horizontal and less hierarchical forms of communication available, and it is the case that a far wider range of people are capable of communicating their views and getting out their messages. We can become aware of Chinese struggles for democracy, the living conditions for Iraqi people or popular protest in South America. This can have a salutary effect on communities which are able to get their views out and to have them reaffirmed by others scattered throughout the world. That said, the reverse is the case because those who seek to destroy a community can use the same media to organize and carry out their destructive activities. Terrorism, crime, drugs have all benefited from globalization. This suggests that the world has not become anything approaching flat (Friedman 2005) as there are still great inequalities, barriers to equal participation and dangers in all sorts of things, including the internet.

A major issue in globalization, as discussed by Ritzer (2004, 2005) is the degree to which it is related to growing homogeneity (becoming the same or 'sameness') or sustained heterogeneity (being diverse and different). This has great implications for communities since the latter would imply the continued survival and vitality of diverse and distinct communities while the former would involve a loss of distinctiveness among communities that would increasingly grow to look more and more alike.

'McDonaldization' is the process by which the principles of the fast food restaurant are affecting more and more sectors of society and more and more societies around the world (Ritzer 2004). It is the latter, of course, that makes this a globalizing process. The idea that more sectors of society and more societies around the globe are being affected by, and are adopting, the *same* principles (for example, efficiency) means that McDonaldization *tends* to be associated with increasing homogenization. At a most basic level many communities around the world look increasingly alike because so many of them have one, or more, McDonald's restaurants (there are over 30,000 of them, most outside the USA), to say nothing of many of its clones in the fast food business (for example, Burger King, KFC, etc.). McDonaldization can have a significant impact on health and social care issues. For example, the rise of obesity and particularly childhood obesity, partly due to increased consumption of fast food, is becoming a major area for concern for health care providers. Fast food has also decreased the social and community involvement of meal times. More generally, more and more organizations operate on basically the same principles, so we can talk about things like 'McUniversities', 'McDoctors', 'McPharmacies' and 'McChurches'. Ritzer (2004) ably discusses the McDonaldization of life and death, where health and social care services such as invitro fertilization are becoming more common place and the use of euthanasia clinics as well as a sanitized and efficient process of funeral has brought McDonald's principles to the end of life.

As powerful as the process of McDonaldization may be, it is a long way from arriving at homogeneous communities, and from wiping out community diversity. Much remains different about communities from one area of a given nation to another, to say nothing of one part of the world to another. Furthermore, McDonaldization produces enemies and counter reactions that lead to more, rather than, less diversity. Individuals, groups, communities and even large global organizations such as Slow Food based in Italy have mounted significant opposition to McDonald's and McDonaldization. Slow Food is particularly important in this regard for its defence of distinctive cities (Slow Cities), local communities, and traditional food and other products. For example, in his defence of locally produced food, José Bové, a modest agricultural farmer, has become an international icon of resistance to global capitalism (Bové and Dufour 2005). The recent global debate on the provision of health care has seen the value of localized provision and the health and social care failing of the USA.

However, there is a deeper kind of homogeneity in the sense that more people become ever more deeply enmeshed in consumer culture. This means that consumption becomes increasingly important to them, perhaps becoming the centre of their lives. We can enjoy sun-dried Italian tomatoes, drinking American cola on Ikea settees whilst watching *Big Brother*. There is a threat to heterogeneity when local, diverse products and practices are eroded by a global consumer culture. Would you rather have cheap standardized shoes made in sweatshop conditions in a distant country by child labour or a bespoke pair of handmade shoes by a local artisan? If the global economy had not made the former so cheap, we might all prefer the latter. These threats to heterogeneity and diversity include communities that grow to be increasingly oriented to satisfying and expediting consumption and which all start to resemble each other. A similar position can be raised in health and social care. The homogeneity of provision has led to a standardized and monolithic provision of services whilst heterogeneity has emerged as a transcultural need from service user groups.

Those who want to sustain communities and their diversity will want to oppose much of what is described above. Heterogeneity at many levels is what makes life and communities interesting and rewarding. Threats to that heterogeneity are regarded by many as leading to less interesting and meaningful lives. More importantly, control shifts from inside the community to external powers that then have the capacity to alter or even destroy that community (as Wal-Mart or Tesco have famously done on a number of occasions). Even more tangibly, these organizations are essentially in the business of making money and very often they do so by exploiting communities and their people, as well as by taking profits to another community, perhaps even to another nation (Klein 2004). All of this can leave a community greatly impoverished, economically, politically and culturally. In terms of health and social care, the control of Big Pharma has seen the provision of certain types of service and the neglect of others. The World Health Organization (WHO) established the Commission on Social Determinants of Health (CSDH) in 2005, on the premise that action on social determinant of health is the fairest and most effective way to improve health for all people and reduce inequalities brought about by globalization.

However, we must not forget that globalization is *not* a one-way street; a unidimensional process. Just as many things flow into any given community, many things flow out, as well. More importantly, globalization can have many positive effects on many things, including communities. Many communities have been greatly enhanced by the entrance of global businesses, the global media, global sports teams, and the like. In assessing the impact of globalization we need to look at *both* a community's gains and its losses. Positive commentators have suggested it is not clear that anything needs to be done about globalization in general, but it is clear that communities need to seek out that which enhances them and to block the entrance of that which threatens them and their integrity, or to limit its impact if it cannot be blocked.

THE FUTURE OF HEALTH AND SOCIAL CARE PROFESSIONS

What of the future? It seems clear that globalization is here to stay and the future will bring an acceleration of it and its effects on everything, including communities and health and social care services. There will certainly continue to be many positives associated with this process, but it is also the case that negatives will continue as well. The thrust of this discussion leads us to worry that the negatives will come to outweigh the positives. After all, the great power and a disproportionate share of the wealth are on the side of the forces that support McDonaldization, consumerism and homogenity. In confrontations with most communities, they have the upper hand (although there are certainly instances where the community 'David' has slain the corporate 'Goliath'). Thus, it is hard to envision a bright future for communities, at least as we have traditionally thought of them. A highly McDonaldized community, one in which much of what transpires is centrally conceived, controlled, and lacking in distinctive content, is a long way from what we have thought of (perhaps over-romantically) as community. We will need to rethink what we may mean by community, but this is far less of a problem than being forced to abandon communities to the larger forces that seek to eviscerate them and to profit from denuding them of what makes them unique and special.

Similarly, the rise in the movement of people is a positive force of migration for more diverse communities such as in the enlargement of the EU, but also presents a bleaker picture of an increase in trafficking, dispossessed populations and the growth of excluded diasporas.

There can be distinctly advantageous bi-products to globalization: the sharing of customs, traditions, ways of life, increased variety and richness in culture, entertainment, sport and the arts, and breaking down of territorial boundaries and insular mentalities. It can give us a vibrant, diverse, dynamic and independent culture that draws from a multitude of sources. On the other hand, globalization can give us a homogenized culture. Cities appear the same with uniform chain stores, global brands and supermarkets. We relax watching Disney films or the insipid Endemol format of *Big Brother*. It can give us a lifeless, alike, static, consumer culture imposed from corporate sources. This suggests we are in a contemporary era of globalization, understood as a positive and negative process that has substantial and significant impact on communities and health and social care wherever they may be.

For health and social care, and the helping services, both positive and negative globalization presents a huge range of challenges. For example, child protection issues are now global concerns with trafficking, exploitation, sex tourism and abuse increasingly coordinated across national boundaries. Adult care services need to account for and be mindful of global dimensions to care, such as respecting and valuing diversity of peoples and culture, and respecting links to geographically distant communities. However, few commentators have focused on how globalization has impacted on health and social care practice. Dominelli and Hoogvelt (1996) demonstrate the significance of globalization on the process of intervention and the labour process in health and social care. As a result of global market forces, needs-led assessments and relationship building have given way to budget-led assessments, increased managerial control over practitioners and bureaucratized procedures for handling consumer complaints. These changes seek to reorient health and social care away from its commitment to holistic provisions and social justice towards technocratic competencies of homogenized and bureaucratic responses. Globalization adds to the pressure for health and social care to abandon its historic mission to promote equality and social justice. It can also accelerate the breakdown of communities and lead to aggravated social problems amongst marginalized and excluded groups.

Dominelli (2007) explores the opportunities and constraints that the dynamics of globalization present for human development in a range of different countries and situations. Arguing that globalization is currently a system of organizing social relations along neoliberal lines, Dominelli examines practical examples of how people respond to significant social changes in their communities. Globalization has collapsed the boundaries of time, space and place in ways that have exacerbated inequalities, at the same time giving rise to unparalleled riches for some and the illusion of equality for all (after all, everyone, at least in the developed world, can commune with a Big Mac).

The challenge to the globalized health and social care worker is to retain the humanity, holism, justice and opportunities that globalization can bring, whilst protecting communities from exploitation and inequalities. Beckett and Maynard (2005) suggest that helping professions, generally, deal with people who in one way or other are marked as different and are, to various degrees, excluded from mainstream society. The challenge for health and social care and helping professions is to operate in a way which, as far as possible, challenges and reduces that exclusion, rather than in a way that confirms and legitimizes it. The danger of the McDonaldization of health and social care in a 'globalized' world is a challenge that is ever more important and central to health and social care and helping professions.

SUMMARY OF MAIN POINTS

You should be able to:

- Discuss the process of globalization.
- Understand globalization's defining features.
- Understand the impact of globalization on communities.
- Understand the impact of globalization on health and social care.

MOMENT OF REFLECTION

1   Consider when you have thought about the global process of health and social care (for example, health and social care services on holiday, holiday tourism, the health and social care of friends and family not in this country). What issues does this raise? What would be the most effective way of dealing with them?

2   Would you be happy with American style health and social care provision? (For example, most American health care is provided by private insurance companies.)

3   Watch Michael Moore's film, *Sicko*.

4   Think about the impact globalization has on your life, the life of your community, and the services that you and your community use. Would you see this as positive or negative?

REFERENCES

Adam, B. (2002) The gendered time politics of globalization: of shadowlands and elusive justice, *Feminist Review*, 70: 3–29.

Appadurai, A. (1996) *Modernity at Large: Cultural Dimensions of Globalization*, Minneapolis: University of Minnesota Press.

Barnett, A., Held, D. and Henderson, Caspar (2005) *Debating Globalization*, Cambridge: Polity Press in association with openDemocracy.

Bayart, F. (2007) *Governance of the World*, Cambridge: Polity Press.

Beckett, C. and Maynard, A. (2005) *Values and Ethics in Social Work: An Introduction*, London: Sage.

Bové, J. and Dufour, F. (2005) *Food for the Future: Agriculture for a Global Age*, Cambridge: Polity Press.

Deacon, B. (2000) Eastern European welfare states: the impact of the politics of globalization, *Journal of European Social Policy*, 10 (2), 146–61.

Dominelli, L. (2007) (Ed.) *Revitalising Communities in a Globalising World*, London: Ashgate.

Dominelli, L. and Hoogvelt, A. (1996) Globalization and the technocratization of social work, *Critical Social Policy*, 16 (47), 45–62.

Drori, G. (2006) *Global E-Litism: Digital Inequality, Social Inequality, and Transnationality*, NY: Worth.

Friedman, T. (2005) *The World is Flat: A Brief History of the Twenty-First Century*, NY: Farrar, Straus and Giroux.

Giddens, A. (1999) *Runaway World: The BBC Reith Lectures*, London: BBC.

Giddens, A. (2002) *Runaway World: The Reith lectures* (2nd edition), London: Profile Books.

Gilroy, P. (1992) *The Black Atlantic: Modernity and Double Consciousness*, London: Verso.

Held. D. (2004) *A Globalising World?: culture, economics, politics* (2nd edition), London: Open University Press.

Held, D. and Kaya, A. (2006) *Global Inequality: A Comprehensive Introduction*, Cambridge: Polity Press.

Hopper, P. (2007) *Understanding Cultural Globalization*, Cambridge: Polity Press.

Kaplinsky, R. (2005) *Globalization, Poverty and Inequality: Between a Rock and a Hard Place*, Cambridge: Polity Press.

Klein, N. (2004) *No Logo; no space, no jobs, no choice; taking aim at the brand bullies*. London: Flamingo.

McLuhan, M. and Powers, B. R. (1989) *The Global Village: Transformations in World Life and Media in the 21st Century*, Oxford: Oxford University Press.

Ritzer, G. (2004) *The McDonaldization of Society* (Revised New Century Edition), Thousand Oaks, CA: Pine Forge Press.

Ritzer, G. (2005) *Enchanting a Disenchanted World: Revolutionizing the Means of Consumption*, Thousand Oaks, CA: Pine Forge Press.

Sassen, S. (2002*) Globalization and the Discontents: Essays on the New Mobilities of People and Money*, New York: The New Press.

United Nations Research Institute for Global Development (UNRIGD) (2007) *Commercialization of Health Care: Global and Local Dynamics and Policy Responses*, Geneva: UN.

Woodward, D., Drager, N., Beaglehole, R. and Lipson, D. (2001) Globalization and Health: a framework for analysis and action, *Bull World Health Organ* 79, 9, 875–81.

Woodward, K. (2003) *Social Sciences: the Big Issues,* Buckingham: Open University Press.

CHAPTER 16

CONTEMPORARY APPROACHES TO LEADERSHIP AND MANAGEMENT

ADRIAN M. CASTELL

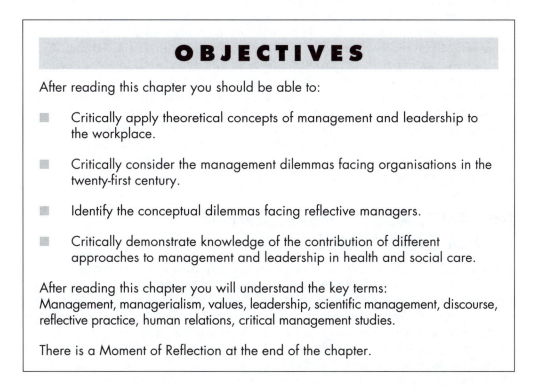

OBJECTIVES

After reading this chapter you should be able to:

■ Critically apply theoretical concepts of management and leadership to the workplace.

■ Critically consider the management dilemmas facing organisations in the twenty-first century.

■ Identify the conceptual dilemmas facing reflective managers.

■ Critically demonstrate knowledge of the contribution of different approaches to management and leadership in health and social care.

After reading this chapter you will understand the key terms:
Management, managerialism, values, leadership, scientific management, discourse, reflective practice, human relations, critical management studies.

There is a Moment of Reflection at the end of the chapter.

INTRODUCTION

The term management is often accepted as having a fixed meaning, shared by members of an organisation and generally uncontested. Images of managers and their forms of action are now deeply embedded in our culture and shape the way we speak about what they do and what we think about what it is to manage. To be a manager, or to act as a manager, suggests a coherent, understood and rational repertoire of skills and knowledge applied to interacting with people in organisations. We will see over the course of this chapter that thinking about what management is and does isn't simple. We will therefore be 'problema-tising' management. This is a term used by some social scientists, not to express something negative, but rather the opposite, as a necessary precondition to genuinely engaging with, and getting behind, what a term or concept really means.

This chapter introduces the concept of management, sets out some key stages in its historical development, indicating how it has changed and illustrates its application in the field of health and social care. However, this is not the main point of the chapter. There are many well written and informative textbooks available which introduce and explain issues such as leadership, organisational behaviour, human resources and postmodern approaches to management, etc., in much more detail than presented here. This chapter seeks to do something different and so only provides a rather loose introduction to the changing management schools of thought. As suggested in the opening paragraph, the idea of management is not fixed or generally accepted, and we will be looking at some of the criticisms that have been made of management theory and practice as well as some of the potential implications flowing from the debates these critiques have engendered.

Such criticisms are particularly germane in the context of an increasing public awareness of failures in management and leadership in health and social care. In the social care arena in particular, problems are not limited to slumps in sales, marketing mistakes or to abstract targets, but have the potential to impact real lives in complex, significant and profound ways. Management failures in the arena of social care are writ large in the popular imagination (from Baby 'P' and Victoria Climbie, Alder Hey Hospital, to the NHS computerised medical record system). We hope that by reading and understanding the material in this chapter you will be better placed to interpret the roots of, and identify for yourself, issues arising from a critical understanding of management, in preparation for your own effective action and intervention.

THE LANGUAGE OF MANAGEMENT AND ORGANISATIONS

It would be difficult to conceive of a life that is not shaped, even dominated by organisa-tions. For most people in developed economies, organisations provide the context for their working lives, their interaction with state service provision and, increasingly, their leisure activities. Organisations are managed, well or otherwise, against a backdrop of constant change, both in terms of the way that people work together and the means that they use, whether it be labelled as 'modernisation', 'restructuring', 'technological advance', or as genuinely framing new possibilities of working that technology may provide (Castells 1999). However, beneath the visible manifestations of such changes often lie unspoken assumptions of what it is to manage and to be a manager, which may be very different things. We will see in this chapter how the forms of change promoted within health and social care increasingly employ and redeploy, borrow and develop a form of language from the business arena, together with the assumptions that this type of language brings with it. Bound up with the use of 'managerial' forms of language is the concept of 'mana-gerialism' itself which rests on certain assumptions about how the world is organised.

Before we return to issues of language and managerialism later in the chapter we will start our journey with previous work on understanding the operation of work based organisations. This is because understanding the approaches, procedures and processes that organisations use to manage people at work and the reasons why people in organisations may behave as they do, plays a crucial role in our effectiveness and well-being at work. Lastly, we will consider issues around the idea of management as a profession, what professions themselves are about, and their relationship with allied and ancillary professions.

In covering the material on management in this way, we hope that you will find answers to existing questions you may have about management and also a corpus of information from which to generate further informed questions about management. Whilst health and social care are very different environments, structurally and culturally, and are subject to different regulatory regimes, the themes presented below are visible in, and common to, both. Whether you are actively considering a career in management, are currently being managed, or like many people find yourself 'acting' in this role, management cannot be avoided. However, developing your knowledge and understanding of management issues, complex or straightforward, will serve to underpin effective action in this underrepresented area of health and social care.

Therefore, in line with the principles reflected in the other chapters of this book, we consider that management is a learning activity and those who practise management can improve their skills by adopting a critical approach to their practice and by engaging in reflective practice.

THE BACKDROP: DEFINING MANAGEMENT

As work in health and social care becomes increasingly specialised the concomitant demands on communication structures increase and the interdependencies between agencies are brought into sharp relief. Modern management is typically considered to be about trying to ensure that interdependencies are organised in such a way as to bring value to the social processes of productive work. By 'social' we are referring to activities involving people, taking place in a particular context, a context which itself is affected by social phenomenon (such as previous failings or the 'credit crunch'). By 'value' we mean something extra that emerges from a transformation, which may be expressed in terms of goods or services and is deemed as such by some stakeholders.

We can begin to get a flavour of the later discussions about the importance of words, of language, in expressing exactly what we mean (or don't mean) by noting that value has a *relative* meaning, that is, what can be considered valuable by one person or set of people (stakeholders) may not be seen so by others. It is this dynamic and contextually located shifting of meanings that we will see emerge as powerful and ubiquitous in this chapter.

Nevertheless, we can all readily conceive of organisations that we think are *well run,* meaning well managed, that is they are providing value to a variety of stakeholders, in perhaps a variety of different ways, such as a hospital or social service department. It is equally easy to think of organisations that are badly managed, and what characterises them can be considered their failure in providing value. However, whilst the notion of value here may provide one index of 'good' management, might there be others? Has the purpose of management always been about 'value', and whose values are 'core', whose 'shared', and whose privileged? We will address these questions in the next section which charts the main waves in management thinking in Europe and the USA over the past 80 or so years.

MANAGEMENT THEORY – A HISTORICAL DASH

Even a cursory look at the proliferation of textbooks covering 'management' provides the reader with a sense of the difficulty of precisely defining this elusive concept (for example, Boddy 2005, Linstead *et al.* 2004, Cole 1998). There are, however, commonalities that emerge from a historical accretion of ideas about management which afford us a coherent way of seeing the development of management thinking. Such a historical perspective typically involves the identification of different stages in the focus of attention of, primarily Western, researchers.

It is informative to consider who was doing the research, and the context in which this story evolves. We can identify two types of writers at the start of the journey, writers based, for the most part, in Europe and the USA. First, those thoughtful managers who reflected on what was happening in their organisations (notable manager-theorists including F. W. Taylor, L. F. Urwick and Henri Fayol) and second, social scientists who undertook formal studies as part of their professional work (for example, Elton Mayo, Abraham Maslow, Douglas McGregor and Fredrick Hertzberg).

The former tended to work inductively, that is to rationalise and make sense of the experiences of being a manager in ways that were organised, or systematised, or which served to regularise patterns of behaviours. In other words it helped them (and others) make sense of their world.

Social scientists on the other hand were more interested in pursuing a way of interpreting and understanding how management actions shape the way that organisations work, by employing the tools of their scientific trade. Perhaps the clearest expression of this form of work is in Mayo's famous Hawthorne Studies in the 1920s, which are often claimed to be the foundation of what is now understood to be organisational behaviour.

The output of both of these two early styles of writers on management differed in their focus. Often labelled the classical school of thought, the practising managers were interested in creating a coherent set of 'rational', in other words scientific, principles which concentrated on the structuring of activities in the work place. Social scientists on the other hand were, as their title suggests, more interested in what humans did, in other words their behaviour.

Scientific managers were primarily concerned with the efficient use of resources, whereas social scientists were broadly interested in a range of human factors, including motivation (what drives people to do what they do), communication, the nature of communication in organisations, and later, what leaders do that makes them leaders. This is why they have been termed human relations theorists: scientists who took as their starting point interrelationships between people and the individuals themselves.

Whilst both sets of early investigators shared commonalities in the rationale for their endeavour and writing, this distinction endures and remains visible. Heavy tomes on management theory by social and managerial 'scientists' continue to fail in the fight for virtual shelf space in bookshops across the globe against books written by professional management consultants and practitioners eager to encourage others to benefit from the remarkable and informative insights that they developed by being 'successful' managers. The echoes of these two approaches, or 'academic lenses', as we will see, still reverberate throughout the literature. It is worth expanding on some tenets, that is the basic assumptions, of the classical school. What was of prime importance here was not the cog in the machine but the machine itself, in other words how organisations could and should be structured to maximise profit and improve worker efficiency. This was no idealised utopian daydream but a considered and systematic attempt to derive and apply genuine scientific principles. The most important early contributor to this school of thought was Frederick W. Taylor, considered to be the founder of scientific management whose approach to making organisations effective was improving efficiency at the 'operative' level, and therefore in contrast with Fayol's focus on the top management level. Taylor believed that a 'best way' of completing a task could be identified and used as the basis for calculating a fair day's pay for a fair day's work, in his view, and importantly, obviating the need for conflict between 'management and men'. The scientific school of management (Sheldrake 1996) brings together four interconnected elements: the systematic analysis of the process of production; the selection of appropriate workers and the training to become a 'first class man' at that task; the forging of a genuine connection between a science at work and a science of work; and a continuous and close cooperation between management and workers.

Scientific management, together with Weber's bureaucracy theory and Fayol's administrative management theory are often considered together as representing the 'traditional' approach to management. In this approach an organisation can be seen as an 'instrument' which is designed to achieve certain objectives, set by those who initiate or control it. A structure can then be set up to best achieve those objectives. Individuals can be fitted into the structure and their behaviour explicitly organised and coordinated.

The emphasis here is on a machine, or engineering, model and the resultant critiques of the traditional model centered around what was missing, or what was impoverished in this view of the organisation. What was insufficiently emphasised was the way in which organisational structure affects and interacts with the elements within that structure, and in particular the role of technology and humans who serve as essential features of that structure, the way that they work in groups and the motivations they possess.

For the human relations writers, understanding human needs was of paramount importance in understanding organisations, and specifically organisations that were effective. Probably the best known of these researchers is Abraham Maslow, whose work on human needs (even though it has been extensively criticised since initial publication) was very influential and continues to be given prominence in curricula of management courses (as well as those of psychology and health and social care), from 'A' level to Masters awards in business schools. Maslow presented the idea of a hierarchy of human needs from satisfying 'basic' physiological needs (food) to the assumed 'higher' needs such as self actualisation, that is fulfilment of the need to achieve what you want to achieve. What ties the diversity of researchers that constitute this school of thought together is the focus on the individual.

From the 1960s onwards we can begin to see the emergence of more sophisticated theories which sought to present and to enmesh a much more complex set of forces operating within organisations. For researchers engaged in this project, organisations were highly complex systems comprising of a dynamic mixture of people, procedures, technology and control. For them, focussing on either technical or social elements (expressed in their terms as subsystems) failed to do justice to the interaction of these forces or elements. Rather, it is the subtle and often hidden ways in which these forces entwine and combine that are the causative agents of organisational behaviour, and, importantly it is these interactions or contingencies that shed light on what makes an organisation effective.

Systems thinking is an important approach, or group of approaches, which emerged to challenge the traditional and human relations approaches to management. For systems thinkers (for example, Jackson 2000) organisations are best thought of as whole systems comprising interrelated subsystems, the interaction of which is more than the sum of their parts, and which display 'emergent' properties. Hence, it is argued, the focus of the traditional and human relations schools is skewed towards those parts of the organisation associated with 'high performance'. Traditional and human relations approaches are therefore seen as reductionist, with the traditional schools of management concentrating on task and structure, and the human relations school on people. Crucially, what is considered to be ignored or given insufficient attention is the interaction of different parts of the organisations that give rise to the whole; constituent parts of organisations are often treated *in vacuo*, or in isolation from the other parts. The systems thinking label is really quite a loose term which encompasses a variety of approaches, including the influential work of the socio-technical systems theorists based at the Tavistock Institute, through to the cybernetic approaches of the virtual systems model. One of the early and most powerful criticisms of these approaches was the way that they dealt with, or rather sidestepped, the real and lived problems of power and conflict because the 'narrative of systems', while appearing neutral, serves to maintain a managerial bias.

It was in addressing these concerns whilst preserving many of the powerful ideas at the heart of the systems approaches, that critical systems thinking emerged. This section ends with a parallel but related strand of contemporary management thought which also places emphasis on the 'critical' – critical management studies – but which also adds postmodern and post-structuralist theory to the critical theory mix.

Let us start examining this mix by looking at critical realists. Critical realists are uncomfortable with the role that positivism affords social phenomenon, whereby they are essentially 'things' to be labelled, measured and counted (formally 'reified') and assumptions are made about the freedom and autonomy that people have over their own actions (formally 'voluntarism'). For them the real world of experience is built upon interaction with real world objects as well as socially constructed artifacts – not just the latter (formally 'social constructionist'). Reflections based on critical reading of situations and power relations form important facets of critical realist approaches. So, whilst adopting a realist ontology (the world is really out there and experienced much as we see it), discursive and socially generated meanings are considered to play a critical role in shaping the way we understand and experience organisational (and extra-organisational) life.

Cunliffe (2009) suggests that adherents of the critical management approaches share the view that reality is not as it seems, and that assuming that it is (formally adopting a realist ontology) remains problematic. Managing, as an example of a social phenomenon, is as much constructed as any other, however uncomfortable the implications. Thus we cannot represent people's realities without answering some difficult questions about the way that *we* represent our own. If we follow this argument further, organisations are also constructed and in fact are being constructed by and through our actions and the language we use. Managers cannot adopt neutral stances with an air of 'scientific' detachment because such a detachment cannot exist. Equally the knowledge that managers bring to management is constructed situationally, that is in the present and in relation to the context in which that management is occurring. The language and practices used in management can construct the very things that are being managed. For example, performance indicators and targets have been seen to drive managerial concerns rather than the quality of patient care or alternative indicators of the effectiveness of service delivery.

The implications of this perspective are profound. If we cannot believe that, for example, evidence based practice is objective, or that information is constructed, then the question of who determines what *is* evidence is moot. Further, who has the power to raise one form of knowledge or evidence over another also has the power to legitimate, prioritise or privilege that knowledge. Often what is privileged is felt to be essentially Western, masculine views of what constitute management practice skills and knowledge, legitimised by, for example, the types of narratives presented above, and reinforced and systematised in the educational domain in university based management development programmes.

A fresh way of considering the changing schools of thought set out above has recently been proposed by Cunliffe (2009), who has identified and characterised a series of academic lenses which are helpful in appreciating changing approaches to management studies. The table below sets out a series of stages which relate directly to the issues of knowledge, power and professionalism set out in this chapter. The first phase relates to the accretion, collection and interpretation of information into a systemic corpus of knowledge discriminable from others. The expertise and power that the deployment of this knowledge has brought in relation to organisational achievement, seen here as effectiveness, legitimated its use and served to increase its value. The framing of this knowledge as the possession of a separate role of professional manager further served to invent and present what a manager does and what a manager is, and to create a management 'class'. Since the 1980s, as indicated above, there have been sets of criticisms from various disciplines and from different points of view which have challenged the idea of a settled notion of manager and the ideology of managerialism. These have been labelled as 'destabilisation' in the figure below because they aim to rock the 'taken for granted', and require us to rethink the ways that we have learned to think about what managers do and what management is for.

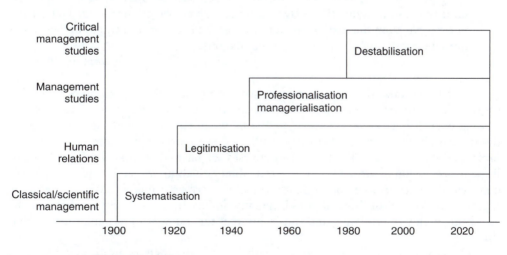

Figure 16.1 A brief history of management
Source: Cunliffe (2009: 13)

SO WHAT DO MANAGERS DO?

Briefly put, management can be considered to be about getting things done using people and other resources, and this is the sense we typically bring to mind when we talk about managing households, children or budgets. Management thus encompasses a very wide range of activities which have in common planning and acting, as well as *thinking about* the planning and acting, and importantly reflecting on the outcome of these activities. Management is also about changing things, about humans as active agents able to make a difference in the world. This task-oriented definition is not, however, sufficient because it essentially integrates the doing of and the managing of work and renders them both under autonomous control. In other words, it appears to assume that people can decide when, where and how, managing is done. Yet if we separate these components, we quickly reveal that it is possible to have some people who only manage and some who only work. The former set of people are attributed a new role and can develop a new occupational niche, plus new titles which frame new responsibilities. These are now 'managers' whose job is to manage, clearly identifiable as separate from those who are managed.

Such a distinction is not without problems, and is neither inevitable nor necessarily appropriate. But this distinction is made, and when it is made its consequences are powerful. Managerial forces are the same forces that have shaped the structure of the organisations that we work in, the work we do in the organisations, and the way we feel about ourselves as part of those organisations and in relation to that work. Management ideas and ideas about management run deep and, many researchers have argued, shaped our thinking about what is desirable and what is possible in organisations.

We will look at this again in a later section, but for now let us consider what may happen when we recombine the two elements, of managing self, and managing others in a role of 'manager'. This quote from Tony Watson picks up and expresses the tensions neatly:

> Managers' work thus involves a double essential task: managing others at the same time as managing themselves. But the very notion of 'managers' being separate people from the 'managed', a notion at the heart of traditional management thinking, undermines a capacity to handle this.
>
> (Watson 1994: 13)

Often when we talk about management we are in fact referring to quite a specific set of behaviours or actions, and in doing so are therefore limiting our ways of discussing what it is to be a manager, narrowing what can be termed the 'discourse' or discussions about what management is. Why is this important? It is important because limiting the number and the type of discourses we have about management leads to limited opportunities, to constraining our ability to think wider or creatively or to consider alternatives, and consequently constrains critical thinking. More worryingly it closes off avenues of thought, and implicitly defines the very words we can use, the two being highly interrelated, and thus reinforces the 'taken for granted', the way that things are.

Perhaps you may be wondering whether this really matters at all, and what this has got to do with the everyday performance of management as 'managers know what they have to do'. Anne Cunliffe (2009) addresses this concern in a pithy manner:

This is not just a semantic or intellectual issue, it's also a practical one, because whether we are aware of it or not, words do things – they influence and play out in our actions and relationships. Consider how a person's actions and ways of speaking and relating to other organisational members change in overt and subtle ways when she or he becomes a 'manager' and part of a management team.

(Cunliffe 2009: 8)

VALUES

This now raises questions of how the values understood or expected in the role of twenty-first century manager are incorporated, that is, become part of your being, and whether values held in a health and social care setting are commensurate with those of being a manager. The values which underpin your motivation to work in the field of health and social care are crucial, but will inevitably be hidden, fuzzy, or partial. Making these values more explicit is important in order that you may be better able to articulate decision making processes, recognise alternative viewpoints, employ critical thinking and gain commitment for your actions and for the way that you explain those actions.

Let us start with the ideology of 'managerialism' which both expresses and reinforces certain values. These values are not necessarily shared with those traditionally associated with what may be seen as 'caring' professions and it is worth attempting to tease out and contrast the two. There is a danger, as indicated by Barnard (2008: 14) of making it appear as though there is some form of enduring static list of values which we can compare. Of course values are dynamic concepts which change, flourish and wither, but nevertheless it is worth attempting to fix them temporarily, as presented in Table 16.1, however arbitrarily, in order to help express and understand that difference, or those contrasts. Even though we can see a new form of managerialism arise, primarily within public sector organisations, the song remains essentially the same. This 'new public management' still concerns taking processes and practices from the commercial environment and applying them with market orientated gusto into the public sector, which includes hospitals, universities, schools and health care.

It is also worth considering the *value accorded to values* in the fields of management and health and social care. Examining the index of most management textbooks for reference to 'values' will typically lead only as far as a discussion of values as part of organisational 'culture', that is a separate discriminable entity. Values here are akin to subjectivity and therefore antithetical to the fair and neutral discharging of the 'managerial function'. Managerialism has little regard for emotions, motivations and the value laden richness of human experience. In fact, managerialism is presented as a proudly value-free modus operandi, untainted by subjectivity.

On the other hand the notion of value has, at present, high currency in the fields of heath and social care, and whilst debate exists about the expression, form and condition of values in this context, they remain central to the field. The NHS and General Social Care Council explicitly present values at the core of their activities. For example, in a 2006 UK Department of Health review of mental health nursing (Department of Health 2006 – mental health nurses (MHNs) currently form the largest profession working in mental health) – values are clearly posited as central to professional development:

Table 16.1 Managerialism and tensions in health and social care

Managerialism	Health and social care tensions
Espoused goal – making organisations effective and efficient	Espoused goal – improving life chances
Means – rational, neutral, scientific	Means – making organisations effective and efficient versus participation in decision making
Value free	Values as core feature of identity
Value neutral	Value led
Values as part of organisational 'culture'	
Functionalism and reductionism	Holism and integration versus centralisation and bureaucratisation
Focus on measurable targets – efficiency, effectiveness, process	Focus on measurable targets versus non-operationalisable targets – quality of service, best practice, best value
Proximal focus – specialisation, professionalisation, knowledge as power	Distal focus – partnerships, advocacy, inter-agency working, knowledge sharing
Task centred	Person centred
Realist ontology	Realist ontology versus critical realism
Focus on quantitative methods – hypothesis testing, controlled experiments, evidence based decision making.	Critical role for both qualitative and quantitative research, including action research and participatory action research. Controlled experimentation as the basis for decision making in the clinical, not the management arena

Mental health nursing will be a profession based on a clear set of values that informs every aspect of practice. Mental health nurses (MHNs) will work in partnership with service users of all ages, their carers and other professionals to improve the service user's experience and outcomes of care. MHNs will value the aspirations of the service user, offer meaningful choice in evidence-based interventions and care, adopt a positive attitude to personal change and support social inclusion.

(Department of Health 2006: 8)

Interestingly the main text of this document makes reference to the term 'management' 14 times. Each time the management referred to was management 'of' something. That something was 'risk' in seven of the references, 'violence' twice, 'medication' twice, and 'care', 'depression case' and 'service users' once each. In other words the meaning of management here refers to something external to the MHN but within their professional expertise, which is skills-based but concerned with ameliorating problems in each of these areas. Managing is interpreted as synonymous with 'dealing with' – the 'what' – and values form part of the 'how'.

Wider professional and developmental conceptions of management which are notably absent here include self management, reflection, growth, as well as the narrative of management as a career path.

However, approaches and language are changing, and more recent policies present much more emphasis on the 'how', notably in relation to person centred support, partnerships, the individual as commissioning agent, and self management. For example, in relation to adult social care the 'Putting People First' (Department of Health 2007) initiative sets out the shared aims and values intended to guide the transformation of adult social care and covers all adult client groups, such that 'Over time, people who use social care services and their families will increasingly shape and commission their own services' (p. 2).

Nevertheless such changes in approach move at very different speeds both within health and within social care and between them, betokening their often very different, heterogeneous cultures. Where the 'new' managerialism appears to accommodate values is often only in terms of a discriminable and operationisable concept, one that can be isolated from other issues, agreed on, measured, and for which there is a 'solution'.

How might we compare the values of managerialism and those present or at least tacitly accepted in the field of health and social care. Table 16.1 illustrates an attempt to compare values across the two domains.

The term 'values' as employed above broadly reflects individual tendencies to act in particular ways according to an internal sense of right and wrong. Ethics can be thought of as a system of standards typically expressing professionally bounded behavioural constraints on action, such as the British Association of Social Workers codes of ethics. Gomm (2004) sets out the problems of ethics by using a clear taxonomy. He proposes that Max Weber's term 'value relevant' is useful in allowing researchers in the social sciences to recognise that research choices about what to research as legitimate questions cannot be disentangled from the personal, political and moral contextual terrain in which the researcher operates, and this need not necessarily be problematic. Difficulties arise, however, post topic selection, after which the values of the researcher need to be removed 'from the conduct of the research except the value of getting at the truth and the values grounding the humane treatment of the people involved in and affected by the research' (Gomm 2004: 14). The use of controlled experiments (quantitative research), whereby the researchers themselves are explicitly removed from the process of research is a good example of this, and one which reflects the tenets of what is known as the familiar hypothetico-deductive method. It is the role of others, not the researcher, to decide what to do with the results; the expertise of the researcher is just to research, such that 'it would be a breach of trust for researchers, as researchers, to allow their desires to change the world, or their personal values or career interests to influence the outcome of the research' (Gomm 2004: 15–16).

However, this position and the assumptions that it entrains, are similar to those which we have seen to be critiqued by later theorists such as those from critical management studies, and in the management domain it is becoming clear from our earlier discussion of discourses and their power relations that such assumptions have been widely attacked. One of the most powerful criticisms centres around the current distribution of power in society. This includes the power to determine what is worthy of research, what will be funded, what in fact constitutes a social problem. Those defining what is the problem, and having the power to disburse funds to allow the study of that problem, effectively shape the contours of social science research. The way that this shaping is seen to operate is in terms of privileging one sort of social arrangement or one set of people. For example, the current phase of service user involvement in health and social care is an attempt to redress a recognised previous imbalance. Gomm (2004: 16) again expresses this problem neatly: 'It can be, and is, argued that current knowledge is biased against women, against poor people, or against members of minority ethnic groups, and in favour of white middle class men and big business, and so on.'

Whilst we might question the omission of disabled people and other groups, the point is well made. The consequence of this problem has been that researchers have identified the need for 'value led', rather than 'value neutral' research based on the identified 'need' to produce knowledge and a critical understanding which balances the inequalities present in society. Much of the work, which may be considered under the umbrella term 'critical research' and in management 'critical management studies', adopts this view and includes feminist research, disability research, anti-racist research and queer theory. It is worth noting that assuming that one has the ability to recognise an imbalance or injustice, to further claim that research is necessary, and then to undertake that research oneself, each reflects moral judgements on the part of the researcher. Managers both commission and undertake research. As managers you may well be expected to interpret research produced internally as well as that produced by external agencies. Understanding the values underpinning the research and affecting the choices of methodology, of scope, and conclusions will be an important step in determining their utility and usability in your situation. Applied more widely, a better awareness of your own values and how they shape what you do as a manager, will help you in interacting with other managers internally and other agencies externally, particularly in terms of what you each expect and why.

The discussion so far has considered the history of management, what managers do, and the way the language of management can construct particular ideas and practices and avoid or distort the value-based nature of health and social care. We will now look at managing with and for others.

MULTIPROFESSIONAL WORKING, PARTNERSHIP AND STAKEHOLDERS

Earlier in the chapter we referred to the work of the classical and scientific management schools of thought and indicated that they were instrumental in bringing a more 'scientific' approach to the study of managers and managing of organisations. There was much more that grew out of this work, and in many ways something more pervasive and enduring than the theories themselves. What emerged from and together with their work was a notion of management as a discrete and valid profession, separate and identifiable, comprising a coherent set of roles and a management cadre or class, possessing and enacting a new form of expertise.

This expertise could be brought to bear on the body of the organisation to render it both more efficient and effective. Moreover, the expertise was modern, scientific and transparent, helping to legitimate this new role of manager whilst rendering management activities as essential forms of control, as necessary to organisations as their raw resources.

Thus a profession was born, and co-varying with the development of that profession over time was the emergence of a set of values or ideology which provided this neophyte profession status and authority for their actions. The idea of an ideology which represented and reflected this role of managers as rational logicians, impartially employing their management expertise in service of achieving organisational goals was attractive, pervasive and remains very powerful. Its self reinforcing beliefs in its own correctness and rationality are mirrored by a patterned sense of self belief in its adherents. Not surprisingly this ideology moved from business quickly into other types of organisations.

A legacy of the responsibility of organisational effectiveness resting on the shoulders of a professional managerial class is that the quality of the provision of services will by turn be improved with the implementation of new managerial roles, and increasingly policy designed to do just that is being introduced in the public arena.

The manager as professional hybrid is not an abstract conception or something happening somewhere else. In the UK its implementation is enshrined in policy and the interplay of its tensions played out publicly in public management, and daily in offices and corridors. A recent example from the National Health Service is in respect to the 'modern matron' initiative. This policy enshrined a new role which was introduced in order to address the concerns associated with an outdated and autocratic idea of what matrons were and did, and also to introduce a clear path for nurses into management.

However, there began to be clear evidence that problems were emerging with this new role, which became the site of action for the abrasion between two professional hierarchies, that of nursing and of management (Savage and Scott 2004), tellingly, even when the managers were previously nurses. The reason, the authors claim, is in large part because of the decoupling of management and nursing practice.

In a fascinating recent study on these modern matrons, Currie *et al.* (2009) make four further points which link this change of role to more profound changes in public service organisations.

> Modern matrons exemplify the introduction of 'hybrid' (professional/managerial) roles associated with government policy concerned to modernise the delivery of public services. Our findings reflect the challenge of introducing new roles within pre-existing but dynamic system of professions that characterises many public service organisations across the world. There are four dimensions of professions that should be considered when introducing new roles. These are: the dynamics of the profession with which new roles are most closely associated; the changing role of those within this profession and its relationship with the new role; the relationship between various professions and power differentials that impact upon the new role; and the relationship between the new role and organisational management. Successful enactment of new roles envisaged by policy-makers requires new roles to converge with existing professional practice and hierarchy.
>
> (Currie *et al.* 2009: 309)

What has been termed 'new managerialism' is rapidly permeating all areas of public service provision, from universities to GP practices. The concerns about what it is to manage and employ professional expertise in such environments raises further debates on new practices, new policies and freshly constructed roles designed to further the implementation of those policies. A key feature of the landscape of new managerialism is the manner in which core management functions are enacted and policy achieved. The tasks and processes of management are now to be performed by particular individuals who do much more in ways which are creative, which inspire and motivate others and which express and articulate the 'mission' of the organisation. These individuals are not just managers, they are leaders.

LEADERSHIP

It is difficult to conceive of people acting as managers without simultaneously think-ing about what it is to lead. The meaning and importance of what it is to be a leader has seen increased attention, emerging from the management literature into the wider area of business, and a plethora of books and articles reflect the levels of interest now generated by the topic of leadership.

As we have seen above, when we assume a more critical stance, these debates can be seen as framed by discourse about the adequacy of definition, the problems of retroanalys-ing and categorising different types of leader and the value of the application of the results of such thinking. Nevertheless, it is instructive to look briefly at the literature with the aim of achieving a sense of what a critical understanding of this branch of management studies may offer. Most introductory management text books will cover the topic of leadership by introducing distinctions that have been drawn between the terms management and leadership, followed by the idea of types, perhaps best described as archetypes, of the most commonly recognised leadership styles, and a discussion of the relationship between situation and style (*see* for example Huczynski and Buchanan 2007), which will often involve some critical questions. However, it is not the difficult questions or their complex answers that get remembered and repeated. Instead, leadership classifications, tables, lists and continuums provide accessible chunks of information to identify leadership styles. The caveats, application constraints, limitations and criticisms are less easy to assimilate and usually more boring. It is much more fun to play 'spot the leadership style' than to question the epistemology on which that classification rests.

The authority of leadership, in large part, is derived from Weber's classification of authority. *Charismatic* leadership is typically introduced by a historical list of char-ismatic leaders who achieve influence by virtue of the 'strength' of their personality and their exceptional nature which sets them apart from those that are led. An important assumption here is that you cannot learn to be this type of leader, it is somehow inher-ent in the traits that are possessed by the individual, but is worth noting that the idea of personality 'traits' is the subject of some serious debate in the field of psychology.

The next type of leader is termed *traditional* and this applies to individuals who are leaders by virtue of history or their birth, a situation which can be contrasted with *situational* leaders whose influence is derived from and limited by the particular contex-tual characteristic in which they find themselves. Traditional leaders gain their authority from doing things in a similar way to how they have always been done, conservatively. Critics of situational leaders suggest that they are unlikely to be able to work across the variety and range of situations that comprise modern working environments.

By contrast, the *appointed* leader derives and maintains influence from the posi-tion that they hold and it can thus be considered a bureaucratic form existing by virtue of a 'slot' in the organisation, regardless of the extent to which they are able to discharge the demands of this role in ways that render them powerful. This is akin to Weber's term 'rational-legal authority'. Lastly, and in contrast, the *functional* leader is in this position because of their very ability to do what is desired in that role, and is therefore well able to change what they do and how they do it in accord with the prevailing and changing demands of the situation.

Leadership is therefore as much about what a person does as what a person is. This has led to procession definitions that are grounded in the situational enact-ment of particular behaviours designed to encourage others to undertake group tasks without coercion and with their consent. The idea here is that there are group goals towards which the leader steers the group and that there are very different ways that an effective manager might choose to select in order to achieve this aim, according to situational variables. Bluntly expressed, management is concerned more with maintaining stability, whilst leadership is about being inspiring, creative, visionary and motivating. Quite a heroic combination for a director of adult mental health in a primary health care trust, let alone the team leader of a hospital cleaning service!

As we might expect the range of approaches to leadership varies according to the school of management. Scientific management may look to an ideal form or type whereas contingency theorists may choose to look at leadership as responsiveness to changes in situations. Cole (1998) identified a tripartite classification into trait schools, style theories and contingency theories.

Identifying particular patterns or tendencies for behaviour in what leaders do, characteristic aims of the trait school, has not proved fruitful. Perhaps the most that can be said is that the most commonly occurring traits that do emerge are energy, resourcefulness and intelligence; this doesn't take us very far.

From a discourse point of view the idea of a leader is constructed, that is manufactured in language, and rooted in ideas about the world that are not shared and constant. Social reality is different for all of us and leadership is just as much a social phenomenon as a 'talent oriented' game show. Why is this important? Because leadership is co-created between leader and follower via the mundane way we talk and act in organisations, how we relate socially. For Fairhurst a discursive approach to leadership 'represents leadership as a process of influence and meaning management among actors' (Fairhurst 2007: 5). Those actors are you and all the people that work with you and who may work 'for' you. It seems strange to think of it in this way but leadership is about working out what it means for you and for your organisation to call someone a leader, to attribute that label to them, and importantly the way they influence others in that role.

PROFESSIONS AND PROFESSIONALISM

The context in which health and social care professionals operate is dynamic and subject to rapid and unpredictable change, and this demands both a change in the way in which professions undertake their practice and the way that they interact. The realm of social care has provided and continues to provide examples of failures sufficiently shocking as to initiate both major changes in the form and nature of professional development as well as changes to policy and procedures enshrined in legislation.

One way of thinking about discourses is in terms of what is allowed to be said and what is not up for discussion; what it is within the remit of the professional and what can be challenged. Discourses are powerful. They shape not only our understanding of social situations, but the very terms we can use to express our understanding and even our lived experience. Understanding how discourses arise, form and are reformed can be broadly termed as deconstructing the notion of professional expertise.

If we consider the most obvious manifestations of professional discourse in the postmodern horizon and the acceptance of the 'market economy', then what is entrained by this apparently simple notion is at the same time complex, elusive and profound. The terminology is of resource allocation and of competencies, of 'things' which have market value. These 'things' include professional skills and professional knowledge, which become 'commodified' and are rendered transparent, substitutable and to be bought at the cheapest rate.

Goods, services and professional expertise are, in effect, all commodities to be purchased from a 'provider' in a competitive environment. It presents an environment in which actions by managers in making purchases reinforce and privilege forms of action which themselves serve to define what it is to manage – in this sense to control power. The words that we use shape and change what we do and, importantly, the way that we make sense of what we do is through the same behavioural lens.

Why does this matter? It matters because it is the performative component of managerial behaviour in the world of work inhabited by health and social care workers, of whatever form, that is important. Effective inter-agency communication and intervention, cooperative working, the sharing of power through partnerships, service user involvement and genuine engagement with different values characterise work in this field. It also matters because of the status implications that, for example, a market orientated view necessarily has for the preservation of what has been argued as the defining characteristics of professions and their specialised knowledge.

Whether professional knowledge is 'legitimate' is a disputed and contested area. What authority does a professional have (which marks them out as embodying especial right to practise), if the ways in which that knowledge is gained can be called in to question? Further, if it is not a professional's right to disseminate that knowledge then, the common sense argument goes, what rights do they have? Importantly, this goes as much for a professional researcher whose rise through the ranks is presaged on the years of engagement with formal theory, as it does for the professional managers and clinicians whose years of experience form the basis for the practical application of knowledge they hold so dearly. What, therefore, is the status of the knowledge possessed by the vast majority of workers in the 'caring' professions whose daily experience is the sustained and continual enmeshing of both theory and practice?

Further questions arise over the relationship between professional managers and professional social workers, or neurosurgeons, or youth workers. If the ability to manage is to be carved out as an 'essential' characteristic of senior positions, does this mean that the domain of individual expertise is reduced (they are going to be spending less time doing it). Or does being a senior specialist require those skills in order to be considered senior. The tensions arising from attempting to answer these questions in ways that enable staff to do their job are real, present and played out daily. Indeed, the fight for power, for control of resources is also a rich site of dispute between different professions and individuals. For example, social workers are 'care managers', but management between levels of staff and management *of* people's care are very different indeed, revealing a complex interplay between potentially competing requirements. In addition, with the increasing growth of user-led organisations supported at policy level, such tensions will not only be more likely to emerge, but to be played out in a more public arena.

The vexed question of the relationship between knowledge and power is given a new dimension here when we consider what we really mean by knowledge. Is it the same as information, something special, or a meaningful collection of data to be accessed on demand? Is it something that managers have, or something they create? Not surprisingly, there are alternative views about what knowledge is, and how we get knowledge about knowledge. The set of ideas about how we get to know anything are termed epistemological questions. In respect to the epistemology of knowledge, Currie and Kerrin (2004) encapsulate a useful and important distinction that links directly with our recurring practice/theory theme:

> in general an epistemology of possession focuses upon what is known – that is, the knowledge possessed by an individual or a group. This includes tacit knowledge, which is significantly different from explicit knowledge. An epistemology of practice takes ways of knowing as its focus and concerns itself with the action of individuals and groups.
>
> (Currie and Kerrin 2004: 11)

Having briefly engaged with critiques of professions, their knowledge claims, status and power relations, it is time to consider how this affects the way we think about two themes which emerge from this chapter: first, the importance that competing claims for legitimacy have for the high degree of inter-profession interaction which characterises the terrain of health and social care, and second, what it might mean for you as a student and worker and potential manager in health and social care.

In terms of inter-professional discourses and their influence on the context of work, potential disputes are perhaps at their clearest in the framing of discourses between professional managers, hired to bring a rational/scientific approach to the process of managing resources effectively, and the reaction of those 'resources' themselves.

For example, popular television hospital drama vignettes illustrating tensions between care workers and managers are a common theme, with bureaucratic professional managers parachuted into hospitals, possessing little experience outside the commercial, affronting and damaging diligent time-served practitioners. However, the implications and results from the playing out of such tensions are real and severe; the failings in gaining commitment from stakeholders in high profile and ambitious IT systems often lead to them being written off after extremely expensive and ill-considered development. The reality of these types of problems is well understood and is in fact a characteristic part of organisation life.

What is less well recognised are the countless instances that remain 'under the wire', hushed by fear of bad publicity and hermetically sealed by out of court settlements. Thus, the potential, the utility and value of consideration of these problems as aids to avoiding repetition remains forever stymied by stringent and enduring gagging clauses. It is not the aim here to provide prescriptive advice on how to avoid poor management decisions; there are plenty of books which seek to do just that, each with its own assumptions and therefore forms of discourse. The hope here has been that you are first alerted to the existence of these narratives, discourses or ways of making sense of organisational complexity and managerial behaviour and, once recognised, are able to make decisions and act in ways that challenge and reformulate these discourses commensurate with your own values and reflective approach to learning.

CONCLUSION

Over the course of this chapter we have briefly charted the rise of different schools of thought and approaches to management since its inception as a site of enquiry. We have seen the focus of the academic lenses move from the concern of managers being to ensure that organisations run effectively and efficiently, through the human relations school where the focus has been on individuals, their actions and internal states, to critical management theorists for whom exposing discourses and deconstructing world views are central to their endeavour. We have seen that each school necessarily has at its heart assumptions about the world and the role of managers in that world. We have looked at critiques of the most ubiquitous form of management ideology, managerialism, and its new guise, 'public managerialism', from the perspective of discourses which shape and alter what we consider the role of managers to be. We have seen the way in which professionalisation has legitimised managerial knowledge and management action.

The chapter has also sought to reveal a number of tensions that exist between professional managers as a class, and constituent professions in the field of health and social care. A critical and open discussion of these issues helps to understand what good management and leadership is and how this can improve health and social care practice.

These tensions are not abstract but stud the everyday interactions of managers with those who are managed, leaders with those who are led. We have also seen that these interactions reproduce as well reflect forms of relations, to the extent that they can mould what it means to be a manager in a particular context as well as what it is to manage in that context, which may not be the same. These tensions are not just expressed in the visible world of individual managerial behaviour, but are played out in the private or internal domain where managers reflect on their own actions, by 'reflection in action', as well as 'reflection on action' (Schön 1983), and try to make sense of what they have done. We have explored the notion of 'values' as an example site of action for the expression of potential dissonance.

The values which drive your motivation to work in the field of health and social care are crucial, but will inevitably be partly obscured or never explicitly articulated. Becoming a reflective practitioner will involve engaging with processes that in part make these values clearer to yourself. This is important in order that you may be better able to articulate decision making processes, recognise alternative viewpoints, employ critical thinking and gain commitment for your actions and for the way that you explain those actions.

We hope that in reading this chapter you have developed a sense of the difference between being a manager and acting as if you were a manager. We also hope that you recognise that there is no simple checklist of good practice nor a comprehensive list of management principles which you can simply apply to your situation – no matter how many airport bookshelf titles scream otherwise. Managing involves understanding that you will undoubtedly make mistakes and you will make poor decisions. That there is no simple or single way to be a 'good manager' is, in a profound sense, related to the acceptance of the notion emerging most notably from the social constructionists and critical management theorists that there is no single 'truth'; an idea which for a large number of managers remains scary, easily ignored and destabilising (Cunliffe 2009).

Being aware that attempting to be sensitive to others' values, figuring out what you should and could do, and why, what impelled you towards a particular course of action, how what you have been asked to do accords with your values, and then attempting to frame this reflection in terms of a critical approach to prevailing ideologies, is going to be difficult. It is much easier not to do so, and accept the prevailing ideology of managerialism.

But if you do engage in at least some of these processes and question the 'taken for granted', your time as a manager is more likely to yield a rich and powerful source of learning and to provide a platform for a happier and more fulfilling role. Managers often experience dissonance, alienation, health problems, exhibit arrogance and develop deep dissatisfaction. Adopting a critical approach may not be preventative, but for many of you the process of seeking to understand 'why' will be a crucial part of the process of changing that 'why'.

SUMMARY OF MAIN POINTS

You should be able to:

- Critically apply theoretical concepts of organisation behaviour and leadership to the workplace.
- Critically consider the managerial dilemmas facing organisations in the twenty-first century.
- Identify the conceptual dilemmas of organisational development.
- Critically demonstrate knowledge of the contribution of different approaches to leadership and human resource management in health and social care.

MOMENT OF REFLECTION

Think of two meaningful encounters that you have had with 'management' in two different organisations. What were the positive and negative moments of that encounter? What did you think about the manager's behaviour and, reflecting on the experience now, what did it make you think or feel about their role?

Do you plan to become a manager? If you do, what do you think will be important discourses for you? If you don't, what is it about the role that dissuades you from wanting to pursue it? What might change your mind?

REFERENCES

Barnard, A. (2008) Values, ethics and professionalisation: a social work history, in Barnard, A., Horner, N. and Wild, J. (Eds) *The Value Base of Social Work and Social Care: An active learning handbook*, Milton Keynes: Open University Press.

Boddy, D. (2005) *Management: An introduction* (3rd edition), Essex: Prentice Hall.

Castells, M. (1999) Flows, Networks and Identities: A critical theory of the Informational Society, in Castells, M., Flecha, R., Fiere, P., Giroux, H., Macedo, D. and Willis. P. (Eds) *Critical Education in the New Information Age*, Maryland: Rowman and Littlefield Publishers Inc.

Cole, G. A. (1998) *Management: Theory and Practice* (5th edition), Gosport: Letts.

Cunliffe, A. L. (2009) *A very short, fairly interesting and reasonably cheap book about management*, London: Sage.

Currie, G. and Kerrin, M. (2004) The Limits of a Technological Fix to Knowledge Management: Epistemological Political and Cultural Issues in the Case of Intranet Implementation, *Management Learning*, 35 (1), 9–29.

Currie, G., Koteyko, N. and Nerlich, B. (2009) The dynamics of professions and development of new roles in public services organizations: the case of modern matrons in the English NHS, *Public Administration*, 87 (2), 295–311.

Department of Health (2006) *From values to action: The Chief Nursing Officer's review of mental health nursing*, London: HMSO.

Department of Health (2007) *Putting People First: A shared vision and commitment to the transformation of Adult Social Care*, London: HMSO.

Fairhurst, G. T. (2007) *Discursive Leadership: In Conversation with Leadership Psychology*, Thousand Oaks, CA: Sage.

Gomm, R. (2004) *Social Research Methodology: a critical introduction*, Hampshire: Palgrave Macmillan.

Huczynski, A. and Buchanan, D. (2007) *Organizational Behaviour: An Introduction* (6th edition), London: Financial Times/Prentice Hall.

Jackson, M. C. (2000) *Systems Approaches to Management*, New York: Kluwer.

Linstead S., Fulop L. and Lilley, S. (2004) *Management and Organisation: a critical text*, Hampshire: Palgrave Macmillan.

Savage, J. C. and Scott, C. (2004) The Modern Matron: A Hybrid Role with Implications for Continuous Quality Improvement, *Journal of Nursing Management*, 12, 419–26.

Schön, D. (1983) *The Reflective Practitioner. How professionals think in action*, London: Temple Smith.

Sheldrake, J. (1996) *Management Theory: From Taylorism to Japanization*, London: International Thomson Business.

Watson, T. J. (1994) *In Search of Management*, London: Routledge.

Weber, M. (1949) *The Methodology of the Social Sciences*, New York: Free Press.

CHAPTER 17

EVIDENCE BASED PRACTICE IN HEALTH AND SOCIAL CARE

MICHELE RAITHBY AND CHRIS RING

OBJECTIVES

After reading this chapter you should be able to:

▪ Examine the nature and forms of health and social care knowledge.

▪ Understand critical appraisal and its application in health and social care.

▪ Examine the theories, methods, interventions and barriers to applying evidence in health and social care.

▪ Examine the contribution of an evidence based perspective to health and social care.

After reading this chapter you will understand the key terms:
Critical thinking, evidence based practice.

There are seven Moments of Reflection to work on throughout the chapter.

INTRODUCTION

Using the best current evidence to inform and improve practice in health and social care is seen as a cornerstone of being a competent practitioner in the helping professions. The ability to keep up with and utilise relevant up-to-date empirical knowledge is now an expectation in multi-professional contexts. This chapter discusses the skills, knowledge and understanding required to do so in health and social care practice, using a variety of settings as examples.

The chapter begins with some case examples and then provides an overview of key debates on the development and use of critical thinking and evidence based practice in health and social care, including ethical issues. The nature and range of research and practice knowledge that can impact on helping services is explored, and sources of credible information and research, including systematic reviews, are discussed. The importance of skills for critical thinking and appraisal, in order to judge relevance and applicability to service needs, is illustrated throughout with examples and exercises that relate to practice and the potential impact on service users.

The concluding section discusses potential gateways and barriers to implementing evidence based practice in the workplace, with suggestions and exercises that can be used by both students and current practitioners. At the end of the chapter, there are further discussion points for individual and group use.

THE CONSEQUENCES OF GETTING IT WRONG

We tend not to live our lives in an evidence based way: the risks of death or serious injury travelling by road are greater than by aeroplane, yet we do not feel the same sense of anxiety when buckling the car seatbelt that we may feel on takeoff. The potential consequences of poor practice in the area of human services can also be catastrophic, as illustrated in the following examples of some high-profile scandals in health and social care.

Case examples

*   In 1987, 121 children were taken into care in Cleveland after two paediatricians used a novel technique to diagnose sexual abuse (reflex anal dilatation test). Three-quarters of the children were later returned to their families (including some under further supervision) after extensive negative media coverage.
*   In 1998, a paper was published in the *Lancet* linking case studies of 12 children with histories of bowel problems and autism with the MMR (measles, mumps, rubella) triple vaccine. After heavy press coverage interpreting this as a causal link, take-up of the MMR vaccination fell considerably, followed by a rise in childhood measles (*see* Goldacre 2008 for further discussion).
*   In 1990–1, nine children were removed from their families in Orkney, suspected of being victims of satanic ritual abuse. The children were returned following a legal ruling that the evidence used by social workers was seriously flawed. Similar cases based on allegations of ritual abuse occurred in Nottingham (in 1987) and Rochdale (in 1990). A government commissioned report found there was no foundation for many claims of ritual abuse, and there had been heavy influence on social workers from evangelical groups (La Fontaine 1994 and 1998).

All of these cases had potentially profound effects on people's lives. As Sheldon and Macdonald (1999) comment, it is perfectly possible for well meaning, dedicated people to cause remarkable harm. The medical ethical impulse of 'Do no harm' crosses disciplines; good intentions are not always enough. Emerging health and social care professions such as social work and nursing are still developing both a recognised knowledge base and ways of applying that knowledge effectively. As part of that effective application, bringing a critical perspective to decision making can be crucial. The following activity centres on the personal criteria that may be used when making decisions around interventions in health and social care practice. If you have not had any work experience yet in a practice setting, think about how you might make decisions in the future.

MOMENT OF REFLECTION

Activity One: Making decisions in interventions

How do you make decisions about how to work with people in health and social care? Imagine you are working with a service user. Which of the following would you rely on to make decisions about how you will work with them?

- Your intuition (gut feeling) about what will be effective.
- What was usually offered at your agency/team.
- What you know by critically reading professional literature.
- What you are most familiar with.
- Your experience with a few cases.

(Adapted from Gibbs and Gambrill 1999)

Now imagine that you have a potentially serious medical problem, and you seek help from a physician to examine your treatment options. Which of the same criteria would you like your physician to rely on when he or she makes recommendations about your treatment?

Were there any differences in your responses to the two scenarios? If so, why?

CRITICAL THINKING

The previous activity introduces the concept of critical thinking in action. Many people may answer the second scenario differently because they have been made to put themselves in the shoes of a service user or patient. The exercise does not try to reinforce stereotypes of medicine and social care (check your own stereotypes here: open toed sandals and woolly, good intentions versus stethoscopes and hard-nosed objectivity). Both professions deal with people in distress, who are experiencing complex interactions between their emotional and physical states. Practitioners in both professions are likely to use intuition as an initial response. However, this is the starting, not finishing point. Imagine presenting evidence in a legal setting such as a court or tribunal. There will be little mercy shown to a professional under cross-examination who claims intuition as the source of their information.

Gambrill (1997: 125) has given a definition of critical thinking as involving:

the careful examination and evaluation of beliefs and actions in order to arrive at well reasoned ones.

As we have seen from the examples of when things go wrong, critical thinking is not necessarily easy to practise: the following activity will help you appreciate why.

MOMENT OF REFLECTION

Activity Two

Look at this extract from the witness transcript in the Victoria Climbié inquiry (2001) of a social worker from one of the local authorities involved in the child's care. The cross-examination centres on whether social workers or the police questioned the diagnosis of a consultant paediatrician (Dr S).

Barrister:	Do you ever in cases seek a second opinion, if you have doubts, on the basis of information you have received about the circumstances of the case, that a diagnosis is correct?
Social worker:	I personally have never disputed a case.
Barrister:	Would you know the mechanism by which you would do that?
Social worker:	Obviously if a junior doctor had seen a child, I may say, "Has Dr S seen the child?", because Dr S was always the person that I felt was a highly respected person at [the hospital] and I would always rely on her diagnosis.
Barrister:	Did you not see it as any part of your role to critically evaluate the information you were presented with?
Social worker:	At that time, no.
Barrister:	So you did not think to explore with her the reason for the diagnosis?
Social worker:	As I said, I did not – I am not medically trained, so I did not feel I could dispute Dr S's findings.

What conclusions do you draw about the perceived relative status of the social worker and the consultant? How has that affected the decision making process?

Gambrill (1997) has outlined a series of potential pitfalls in individual thinking, a few of which are outlined in the following activity.

MOMENT OF REFLECTION

Activity Three

Here are some fallacies in thinking. Try to give some examples of how these fallacies can appear in practice from your learning so far:

- Relying on emotional reaction or 'intuition' alone.
- Relying on the status of the speaker.
- Relying on the popularity of a theory.
- Focussing only on success.
- Relying on a few unrepresentative case examples.

Can you give examples of how these fallacies can operate in practice? Can you think of other fallacies?

Munro (1999) has applied knowledge of these cognitive biases to errors in thinking in child protection. From her analysis of child death inquiry reports, she illustrates tendencies in workers across health and social care only to seek information that supports their own views.

It is important to ask sceptical (*not* cynical) questions when considering how crucial decisions are being made that may affect people's lives profoundly. In other words to consider whether you could be wrong in assumptions or thought processes as being open-minded does not have to mean being empty-headed. It is a humbling experience to ask yourself the question 'Could I be wrong?', and indicates a willingness to challenge not only the assumptions of others, but of oneself as well. The next section moves from developing these habits of individual thinking that can be practised and developed, to the development of evidence based practice.

WHAT IS EVIDENCE BASED PRACTICE IN HEALTH AND SOCIAL CARE SERVICES?

Evidence based practice (EBP) in medicine is a relatively recent concept. Doctors have raised their status enormously from that of Dickensian 'sawbones'. Nevertheless, hospitals may still be viewed with some trepidation by patients in the modern era of MRSA and other infections, but these pale beside the perils of the mid-nineteenth century Vienna lying-in hospital, where one in six women giving birth died from the infection puerperal fever (*see* Nuland 2004). A physician at the hospital, Semmelweis, correctly concluded that the habit of doctors moving directly from dissecting cadavers to assisting at births, without washing their hands, was a primary route of this infection. He introduced hand washing in the hospital, and cut deaths by a factor of ten.

Sheldon and Chilvers (2000: 5) provide a working definition of evidence based social care, derived from a definition of evidence based medicine by Sackett *et al.* (1996), substituting 'service-users and carers' for 'patients':

> the conscientious, explicit and judicious use of current best evidence in making decisions regarding the welfare of service-users and carers.

Conscientious refers to the idea discussed earlier of an ethical obligation to justify professional expertise. *Explicit* means being open and transparent with service users and other professionals on how decisions are arrived at, and *judicious* means using sound judgement in making those decisions. Gibbs (2003: 6) provides another definition that emphasises that this is a process that should continue throughout the professional life of practitioners:

> Placing the client's benefits first, evidence based practitioners adopt a process of lifelong learning that involves continually posing specific questions of direct practical importance to clients, searching objectively and efficiently for the current best evidence relative to each question, and taking appropriate action guided by evidence.

Note 'guided by evidence': the implication is that this is one of a number of resources available to the skilled practitioner to maximise what they are able to offer.

WHAT ARE THE CLAIMS FOR STRENGTHS OF EBP?

For proponents of EBP, the potential benefits include improved outcomes for service users, credibility of services, enhanced accountability and cost-effectiveness. The ideal is that the principles of evidence based medicine can – and should – be applied more rigorously across other professions. These aims are consistent with professional ethics, can bridge the gap between research and experience and may provide common ground across helping professions (Gibbs 2003). The extent of inter-professional work in organisations such as Care Trusts demands a common understanding of the place of empirical evidence in practice, if this is to contribute effectively to deciding on and delivering health and social care. For example, in mental health care a shared approach to the use of specific medication in particular conditions such as bipolar disorder, is vital for its appropriate use in treatment plans. Empirical evidence of a medication's effectiveness in symptom control, and users' accounts of receiving this, can assist a reasoned decision, involving all parties, on whether and how to use it. In other areas of practice, for example social work, a growing number of 'how to do it' guides have been published (*see* for example Gibbs 2003; Newman *et al.* 2005).

Inherent in all these ideas of EBP lies the existence or accessibility of empirical knowledge – or research evidence – which can be brought to bear upon a problem. Professional codes of conduct now generally demand that health and social care practitioners access and draw upon this when seeking to understand and intervene in the problems they are presented with. However, knowledge is more widely available in some areas than others. Emerging professions in health and social care have a particular struggle, as EBP is a relatively new concept. Swinkels *et al.* (2002) examine the challenges physiotherapy, midwifery and nursing face with developing their own distinctive knowledge base and models of practice. Professionals are suspicious of audit, loss of perceived autonomy, and the mechanisation of practice. However, being compassionate does not preclude being hard headed. The consequences of not being so are potentially catastrophic (*see* previous scandals).

WHAT COUNTS AS KNOWLEDGE?

What counts as knowledge is a highly contested area: the aims and assumptions of EBP current in health care have not been accepted uncritically by practitioners or academics working in the field of social work (*see* Webb 2001, and the response by Sheldon 2001, for an example of the debate). One objection is that evidence based approaches are associated with methods common in natural sciences such as experiments. Commentators such as Webb claim that such methods are not appropriate for examining the complexity of human relations embedded in social welfare interactions and interventions.

Within the health professions, however, the empirical methods of the natural sciences attract considerably more respect than in social work. These have been successfully applied to understanding and addressing a very wide range of health problems, such as the infectious diseases (in the late nineteenth and twentieth centuries as we have seen above) and more recently heart disease and stroke. Although the knowledge accumulated through the health sciences such as physiology, biochemistry, pharmacology and pathology is not (in most cases) expressed in the same form as the laws forming the foundations of physical sciences, it provides practioners with comparable power at least in some settings. Medical sciences provide an enormous variety of models, capable of explaining disease processes, informing the development of means to address these, and evaluating their effectiveness.

The methods and findings of medical and allied health sciences have therefore come to command respect partly because of their practical utility. Initially in public health and medicine (nineteenth century), rapidly followed by nursing and psychology, these methods have been used effectively to achieve major advances in the understanding and treatment of a wide variety of problems. Essentially, this constitutes the knowledge base of the health professions. EBP has achieved considerable credibility in health care, which is apparent in the widespread availability of clinical guidelines, and the use of 'clinical audit' of routine performance against these.

The potential benefits of applying a comparable approach (based upon the approaches of both social and natural sciences) to social work, social care, and related areas such as offending behaviour, have attracted increasing attention this century. The development of an equivalent knowledge base for these forms of work appears to be limited by several factors, such as scepticism about the validity of the positivist paradigm underpinning health and (to a lesser extent) social sciences. Considerable doubt exists about how far the latter can be applied to construct models that enable us to explain and effectively address social problems, because the social world differs from the material world, where the positivist approach has proved its value.

Many of the methods and language of social science attract considerable scepticism. Doubt exists about their power to generate robust, testable explanations of social problems, or to evaluate interventions.

Case example: Evidence or hoax?

In 1994 a physicist 'Alain Sokal' submitted an article to the cultural studies journal *Social Text*, in which he proposed links between quantum gravity and psychoanalysis (among other things). The article was duly published, but then exposed as a hoax, with the aim of demonstrating that nonsense could be 'dressed up' in scientific-sounding language and be accepted uncritically (Sokal and Bricmont 1998).

There are debates about 'attributive confidence' in research methods, and how robust they may be. Not all research designs carry the same weight. For example, the design of randomised control trials (RCTs) is to control for selection and other external sources of bias. However, non-experimental designs can also highlight issues that are excluded by the design of RCTs, particularly if a number of studies in different circumstances give similar results. Opinion surveys and focus groups are very valuable to hear the experience of service users, but have the limitations of small, self-selecting sample sizes.

RCTs are often regarded as the 'gold standard'. However, they may not always be conducted according to the ideal. For example, Aisenberg (2008) points out the lack of cultural competence in the way randomised control trials are carried out in mental health, as black and minority ethnic groups are severely under-represented. On the other hand, experimental designs are not exclusive to the 'natural' sciences. Oakley (1998) provides a reminder that there is a forgotten history of a tradition of experiments in social science. Some unhelpful dichotomous positions have therefore emerged in health and social care research as a result of entrenchment in favoured methodologies. An anti-intellectualism has been identified in the ethos of nurses (Swinkels *et al.* 2002) with a perception that researchers are divorced from the 'real world' of practice. One consequence of claiming firm allegiance to a particular stance has been the placing of qualitative and experimental research at opposite ends of a spectrum of methodological approval. Yet such an uncritical rigidity may lead to a false debate based on stereotypes rather than the appropriateness of a particular method in context. There are shifts towards less oppositional stances occurring within social work research, however, which acknowledge the role of exploratory research and combining qualitative and quantitative approaches (*see* for example Sinclair 2000).

As Sheldon and Macdonald assert (1999: 13):

> We know of many examples of rigorous, representative, qualitative research, which very usefully reveals the highs and lows of what it is like to *be* dependent on social services. But we also know of many nicely controlled, sensitively conducted, randomised control trials. (...) Let us be clear, there is no single research methodology that is always better than any other, it all depends on what one is hoping to learn.

Case example: Effective parenting

Between 1995 and 1999, 141 children between the ages of three and eight, referred because of their anti-social behaviour, were assigned to a parenting programme based on the Webster-Stratton behavioural programme or to a waiting list for future intervention as a control group. The results of the trial, published in the *British Medical Journal* (Scott *et al.* 2001), were very encouraging. Among the intervention group, the ratio of praise to ineffectual commands increased by three times, and this change in fundamental behaviour translated into significant reductions in anti-social behaviour among the children and in levels of parental strain. The costs were similar to those of a standard mental health response for which there was no equivalent proof of impact on well-being.

The original developer of the programme, Carolyn Webster-Stratton, commented on the results of the trial, saying that the study had helped to narrow the gap between the theory and practice of mental health for children.

WHAT EVIDENCE DO WE HAVE?

There is a limited range of empirical evidence available to underpin the social work knowledge base (SCIE 2005). This is compounded by the relatively low level of funding provided for research in social work (by comparison with the health professions), as well as the limited interest, skills and support available for primary research within social work agencies.

However, within health care, it is apparent that a very large knowledge base exists. That relating to social work is much more limited, reflecting the relative priority given to research in the two communities The overall annual spend per workforce member stands at about £25 in social care compared with £3,400 in health (SCIE 2005). As a consequence:

> The vast majority of interventions [in social care] are not evaluated before they are introduced, and ... much of the work we do with children has the status of an uncontrolled experiment.
>
> (Macdonald and Roberts 1995: 5)

While there is quite extensive empirical evidence in some areas of practice, this is of variable quality. This is illustrated by the review of 95 studies published in professional social work and allied journals between 1979 and 1991 (Macdonald *et al.* 1992). Macdonald and colleagues found that 75 per cent of the studies gave clearly positive results; 17 per cent were more mixed but worthwhile; and only two studies appeared wholly negative. This appears to give a reassuring picture, particularly in contrast to evaluations of effectiveness in the 1970s. However, there were problems with the methodology and scope of the studies. These included little evaluation of routine work, failure to give basic information such as the frequency of intervention, where or how long the help was offered. There was also little information on ethnicity or the social class of clients. Overall, 41 per cent did not give enough detail for replication. This underlines the necessity to scrutinise critically the claims being made.

Much of the value attributed to an evidence based approach lies in its potential to inform action, helping practitioners to make better decisions in a given situation. However, social work research and qualitative research methods have led the way in extending our understanding of what it is like to experience social and health problems, and to use the corresponding services.

For instance, the use of narrative methods in mental health research has highlighted the differing meaning attached to 'recovery' by people with mental health problems, and what helps and hinders this process (Ring 2007). Elsewhere, empirical qualitative research has highlighted how parents of disabled children experience this role – often rejecting the label of 'carer', seeing themselves first and foremost as parent, but despite this needing child-support services, sometimes reluctantly accepted (Beresford 1996).

These insights are supporting development of good practice in several ways. They highlight the value of taking a holistic approach to problematic situations; they allow for negotiation of a common understanding of the nature of a problem; and they open up more options to address this.

WHAT SKILLS AND KNOWLEDGE DO STUDENTS AND PRACTITIONERS NEED?

There are a number of 'how to do it' guides available on the process of EBP. One (Newman *et al.* 2005) proposes the following ideal model:

1   Formulate question.
2   Search.
3   Retrieve.
4   Appraise.
5   Implement.

However, this is deceptively simple and putting this into practice is more complex. The first task is to be able to formulate a question that is answerable, relevant, and amenable to conducting a search for the best current information. Gibbs (2003) calls these client-oriented, practical, evidence-search questions (COPES). In order to search for evidence, knowledge of the most appropriate resources and how to navigate them is required. Understanding how to read academic sources critically and distinguish good quality research from less rigorous work is needed to make sense of the material obtained. Interpersonal and change management skills are essential to implement evidence and more effective models into routine practice in health and social care, for the benefit of those who use the services. Evaluation requires the willingness to review objectively outcomes in the light of aims and interventions provided.

MOMENT OF REFLECTION

Activity Four

Do an audit of your own knowledge and skills of the stages of evidence based practice, from posing relevant questions to translating them into practice. What do you need to learn more about?

WHAT KEY RESOURCES ARE AVAILABLE?

There are well established and credible sources of information available that are designed to help busy practitioners. An indicative list of useful resources is included at the end of the chapter. For example, the Cochrane Collaboration in health care and the Campbell Collaboration in social care are international partnerships that commission systematic reviews of published research, which are then searchable in their databases. Such reviews, as the name suggests, involve teams trawling systematically through all published research on a given topic, applying thresholds to the research to exclude those of poor quality, synthesising the results and publishing overall conclusions. These summaries provide a service to time-pressed practitioners who want to survey the current state of knowledge in a particular area, and are an effective means of coping with the growing mountain of information, which is very difficult for an individual to find and read, let alone analyse and absorb. Professional organisations such as the Social Care Institute of Excellence also produce searchable databases of published information and practice guides that are aimed at staff and service users, rather than specialist academics. Such organisations demonstrate the expectation that practitioners in health and social care are expected to keep themselves updated as part of their professional codes of conduct. Sweden's Institute for Evidence Based Social Work Practice is an international example of how governments in other countries may use their power to induce organisational change toward EBP in social work.

MOMENT OF REFLECTION

Activity Five

Choose some of the resources at the end of the chapter that are relevant to your interests and familiarise yourself with how to use their databases, guides etc.

PUTTING IT ALL INTO PRACTICE – BARRIERS AND GATEWAYS TO IMPLEMENTATION OF EBP

Let us take an example from the area of mental health. Family members frequently experience considerable difficulty in knowing how best to cope with the behaviour of a person diagnosed with schizophrenia. There is good evidence that 'expressed emotion' – critical attitudes and inconsistent behaviour towards the affected person – increases the likelihood of relapse. Families can be taught how to respond differently to problematic behaviours: doing this has consistently been shown to reduce the risk of relapse. Social workers and other mental health professionals can learn to do this, and the value of this intervention has been consistently demonstrated (National Institute for Health and Clinical Excellence 2010). However, Fadden (2000) and Sheldon and Macdonald (2008: 306) have drawn attention to how few families are offered this form of help: 'Such interventions, though known about for some years, are not routinely available in the UK outside specialist centres.' This seems scandalous given their recognised effectiveness.

Other opportunities offered by EBP are frequently disregarded. Bradshaw *et al.* (2000) discuss the difficulties of getting well-evidenced psychosocial interventions into practice. In other areas of mental health, however, EBP is more flourishing. The 'Individual Placement and Support' approach to enable people with a mental health problem to return to work is widely regarded as best practice for this purpose. It will be interesting to see whether this proven approach becomes increasingly embedded in policy and practice, or whether (as in the case of family interventions) practice continues only in a small number of 'centres of excellence'.

Some commentators, such as Webb (2001) take the view that the models of EBP espoused in social care offer little scope for improving social work practice, but serve the interests of performance management. He argues that established interests will circumscribe the use of EBP, according to the extent to which this serves policy objectives (such as harm minimisation) while offering little to professional aims such autonomy and self-determination.

Sheldon and Chilvers (2000), surveying social workers' use of evidence in their daily work, found that 90 per cent of a large sample thought research relevant to practice (which could be seen as heartening), and were enthusiastic about the idea of EBP. However, slightly over 50 per cent thought that their day-to-day practice was informed by research. Some of the barriers cited included inadequate access to research evidence, lack of time and skills to make sense of this, and lack of organisational support to apply this to practice. In a more recent survey, the professional magazine *Community Care* undertook a survey in 2009 of social workers' use of information resources in their routine work. Of the 450 respondents, 82 per cent reported difficulties with having adequate resources to make informed decisions. In terms of sources of information, most (88 per cent) asked colleagues, and 29 per cent used journals and other publications. Google was the most popular source for facts and figures, despite a lack of trust in it as an information source.

The example which follows highlights one more lost opportunity to apply good evidence to securing the best outcomes for parents and children.

A case example from social care

The RCT evaluating a model of parenting programmes conducted by Scott *et al.* (2001) has already been used as an example of rigorous research on effective practice. 'Incredible Years' is the international network and training provider that promotes application of that research in routine childcare practice. Nevertheless many parenting programmes are created with no reference to published literature on projects such as Incredible Years.

It has been estimated that there is a two-decade gap between the emergence of best clinical research and the use of these research results in the American health and mental health care systems (Soydan 2007). In the UK, organisations such as Research in Practice (specialising in childcare) have also instigated change projects, which are partnerships between provider agencies over a three- or four-year cycle to explore aspects of using evidence in application to policy and practice. The change projects produce action packs and guidance for implementation. They also include web resources such as blogs with tips for embedding evidence in practice. Service users are also powerful agents in their demands for responsive and effective services that achieve individual outcomes. Networks like 'Involve' in the health services and collaborations with patient networks and the Cochrane Collaboration help to understand how EBP can be applied from user perspectives.

MOMENT OF REFLECTION

Activity Six

If you are studying to become a health or social care practitioner (or are already in practice) consider what steps you might take to practise in a more evidence based way.

Devise an action plan.

CONCLUSION

In conclusion, we have seen how the principles of evidence based practice can produce lifelong learners who draw on research findings and involve service users in order to provide more effective services. There are issues of individual and organisational responsibility here; competent practitioners and competent workplaces are both necessary. To achieve these, a 'culture of thoughtfulness' (Gambrill 1997) should be cultivated. This emphasises individual critical thinking skills and habits of mind, integrity and honesty, as well as work-based organisational issues of access to knowledge bases, ways of sharing information (such as journal clubs), continuing professional development and time to reflect.

MOMENT OF REFLECTION

Activity Seven

Go back to Activity One. Consider again the scenario about making decisions, but from the following perspective: How would you want your social worker, doctor, community psychiatric nurse, etc. to make decisions if you were a user or patient?

SUMMARY OF MAIN POINTS

You should be able to:

- Appreciate the nature, forms and sources of evidence applicable to health and social care.
- Distinguish, explain, and evaluate research approaches applicable to health and social care.
- Appreciate the contribution of empirical evidence to enhancing and evaluating health and social care practice.
- Discuss the factors which promote or hinder evidence based practice.

REFERENCES AND FURTHER READING

Aisenberg, E. (2008) Evidence-based practice in mental health care to ethnic minority communities: Has its practice fallen short of its evidence?, *Social Work*, 53 (4), 297–306.

Barratt, M. (2003) Organisational Support for Evidence-based Practice within Child and Family Social Work: A Collaborative Study, *Child and Family Social Work*, 8 (2), 143–50.

Beresford, B. (1996) Coping with the Care of a Disabled Child, *Health and Social Care in the Community*, 4 (1), 30–40.

Bonner, L. (2003) Using theory-based evaluation to build evidence-based health and social care policy and practice, *Critical Public Health*, 13 (1), 77–92.

Bradshaw, T., Lovella, K. and Richards, D. (2000) PSI and COPE, *Mental Health Nursing*, 20 (8), 10–14.

Brown, K. and Rutter, L. (2008) *Critical Thinking for Social Work* (2nd edition), Exeter: Learning Matters.

Community Care (2009) *Support Shortfall Leaves Staff on Brink of Burnout*. 23rd April.

Fadden, G. (2000) Family Intervention, in Brooker, C. and Repper, J. (Eds) *Serious Mental Health Problems in the Community*, London: Bailliere Tindall.

Gambrill, E. (1997) *Social Work Practice: A Critical Thinker's Guide*, New York: Oxford University Press.

Gambrill, E. (2000) The Role of Critical Thinking in Evidence-based Social Work, in Allen-Meares, P. and Garvin, C. (Eds) *The Handbook of Social Work Direct Practice*, London: Sage.

General Social Care Council (GSCC) (2001) *Code of Practice for Social Care Workers*, London: GSCC.

Gibbs, L. (2003) *Evidence-Based Practice for the Helping Professions: A Practical Guide with Integrated Multimedia*, London: Thomson Learning.

Gibbs, L. and Gambrill, E. (1999) *Critical Thinking for Social Workers: Exercises for the helping professions*, Thousand Oaks, CA: Pine Forge Press.

Gibbs, L. and Gambrill, E. (2002) Evidence-Based Practice: Counterarguments to Objections, *Research on Social Work Practice*, 12 (3), 452–76.

Goldacre, B. (2008) *Bad Science*, London: Fourth Estate.

Greenhalgh, T. (2001) *How to Read a Paper: The Basics of Evidence Based Medicine* (2nd edition), London: BMJ.

Kirk, S. and Reid, W. (2002) *Science and Social Work: A Critical Appraisal*, New York: Columbia University Press.

La Fontaine, J. (1994) *Extent and Nature of Organised and Ritual Abuse: Research Findings*, London: HMSO.

La Fontaine, J. (1998) *Speak of the Devil: Tales of Satanic Abuse in Contemporary England*, Cambridge: Cambridge University Press.

Lewis, J. (2002) The Contribution of Research Findings to Practice Change, *Managing Community Care: Building Knowledge for Integrated Care,* 10 (1), 9–12.

Macdonald, G. (2001) *Effective interventions for child abuse and neglect: An evidence-based approach to planning and evaluating interventions,* Chichester: Wiley.

Macdonald, G. and Roberts, H. (1995) What Works in the Early Years?, Ilford: Barnardo's.

Macdonald, G. and Turner, W. (2005) An Experiment in Helping Foster-Carers Manage Challenging Behaviour, *British Journal of Social Work,* 35, 1265–82.

Macdonald, G. M., Sheldon, B. and Gillespie, J. (1992) Contemporary Studies of Effectiveness of Social Work, *British Journal of Social Work,* 22 (6), 615–43.

Munro, E. (1999) Common Errors of Reasoning in Child Protection Work, *Child Abuse and Neglect,* 23 (8), 745–58.

Munro, E. (2008) Lessons learnt, boxes ticked, families ignored, *The Independent,* 16 November.

Newman, T., Moseley, A., Tierney, S. and Ellis, A. (2005) *Evidence-Based Social Work: A Guide for the Perplexed,* Lyme Regis: Russell House.

National Institute for Health and Clinical Excellence (NICE) (2010) *Schizophrenia: Core Interventions in the Treatment and Management of Schizophrenia in Adults in Primary and Secondary Care,* British Psychological Society and the Royal College of Psychiatrists.

Nuland, S. (2004) *The Doctor's Plague: Germs, Childbed Fever and the Strange Story of Ignac Semmelweis,* London: Norton.

Oakley, A. (1998) Experimentation and Social Interventions: A Forgotten but Important History, *British Medical Journal* 317, 1239–42.

Raynor, P. (2003) Evidence-based probation and its critics, *Probation Journal,* 50 (4), 334–45.

Ring, C. (2007) How can mental health services promote recovery from severe mental illness?, *Research in Practice for Adults Outline 9,* Dartington: Ripfa.

Sackett, D., Rosenberg, W., Muir Gray, J., Haynes, R., and Richardson, W. (1996) Evidence Based Medicine: What it is and what it isn't, Editorial, *British Medical Journal;* 312: 71–2.

Scott, S., Spender, Q., Doolan, M., Jacobs, B. and Aspland, H. (2001) Multicentre controlled trial of parenting groups for childhood anti-social behaviour in clinical practice, *British Medical Journal ,* 323, 28 July.

Sheldon, B. (2001) The Validity of Evidence-Based Practice in Social Work: a reply to Stephen Webb, *British Journal of Social Work,* 31, 801–9.

Sheldon, B. and Chilvers, R. (2000) *Evidence-Based Social Care: A study of prospects and problems,* Lyme Regis: Russell House.

Sheldon, B. and Macdonald, G. (1999) *Mind the Gap: Research and Practice in Social Care,* Exeter: CEBSS/School for Policy Studies, University of Bristol.

Sheldon, B. and Macdonald, G. (2008) *A Textbook of Social Work,* Abingdon: Routledge/ Taylor and Francis.

Sinclair, R. (2000) Young People's Participation, ECM Research and Practice Briefing, London Research Practice.

Smith, D. (Ed.) (2004) *Social Work and Evidence-Based Practice,* London: Jessica Kingsley.

Social Care Institute for Excellence (SCIE) (2005) *Developing the evidence base for social work and social care practice: Report 10,* London: SCIE.

Social Care Institute for Excellence (SCIE) (2009) *Using SCIE Resources: Guide 28,* London: SCIE.

Sokal, A. and Bricmont, J. (1998) *Intellectual Impostures,* London: Profile.

Soydan, H. (2007) Improving the Teaching of Evidence-Based Practice: Challenges and Priorities, *Research on Social Work Practice,* 17 (5), 612–18.

Swinkels, A., Albarran, J., Means, R., Mitchell, T. and Stewart, M. (2002) Evidence-based practice in health and social care: where are we now?, *Journal of Interprofessional Care,* 16 (4), 335–45.

Webb, S. (2001) Some Considerations on the Validity of Evidence-Based Practice in Social Work, *British Journal of Social Work,* 31, 57–79.

USEFUL WEBSITES

Barnardo's – includes the 'What Works' series in children and young people research.
http://www.barnardos.org.uk/

Campbell Collaboration – a development from the Cochrane Collaboration. Systematic reviews of effectiveness of interventions in social and educational practice.
http://www.campbellcollaboration.org/

Centre for Evidence-Based Child Health – linked to Great Ormond Street Hospital.
http://www.ich.ucl.ac.uk/ich/html/academicunits/paed_epid/cebch/

Centre for Evidence-Based Mental Health, Oxford University – searchable database, and developing the Electronic Library for Mental Health (ELMH).
http://www.psychiatry.ox.ac.uk/cebmh/

Centre for Reviews and Dissemination – part of the National Institute for Health Research, and produces systematic reviews of evidence.
http://www.york.ac.uk/inst/crd/

Cochrane Collaboration – systematic reviews of effectiveness of health care interventions.
http://www.cochrane.org

European Research Institute
http://eris.osu.eu/index.php?kategorie=35175&id=5161

Evidence-based Medicine
http://www.evidence-based-medicine.co.uk/What_is_series.html

Evidence Based Mental Health
http://ebmh.bmj.com/

Evidence Based Practice in the Helping Professions
http://www.evidence.brookscole.com/

Evidence Based Practice and Policy, Online Resource Training Center, Columbia University School of Social Work.
http://www.columbia.edu/cu/musher/Website/Website/EBP_CtrBib.htm

Evidence Network – Economic and Social Research Council funded centre for evidence-based policy and practice. Includes a searchable bibliography.
http://www.evidencenetwork.org/

Home Office Research Development and Statistics
http://www.homeoffice.gov.uk/rds/

Incredible Years – evidence-based parenting programme.
http://www.incredibleyears.com/

Intute virtual training
http://www.vts.intute.ac.uk/he/tutorial/social-worker/?sid=3015178

Making Research Count – a consortium of universities and social care providers. Produces events on various topics and briefings on aspects of Quality Protects.
http://www.uea.ac.uk/menu/acad_depts/swk/MRC_web/public_html/

National Mental Health Development Unit
http://www.nmhdu.org.uk/nmhdu/

NHS Centre for Reviews and Dissemination at York University – systematic reviews of health care available online, including effectiveness reviews in child health.
http://www.york.ac.uk/inst/crd/

NHS Specialist Libraries
http://www.library.nhs.uk/SpecialistLibraries/

Personal Social Services Research Unit – sites at the University of Kent, LSE and Manchester – texts of reports available online.
http://www.pssru.ac.uk/

Practice Based Evidence – messages from user and practitioner views in mental health.
http://www.practicebasedevidence.com/

Prevention in Action – online news publication reporting internationally on innovation and effectiveness among programmes for improving children's health and development.
http://www.preventionaction.org/about

Research Mindedness – funded by SCIE to help practitioners and students make better use of research findings.
http://www.resmind.swap.ac.uk/

Research in Practice – resource for evidence-based childcare practice and research. Over 75 participating local authorities in conjunction with universities, research institutions and SCIE.
http://www.rip.org.uk/

Research in Practice for Adults – resource for evidence-based practice and research in adult care. Now incorporates archive of CEBSS.
http://www.ripfa.org.uk/index.asp

Sainsbury Centre for Mental Health – reports, briefings, etc. available online.
http://www.scmh.org.uk/

Social Care Institute for Excellence (SCIE) – headed 'Better Knowledge for Better Practice'. Has crucial role in gathering and publishing evidence for better practice. Includes practice guides and knowledge reviews. Hosts Social Care Online database (see below).
http://www.scie.org.uk/

Social Care Online – the UK's most extensive database of social care information (replaces previous electronic Library for Social Care). Includes knowledge base of searchable abstracts of journal articles and books (also available in 'electronic databases' section of NTU Libraries and Learning Resources online), good practice guides, links, etc.
http://www.scie-socialcareonline.org.uk/

Social Policy Research Unit at York University – 'Research Works' series of reports.
http://www.york.ac.uk/inst/spru/

Social Services Research Group – publish the journal *Research, Policy and Planning*, with full texts available online.
http://www.ssrg.org.uk/

Swedish Evidence Based Practice Institute
http://www.sos.se/socialtj/cus/cuse/imse.htm

WHO Health Evidence Network
http://www.euro.who.int/HEN

CHAPTER 18

CONTEMPORARY MENTAL HEALTH CARE

KIRSTY BEART

OBJECTIVES

After reading this chapter you should be able to:

▓ Discuss perspectives and conceptual models of mental health.

▓ Consider community based services.

▓ Critically review community care.

▓ Have an awareness of mental health legislation, policy and practice.

▓ Discuss assessment and interventions.

▓ Be aware of distortions and discriminations in mental health.

▓ Understand interagency work.

After reading this chapter you will understand the key terms:
De-institutionalisation, community care, needs, positive practice, mental illness, humanistic theory, medical model, integrative model.

There are five Moments of Reflection to work on throughout the chapter.

INTRODUCTION

This chapter explores a range of perspectives in contemporary mental health and social care. This includes conceptual models (medical, social and user), assessment, policy and practice frameworks. It aims to enable you to develop a critical awareness of current provision, policy and legislation, and ultimately to provide you with an opportunity to examine the implications of working with people who have mental health problems and illness. The chapter will introduce you to the nature, role and purpose of 'care' in current service frameworks.

This will be achieved by consideration of:

- Defining mental health and ill health in society and using these concepts to consider the philosophical basis of historical and contemporary care.
- How professionals in statutory and non-statutory services, service users and carers can combine their own individual expert knowledge and philosophies into a plan which meets people's needs and wants.
- Working collaboratively as the key to ensuring that outcomes of care are set appropriately and are achievable, accountable, ethical and effective.

HISTORY OF MENTAL HEALTH IN BRITAIN

The history of society and its behaviour, attitudes and feelings is significant in any context of research. Consideration of this offers the learner a chance to see the progress and changes that have influenced the field of study so far. Allowing the mind to explore the topic in this way encourages perspective and an awareness of the vulnerability of individuals in an ever changing and influential society.

The time periods considered here offer some idea of the kind of attitudes around mental illness over time. This offers us a chance to consider how the person with a mental health problem may have lived in the past as well as the present.

Until the eighteenth century families were still ashamed of relatives who exhibited mental health problems and kept them hidden from society or excluded them from the family. This had the obvious effect of more mentally ill people living on the street who were demonstrating behaviours which were seen as abnormal.

Individuals were considered to be witches or possessed by the devil during the period from the fourteenth to eighteenth centuries. They received treatment seen as appropriate to these 'crimes', such as burning, leeching and exorcism (Darton 2004). Non-therapeutic asylums began to be identified as a means of incarcerating individuals and protecting society from them. Insanity was attended by individual physicians but before the end of eighteenth century there was no actual formal psychiatry or therapy (Norman and Ryrie 2004). Social control was the dominant theme of the time and people were kept in these institutions under potentially terrible conditions. The 1844 Lunacy Report and census of the insane identified inhumane living conditions for people living in asylums. People were reported to be living in cold, dark rooms with stone floors, with walls covered in dirt and excrement (Roberts 2009). However, William Battie and some other reformists developed the concept of institutionalisation as being curative rather than just incarceration for the protection of society (Darton 2004).

Following on with the work of the reformists the early nineteenth century saw the introduction of trained staff in the institutions and the beginnings of looking for treatments and cures (Roberts 2008). Some of the treatments introduced at that time included water immersion. This involved keeping the person under water as long as they could physically stand it before they passed out. Another therapy was to spin the person on a chair with the purpose of shaking the brain into its proper position (Darton 2004). Despite these cruel approaches this era can be seen as a positive turning point for people with these types of issues towards therapeutic care. However, conditions were still poor by today's social standards and therapy was not ethical by any standards applied in current services.

In the 1790s William Tuke identified a new way forward for people with mental health problems/illness and called it moral therapy (Borthwick *et al.*). This technique was about strengthening patients' self control and providing calming environments which were an early attempt at therapeutic intervention.

The attitudes of society towards mental illness started to take another turn during the First World War, with returning heroes who were suffering from 'shell shock' (Roberts 2008). The symptoms of shell shock were similar to those often used to define a person as mentally ill. It was apparent that officers as well as privates, upper as well as lower social classes were suffering from mental illness. Despite mental illness previously being considered a disease of the poor, heroes of war were suffering in similar ways regardless of their social or financial status. Attitudes were changing slowly.

Services began to change and develop based on care rather than just isolation. Outpatient treatment started and in the 1930s the Mental Treatment Act legislated that medics should have more rights to medicate people with a view to containing them more effectively. This is of course not seen as appropriate in contemporary social views but at the time could be seen as quite groundbreaking in its efforts to contain illness and its disturbing effects. Treatments were developed such as tonsillectomy, insulin comas, psychosurgery, chicken soup, cold baths and use of prostitutes. Increases in patient deaths also increased at this time possibly related to the treatments, or continued poor living conditions.

Psychology began to develop in the eighteenth century offering recognition that there is more to mental health than just biology (Darton 2004). Sigmund Freud (1856–1939) founded the school of psychoanalysis. The start of psychometrics, small group psychotherapy and therapeutic communities was evident. In 1948, the advent of the NHS encapsulated the asylums but had little to do with them giving control to different local authorities. The Mental Health National Institute in the 1950s meant that services would be considered in a right of their own. The introduction of psychotherapeutic drugs around this time assisted the care of the mentally ill although it can also be considered a continuation of the dominant medical control. The emphasis in mental illness changed from just rounding up problems into the institutions to encouraging society to use the facilities to help their relatives and keep them well. A massive mental health movement began with the building of state hospitals and the beginnings of psychoanalysis. More legislation followed, deinstitutionalisation and community care, and the prevention approach and holistic philosophies of care became prominent by the end of the twentieth century. Despite the positive changes of the last century the emphasis of mental health services could be said to have remained in the culture of containment and control within the Mental Health Acts of 1959 and 1983. There was still not enough emphasis on empowerment and self determination until the 1990s into the 2000s. The Griffiths Report (1989) led to the Community Care Act (1990) and in mental health this meant the emergence of the Care Programme Approach. Individuals who had been in institutions for many years were assessed for their ability to function in the community as the asylums were being closed. This resulted in a rise in group homes, supportive living and the need for crisis shelters (Norman and Ryrie 2004).

The twenty-first century arrived and with it came the potential for a bigger shift towards patients' rights, and advocacy in the legislation of the Mental Health Act 2007. The Human Rights Act 2000 paved the way in changes with an emphasis of care to meeting basic human rights in legal and ethical standards of consent and capacity, and the National Service frameworks (2000/2001) identified national standards of care based on best practice.

In the contemporary services culture, best practice examples include evidence of empowering environments where consent is actively sought and capacity actively determined. This is directly related but not responsible for the onset of the service user movement which is increasing all the time. The service user movement has developed and Wallcraft and Bryant (2003) identified 300 separate user groups in England. As a result of this more structured approach to self help and pressure group formation Campbell (2005) agrees that mental health service users have a much more prominent involvement in service provision and planning.

MOMENT OF REFLECTION

To make sense of learning from history the current treatments, legislation, practice, philosophies of care and services need to be examined in the context of contemporary culture. There is a need to remember that when looking back at some of the treatments of historical eras there is a tendency to judge the ethics of such practice. Knowing this arms current thinking with the forethought of the following question to relate to your own experience:

What will future generations think of our contemporary practice?

This question should fundamentally remind professionals of the need to keep considering the context of the situation and that society changes and with it changes attitudes, expectations and values. Therefore, all practice must be sound and based on evidence which justifies its use.

The key points of legislation in current services are:

- Deinstitutionalisation – from the 1970s there was a move from hospitals to community with the intention to treat and care rather than incarcerate people in institutions.
- Mental Health Act 1983/Code of Practice 1993 – move from the custodial 1959 Act to community focused treatment and consent.
- Community Care Act 1990/Care Programme Approach – Griffiths Report (1989) identified the need for changes in the structure of the mental health system.
- Community Mental Health Act 1995 – comes from the Ten Point Plan (1993) and the emergence of evidence that there was a need for supervision in the

community. The Act highlights the need for supervision and support of patients following admission and detention in hospital.

- National Service Frameworks (2000/2001) – mental health for adults, and later, older persons, with a section on mental health highlighting areas of best practice for services preventing exclusion or isolation and combining of services.
- Health Act 1999/Health and Social Care Act 2001 – formal structures were put in place to link professionals and service users and non-professional carers to work together better.
- No Secrets 2000 – introduced national standards for protecting vulnerable adults.
- Human Rights Act 2000 – ensured the need for review of mental health law.
- Mental Capacity Act 2005 – presumption of capacity, personal choice and best interests regardless of diagnosis was a significant development in mental health care.
- Mental Health Act 2007/Code of Practice 2008 – current Act of England and Wales. Includes many changes from 1983 but significantly is meant to be much more focused on service users' human rights and individuality.
- New Horizons Consultation 2009 – the Department of Health are currently constructing a new service standard based on the progress or issues arising from the National Service Frameworks. This will be the new national strategy.

MOMENT OF REFLECTION

Consider the three time periods below and the ethical and legal aspects of care of people with mental illness in each. Use the preceding summary to evaluate the changes in attitudes and care:

- pre 1700
- 1900s
- 2000s.

MEETING THE NEEDS OF PEOPLE

Defining mental ill health and devising a relevant plan of care requires expertise, skills and knowledge. The professional role of anyone working in mental health services may vary significantly depending on the basis of training or experience. As will be discussed there are many different ideals, values and functions on the part of the variety of people involved as professional, carer, supporter or service user services. Each group also has defined roles which will mean that all the individual perspectives can and should be considered and valued. The integration of collaboration or joined up working into services has meant that people with mental health problems should have access to a much more integrated support network. However, an audit of service user groups across the UK (Wallcraft and Bryant 2003) identified gaps in service user involvement. This included lack of service user consultation in developing national standards, gaining the voice of people from ethnic minority groups and a lack of investment to implement collaborative practices legislated in the Health and Social Care Act 2001. The development of service users expressing their voice has increased significantly from just a dozen groups across the UK. Wallcraft and Bryant (2003) identified 300 separate user groups in England and Campbell (2005) estimates in excess of 500 groups. The service user involvement is complicated by its necessity to overcome the power dynamics of the traditional services and structures. Whilst trying to achieve this, as is recommended by legislation and contemporary philosophies of care, individuals are faced with the ongoing covert battle of power which dominates UK society's attitude to mental illness. Trivedi and Wykes (2009) demonstrate this by describing a research project that involves the experience and problems of putting collaboration into practice. They describe issues such as the incongruences between the professional's intentions and the services user's ideals. Participation in prescribed therapies for example can be perceived to be simply a further assertion of control by the professional. The service user's consequent lack of willingness to participate can be seen as obstructive or relapse behaviour. An individual's ability to define what they need and want is called into question immediately that mental illness is defined or alluded to. Current changes to the law in the Mental Capacity Act 2005, the Mental Health Act 2007 and much more focused training of professionals are leading towards a less paternalistic approach. This means that professionals can remove the shackles of traditional controlling service provisions and engage in collaboration with service users and their communities. The overarching aims of the new culture seem to lie in effective engagement between professionals and service users. Professionals in the statutory and voluntary sectors can have varying priorities but the agenda of collaboration provides an opportunity to bridge these gaps in mental health care. Thurgood (in Norman and Ryrie 2004: 650) said that true engagement will occur when an organisation is 'providing a service that is experienced by service users (including carers) as acceptable, accessible, positive and empowering'.

This offers a succinct definition of engagement to aim for when trying to establish a common ground between different parties. The main issue is trying to understand what professionals are trying to achieve when engaging people into the services. Bryant (2001) identifies findings from service user research which imply that service users see little to entice them to engage with the services unless they have to.

MOMENT OF REFLECTION

What do you as a professional need to consider when trying to engage individual people with the service you provide?

The need to consider the background to the dynamics of a relationship and how this impacts on a person is essential. Problems with accessing and utilising services are strongly related to this relationship and developing it is a key skill. This kind of self awareness by professionals can be so significant that it influences the traditional norms of control. The risk factors change when this relationship changes and this ensures that individuals make their own decisions and understand the risks. Professionals and carers in all sectors of health and social care are in a position to research and develop their own care approaches. The ten essential shared capabilities (Hope 2004) suggest that comprehensive education and training would help overcome the professional status barriers by ensuring each has the same priorities.

Issues that influence service users' approach to the services and control of their own decisions are influenced by many things and professionals must be conscious of the multi-dimensionality of dealing with mental ill health and all of the issues around it.

Use the scenario below to try and identify key areas which may impinge on a service user's engagement with support services.

MOMENT OF REFLECTION

Jane is a 22-year-old woman. She has been self harming for approximately six years and has been avoiding all contact with support services. She has contacted the Samaritans but has otherwise managed to keep it all to herself. Her experience is a typical one and she experiences the following:

- feeling isolated
- family problems, including parental separation or divorce
- being bullied
- low self-esteem.

SCMH (2006)

What kind of concerns might Jane have in trying to access some support for this problem? Professional control overtaking her control of her own decisions? Fear of being labelled as a self harmer? Lack of understanding of the support available?

What kind of choices does Jane really have with regards to her care? How will the power balance in the professional/service user relationship impact on her decisions? Will the legislation and traditional manner of the services take over her free will?

Lester and Glasby (2006) identify positive practice as a way forward. The main emphasis of this model is about active involvement as opposed to passive service users. It includes:

- Active involvement in research and learning.
- Active involvement in recruitment of staff.

- Implementation of support time and recovery workers strategy – employ service users in teams.
- Active involvement in collaborative provision teams.

Lester and Glasby (2006) offer a useful way to consider these issues of control and domination by the services. They suggest that by considering the service user in a different light, as a consumer, this changes the power balance between the parties involved. If the user is considered in light of their contribution to society as tax payer, the professional can facilitate the patient choice agenda and their own accountability for this, and Lester and Glasby argue that the relationship will therefore be different. To consider this in any relationship dynamic would perhaps eradicate the issues faced by all service users dominated as a result of key factors. Examples of this can be found in race and culture: young black men are often misrepresented as difficult and are likely to be over-medicated (Golightley 2006). Females are often associated with depression and mental illness much more than men (Pilgrim and Rogers 2005). Poverty and education are also closely associated with mental ill health and this has been demonstrated to be true on many occasions, but more recently by Freidli (2009). These factors may be statistically true in diagnosis; however, the basis of these figures comes from the very labelling and social construction theory influence discussed in this chapter. If these influences changed they may well change rates of diagnosis in different race, gender or class groups.

Questions of power: An example

In a supermarket the customer can vote with their feet and choose to go to another supermarket easily. A mental health service user does not have that flexibility. However, that in itself is not the issue. The biggest issue is that the power dynamic in the comparisons is different. The supermarket is not the only answer or shop the consumer can go to but the health and social care services can *appear* to be the only option for the service user within the current disease model structures. The typical power balance is based on who needs who the most.

How can professionals acknowledge the reality of these situations and still ensure people's human rights are upheld? The use of key concepts such as empowerment and advocacy can help to develop self awareness. This in turn engenders a technique of consideration to the individual when approaching and planning care, and avoidance of disempowering behaviours and the institution of Positive Practice as advocated by Lester and Glasby (2006). They offer an example of professionals providing wider service goals and being part of breaking down the old hierarchies of power.

Overall the progress of legislation and direction of service provision is towards collaborative care. This has significantly changed from the beginning of the 1970s and as a society there have been changes to attitudes about mental illness by the use of mental health promotion, media portrayal and informative journalism. These means have increased the profile of the issues of mental illness in positive ways as well as negative. Perhaps the most important aspect of this kind of publicity is the development of awareness in the general public consciousness that mental illness is around and needs to be acknowledged. The improved and encouraging development of more focused programmes that are collaborations of professionals and service users highlights demonstrations of this and how genuine consultation and team development can be enhanced. Shelter homeless charity has a project with Westminster City Council to jointly assess individuals for housing. This brings together the service users with representatives, support and the housing/social services professionals who can offer the services (Hurll 2009). The implications of this are significant as service users can be involved in the actual planning of any future living accommodation with advice and support from professionals who know the system intricacies.

Collaboration is a key area of development in mental health care. Individuals both demonstrate a will and expertise in being part of their own care planning as well as taking on the service provision and the research aspect of working together.

There is a need to briefly discuss the philosophical understandings of what mental illness actually is. Considerations of where it comes from and how it is defined and managed are essential for the reader to be able to recognise the issues professionals and service users deal with daily. The main outcome for all is to overcome issues and ensure the collaboration between them is equal and empowering for both.

WHAT IS MENTAL ILLNESS?

Mental illness is often seen as a socially controlling label and/or a socially constructed entity. These are both theories which have changed significantly over the years. Bowers (1998) identifies classic labelling theory as the process in which society makes rules about deviant behaviour, implying that anyone who breaks those rules with implications for others will be labelled deviant, mentally ill. This is not a measurable concept; different rules apply in different cultures, families and social groups. The implications of this assertion that deviancy is not definable means that all diagnosis is subject to professional opinion. This means that the practitioner's word is final as they are the professional specialists who are able to identify the criteria as well as apply it to individuals. The medical model which will be explained in more depth later, generally asserts that the appearance of symptoms is the result of a biological or chemical imbalance in the body. The problem with mental illness is that its general appearance is not a physical certainty. The example of being able to see pneumonia on a chest X-ray demonstrates the difference between definable physical evidence of illness and the non-visible mental illness. Mental illness is defined by symptoms but these are based on key criteria of aggregated evidence from years of research and definition of people's experience of mental illness. The classification of illness into groups which identify the 'label' appropriate to these symptoms is an international standard. These sources can be found in a diagnostic manual such as the WHO *International Classification of Diseases-10 (ICD-10)*(1992) or *Diagnostic and Statistical Manual of Mental Disorders (DSM IV)* (1994) (Norman and Ryrie 2004). These are the statutory tools used by clinicians in the UK to define and diagnose mental illness. There are many issues with this kind of labelling, not least cultural differences in definition of symptoms, variability and lack of concrete conclusions and the basis of the labels coming from a purely medical research basis. Another issue with this type of labelling is that it categorically ignores the mental health problems people have in day-to-day life, only acknowledging the most severe of illnesses such as psychosis or psychopathic behaviour.

The push towards user led care is a direct resistance to this view. Sayce (2000) discusses many attitudes towards mental illness including society's attempts to remove discrimination and improve the lot of the community by protecting itself from the mentally ill. This change in approach is demonstrated in the moral treatments era, the control and restraint cultures of the 1920s–1980s, and moving forward to more informed and potentially liberating beliefs. Lester and Glasby (2006) highlight key models of care which have benefits but also problems in their implications:

> The Brain Disease model states that people with mental illness should be seen as suffering from a disease which would remove the implication of moral weakness. However, this theory indeed ignores clear evidence that mental illness occurs in certain patterns and higher incidence occurs in certain socio-economic groups based on these labelling definitions. So, moral weakness cannot be the only reason if it occurs in certain circumstances. The current expansion of the medical or disease model is still the most dominant in contemporary health and social care culture today.
>
> (Lester and Glasby 2006)

The alternative models that have challenged this come back to a more sociologically based theory about individual experiences and environments. Sayce (2000) also identifies the 'individual growth model', the 'libertarian' and the 'disability inclusion model'. Norman and Ryries (2004) describe these approaches as general social models that range from the need to consider mental health and illness as part of normal life, to separate it from criminality and deviance and to ensure that people are not disabled by the approaches used in their society and care services. The individual growth model explores what can be seen as a psychodynamic approach in current care, the emphasis being on having no distinct disease categories with a user led continuum of measurement ranging from 'emotional well-being' to 'ill health'. Along the process, markers are identified and offer guidance on key issues that affect a person's equilibrium. The range includes capacity to learn, to achieve autonomy, be self aware, enjoy relationships up to meeting challenges. This theory asserts that all individuals are moving back and forth on this line all the time. This offers a meaningful definition of mental illness rather than the biological reductionism of the medical/disease model and implies that mental illness and health are part of normal life rather than abnormal. Individuals can explore their views, values, ideas, etc. with a view to examining what is causing them the distress they are feeling.

The need to consider the cognitive, behavioural and the psychoanalytical models is a further extension of this discussion. These models consider more intricate elements of cognition and behaviour as learned which can therefore be unlearned. Lastly, the influence of the psychodynamic model contains an assertion that a person's life is controlled by their own experiences from early life. Based on these models the decisions of how to label or not are put into the hands of professionals who use the *ICD-10* (1992) or *DSM IV* (1994) as described earlier. To define abnormality is perhaps the aim of using this tool, with its disease labelling basis, and using it suggests that as a culture we are still entrenched in the labelling of people as rule breakers. The alternative does require a more individual approach. The professional, non-professional carer and service user will need to compromise and develop a combination. Although there may be a need for medicalisation, priority is also given to the individual's perspective and views.

Some issues with this psychosocial approach are that the relevant therapy requires long-term input and expensive manpower. The provision of services and specialists is based on national standards and therefore key standard services are generally only available. However, this can vary in different regions as authorities and trusts control the spending in certain specialities based on local need. Despite the potential implications of this the Layard Report (2006) has led to a Government initiative to train 10,000 new therapists.

Lester and Glasby (2006) discuss social models as the approach that acknowledges psychological and social influences as significant in a person's perceptions of their own illness. This seems to be a common ground and basis to work together for the medical/disease model approach and the more humanistic approach of person centred care. However, it is not clear that this is indeed the reality of this mix and further research in this area would help to establish its theoretical viability. Mental illness can therefore be defined by use of one or all of these models but most professionals and informal carers have focused strategies and use the models appropriate to the service user they are working with.

The integration of professionals, service users and non-professional carers means there is ample expert knowledge in any team. The use of the combined approach based on the amalgamation of fundamental beliefs and values about mental illness can be productive.

The issue faced by service users now is whether these changes have in reality taken the field or area of mental health and illness into a new era of care and better understanding.

THE MOVE TO CARE WITH BETTER UNDERSTANDING

The current move towards person centred care in mental health has its root in humanistic theory and Rogers (1961). This is very in tune with Sayce's (2000) theories of 'libertarians' and 'disability inclusion' as it considers the individual's rights as paramount and important. This is in contrast to previous models which have placed the power of decisions in those trained and qualified to make informed decisions, for example the rule makers and professionals. The person with a mental disorder needs to be an integral, functioning part of society to be able to influence it. However, various processes like unemployment, illness and bereavement can lead a person to become socially excluded (Byrne 2005), and when mental illness is included in this mix then discrimination, isolation and a lack of understanding compound this even more (Sayce 2000). As a result of this exclusion many service users are not able to be involved in their own care or the planning of service provision generally. The person centred approach has influenced many models of care used by practitioners today because of its facility to change the relationship between the service user and professional to a more equal one.

The humanistic approach can be seen in assessment and Watkins (2001) identified the person centred assessment as a means of gaining information and understanding about a service user by looking at their situation from their perspective.

Kitwood and Bredin (1992) also used this foundation to revolutionise care of people with dementia. They identified the need to see the person and not the disease, therefore encouraging carers and professionals to find a way through the frustrations of conflict and meet it with understanding and empathy (Beart 2006).

Rethink (2009) identify key therapies in two categories, medication and talking therapies. This is significant in the area of care of people with psychotic illness such as schizophrenia who were traditionally offered medication as the main treatment.

The development of the tidal model (Barker 2000) is another significant move towards the perceptual understanding of mental illness and problems. This model offers an alternative approach for service users to describe and be listened to based on their own perceptions of their own experience.

Professionals need to listen and use their own experience and skills to participate in a caring relationship. The emergence of person centred approaches in the services is demonstrated in each of these categories of illness and is ever developing.

The influence of all of these classic determining factors about defining, labelling or diagnosing mental illness is directly related to the current development of care. These developments include a move into a culture of empowerment and person centred care. Consent and capacity are the criteria driving the decisions; learning to live with mental health disturbance rather than trying unsuccessfully to cure it. Joined up working and collaboration of all the services make access easier and more consistent. In conjunction with improving these issues in the services, the service users need to be able to develop as individuals as well as develop the movement they need to represent them. However, there is evidence to suggest that some key areas of empowerment and engagement are still an issue, such as having no national forum, and women and black people not being represented well by the movement (Wallcraft and Bryant 2003). This of course has implications for under-representation as a body of people advocating their rights. Golightley (2008) also identifies issues in the rights of children to determine or influence the mental health care they receive. He argues that this slow move to empower children in this setting contradicts the Richardson committee recommendations to consider capacity from the age of 10–12 years using the Gillick competences.

DEFINING MENTAL ILLNESS AND AN INDIVIDUAL'S CARE IN CONTEMPORARY CULTURES

As a result of the changes and theoretical perspectives highlighted in the previous section, the services in the UK are changing and are potentially liberating, ethical and effective. However, despite the development of theoretical advancement in definitions and care, the fact is that currently labels are used and mental illness is categorised and classified into the following structures using *ICD-10* or *DSM IV*:

- organic including dementias and delirium
- mood disorders – depressions, mania
- schizophrenia, psychosis
- substance misuse
- neuroses – phobias or obsessions
- behavioural disorders
- personality, psychosomatic, eating disorder, post traumatic, etc.

The move to better understanding requires active change and the models above form the basis of thinking in this area. It is from this that contemporary labelling can take place. This is how society and professional groups take the philosophical under-standings of care and identify care strategies. The professional needs to consider the potential for practice as a variable. People are different, organisations have different priorities and funding, and professionals have different types of training.

The ways of understanding what illness actually is and how care can be planned lie in where an individual stands on the debate.

MOMENT OF REFLECTION

The medical disease model combined with the social and psychological models could be considered the future path of definition. This amalgamation would con-sider a person's individual journey in life in relation and in conjunction with any biological/chemical imbalances.

Try and think of medical, social and psychological aspects of a mental health difficulty/illness.

The basis of any plan then can be a combined effort and follow a much more integra-tive model:

Integrative model of mental health

1	Social Constructs +
2	Psychological interpretation of experience +
3	Biological/actual physical changes (for example, organic brain damage)

1   Social norms, problems including cultural conflict or clashes, societal and indi-vidual ability variation are combined into statistical evidence of norms. This offers guiding but not definitive pictures of contemporary issues.
2   This can be used in conjunction with an individual's identification of feelings, behaviours, distress and the physical assessment. This can be used to establish any other cause and provide a collaborative and empowering approach to assess-ing an individual's needs.
3   The need for a disease could be mistaken as almost redundant but it should not be ignored. All changes in a person's normal pattern are relevant including physical. Medical intervention offers treatments and relief from symptoms.

The process of identifying and measuring in this way could mean care and treatment can be more targeted and focused. The rights of the individual are enhanced by the professional approach which means more than just treating the possible disease. The individuals tackle self-defined problems, despite the over-riding legislative control, for example the Mental Health Act 2007. The integrative model approach allows the acceptance of the disease and control perspective whilst allowing influence of the individual's perspective and social influences. So the integrative model of care that is already a part of the professional's skills of care offers a technique which harnesses the benefits and counters the pitfalls of each as an individual perspective or approach.

CONCLUSION

In conclusion it is always useful to reflect on what was intended to be the message, as well as consideration of what was learned. To do this, take a moment to reflect on how the outcomes set at the beginning of the chapter, repeated below, have been considered and in what ways can they enhance your understanding of a very complex, diverse and evolving area of health and social care.

*   Defining mental health and ill health in society and using these concepts to consider the philosophical basis of historical and contemporary care.

The changes in care from the eighteenth century to present day are significant. They can be seen as moving from a complete lack of understanding to a much more evidence based and ethically guided approach to care and treatment. The change from the fourteenth century when individuals were dealt with as witches up to present day user and professional collaboration in dealing with symptoms of illness or problems demonstrates this (Campbell 2005). The changes in care are encapsulated by the emergence of new therapeutic approaches and the ever changing definitions of mental health, illness and legislation. It is vital for professionals and carers to understand the implications of this practice so that they can reflect upon the actions they take when working with people with vulnerabilities such as mental illness. Moving on from an evidence based, ethical, philosophical approach towards problems or concerns that the individual has identified themselves leads the professional onto the next outcome, which is to identify the problem itself:

*   How professionals in statutory and non-statutory services, service users and carers can combine their own individual expert knowledge and philosophies into a plan which meets people's needs and wants.
*   Working collaboratively as the key to ensuring that outcomes of care are set appropriately and are achievable, accountable, ethical and effective.

So what is mental health or illness and how does it affect the way in which our expert knowledge assists people to plan and recover? The labelling and definition of mental illness is structured in its approach to research and in the search for cures and treatments. However, the advent of different approaches to mental health care has meant that the traditional medical labelling system cannot continue independently of all other approaches or models of care. The development of the previously dominant medical attitude to more integrated social models of contemporary services has meant there is scope for care to be structured in a much more individualised way using all the appropriate techniques available. The use of the social and psychological models and appropriate person centred care encourages inclusion and less paternalistic approaches. Examples of dementia and schizophrenia care are offered in the chapter to demonstrate that this move is a positive one.

An awareness of the effect a professional relationship has on the care and service user engagement is important to ensure ethically guided care and practice. The changes in legislation and development of new therapeutic approaches into statutory services is allowing this; professionals just need to adopt it. The use of philosophies and models like Positive Practice and the integrative model offered here may well be a useful starting point.

The professional perspective is constantly changing in conjunction with society, environments and services. The focus of how transitions are made is based on the individual's approach to these issues. The practitioner must take responsibility for their own actions. They must define their own professionalism based on knowledge of the history and changes to understandings of mental health and illness. Awareness of the impact of how we define mental ill health and where these definitions are situated in the power dynamic of any relationship is essential. Understanding what this means within the statutory system and beyond is an essential foundation of knowledge for anyone working with people who have mental health issues.

REFERENCES

Barham, P. and Hayward, R. (1995) *Relocating madness – from the mental patient to the person*, London: Free Association Books.

Barker, P. (2000) *The Tidal Model* [online], S. L. Clan Unity Ltd. Available at: http://www.tidal-model.com/ (Accessed June 2009).

Barnes, M. (2001) *Taking over the Asylums: empowerment and mental health*, Palgrave, London: Palgrave.

Barry, P. D. (2002) *Mental health and Illness* (7th edition), Philadelphia: Lippincott-Raven.

Beart, K. (2006) *Fundamental aspect of caring for a person with dementia*, London: Quay Books.

Bell, A. and Lindley, P. (2005) *Beyond the water towers: The unfinished revolution in Mental health services 1985–2005*, London: Sainsbury Centre for Mental Health.

Borthwick, A., Holman, C., Kennard, D., McFetridge, M., Messruther, K. and Wilkes, J. (2009) The relevance of Moral treatment to contemporary mental health care, in Reynolds, J., Muston, R., Heller, T., Leach, J., McCormick, M., Wallcroft, J. and Walsh, M. (2009) *Mental Health Still Matters*, UK: Palgrave Macmillan/Open University.

Bowers, L. (1998) *The social nature of mental illness*, London: Routledge.

Bryant, M. (2001) *Introduction to user involvement* [online], London: Sainsbury Centre for Mental Health. Available at http://www.scmh.org.uk/pdfs/introduction+to+user+involvement.pdf (Accessed 4 April 2009).

Byrne, N. (2005*) Social Exclusion* (2nd edition), Berkshire: Open University Press.

Campbell, P. (2005) *From Little Acorns – The mental health service user movement* [online], London: Sainsbury Centre for Mental Health. Available at: http://www.scmh.org.uk/pdfs/mental+health+service+user+movement.pdf (Accessed 1 April 2009).

Carnwell, R. and Buchanan, J. (2005) *Effective Practice in Health and Social Care: A partnership approach*, Berkshire: Open University Press.

Darton, K. (2004) *Notes on the history of mental health care* [online], London: MIND. Available at: http://www.mind.org.uk/Information/Factsheets/History+of+mental+health/Notes+on+the+History+of+Mental+Health+Care.htm (Accessed June 2009).

Department of Health (1989) *Griffiths Report*, London: HMSO.

Department of Health (1999) *No Secrets: The protection of vulnerable adults*, London: HMSO.

Department of Health (2000) *National Service Framework*, London: HMSO.

Department of Health (2001) *National Service Framework for older people*, London: HMSO.

Fernando, S. (2002) *Mental health, race and culture*, Basingstoke: Palgrave.

Freidli, L. (2009) *Mental Health, Resilience and Equalities* [online]. Geneva: World Health Organisation. Available at: http://www.mentalhealth.org.uk/publications/mental-health-resilience-and-inequalities-report/ (Accessed 4 April).

Golightley, M. (2006) *Social Work and Mental Health* (2nd edition), Exeter: Learning Matters.

Golightley, M. (2008) *Social Work and Mental Health* (3rd edition), Exeter: Learning Matters.

Hope, R. (2004) *The Ten Essential Shared Capabilities: A Framework for the Whole Mental Health Workforce* [online]. London: Department of Health. Available at: http://www.dh.gov.uk/en/Publicationsandstatistics/Publications/PublicationsPolicyAndGuidance/DH_4087169 (Accessed June 2009).

Hurll, E. (2009) *People with mental health problems*, London: Shelter. Available at: http://england.shelter.org.uk/professional_resources/good_practice/vulnerable_groups/people_with_mental_health_problems (Accessed 4 April 2009).

Illovsky, M. E. (2003) *Mental health professionals, minorities and the poor*, Hove: Brunner-Routledge.

Kitwood, T. and Bredin, K. (1992) Towards a theory of dementia care: Personhood and well being, *Ageing and Society*, 12, 269–287.

Layard, R. (2006) *The Depression report: A new deal for depression and anxiety disorders* [online], London School of Economics. Available at: http://cep.lse.ac.uk/textonly/research/mentalhealth/depression_report_layard.pdf (Accessed 2 April 2009).

Lester, H. and Glasby, J. (2006) *Mental Health Policy and Practice*, Hampshire: Palgrave Macmillan.

Morrall, P. and Hazelton, M. (2004) *Mental health: global policies and human rights*, London: Whurr.

Norman, I. and Ryrie, I. (Eds) (2004) *The Art and Science of Mental Health Nursing: A Textbook of Principles*. Berkshire: Open University Press.

Pilgrim, D. and Rogers, A. (1999) *A Sociology of Mental Health and Illness* (2nd edition), Buckingham: Open University Press.

Pilgrim, D. and Rogers, A. (2005) *A Sociology of Mental Health and Illness* (3rd edition), Buckingham: Open University Press.

Rethink (2009) *Treatment and therapy* [online], London: Rethink. Available at: http://www.rethink.org/living_with_mental_illness/treatment_and_therapy/index.html (Accessed 31 March 2009).

Reynolds, J., Muston, R., Heller, T., Leach, J., McCormick, M., Wallcroft, J. and Walsh, M. (2009) *Mental Health Still Matters*, Buckinghamshire: Palgrave Macmillan/Open University.

Roberts, A. (2009) *Mental Health History Timeline* [online], London: Middlesex University, Available at: http://www.mhhe.heacademy.ac.uk/links/mental-health-history-timeline/ (Accessed 20 April 2009).

Rogers, C. (1961) *On becoming a person,* London: Constable.

Sainsbury Centre for Mental Health (2006) *Self Harm* [online]. Available at: http://www.mentalhealth.org.uk/information/mental-health-a-z/self-harm/ (Accessed 4 April 2009).

Sayce, L. (2000) *From psychiatric patient to citizen – Overcoming discrimination and social exclusion*, London: Macmillan Press Ltd.

Thomson, T. and Mathias, P. (2000) *Lyttles Mental Health and Disorder* (3rd edition), London: Balliere and Tindall/RCN.

Trivedi, P. and Wykes, P. (2009) From passive subjects to equal partners, in Reynolds, J., Muston, R., Heller, T., Leach, J., McCormick, M., Wallcroft, J. and Walsh, M. (2009) *Mental Health Still Matters*, Buckinghamshire: Palgrave Macmillan/Open University, Ch. 41.

Wallcraft, J. and Bryant, M. (2003) *The mental health service user movement in England, Policy Paper 2* [online], London: Sainsbury Centre for Mental Health. Available at: http://www.scmh.org.uk/publications/mh_service_users.aspx?ID=537 (Accessed 1 April 2009).

Watkins, P. (2001) *Mental Health Nursing: The art of compassionate care*, Oxford: Butterworth-Heinemann.

Woodside, M. (2002) *Inside my head (Videorecording)*, London: Channel 4 Television.

World Health Organization (1992) *International Classification of Diseases* (10th edition), Geneva: WHO.

CHAPTER 19

THE PRACTICE OF COUNSELLING

GRAHAM WHITEHEAD

OBJECTIVES

After reading this chapter you should be able to:

■ Discuss the application of counselling, including: boundaries and ethics; assessment and referrals; supervision and support; managing the helping relationship.

■ Consider counselling skills: the core conditions in action; giving and receiving feedback; reflection on practice.

■ Understand self awareness: personal barriers to the core conditions, for example, prejudices; stereotyping.

After reading this chapter you will understand the key terms:
Therapeutic relationship, ethics, confidentiality, assessment, referral, supervision.

There are six Moments of Reflection to work on throughout the chapter.

INTRODUCTION

The practice of counselling explores the application of counselling skills in contemporary Britain. The chapter includes discussion of the ethics, principles and purpose underpinning counselling practice; discusses practitioner development of counselling skills; explores the dynamics of the therapeutic relationship and encourages an active process of self-exploration and enquiry. Practice issues explored include discussion of counselling settings; boundaries and ethics; assessment and referral; supervision and support; and consideration of how to manage the helping relationship. Case studies are offered to give an understanding of the contribution of counselling practice to the study of health and social care. Throughout the chapter there are activities aimed to generate discussion, involving group and reflective exercises.

THE PRACTICE OF COUNSELLING

The development of the practice of counselling in the UK since the 1970s has been dominated by a proliferation of therapeutic approaches in both training and delivery. The theoretical models discussed earlier in Chapter 12, *Theories of counselling* have evolved to meet the cultural needs of specific groups and settings across a wide spectrum and hence are of particular significance in the education of health and social care professionals.

McLeod (2003: 3–5) comments on counselling as a twentieth century invention and charts the evolvement of counselling as an occupation, discipline and profession. These include the formation of professional groups such as the British Association for Counselling and Psychotherapy (BACP) and the British Association of Behavioural and Cognitive Psychotherapies (BABCP) since the early 1970s, which have developed to represent the professional interests of those entering capacities involving a therapeutic response. Pilgrim (2002) cited by Feltham in Dryden (2007: 13) offers a discussion of three distinct phases of the development of counselling in Britain. These are identified as:

> psychoanalysis and behaviourism as co-existing and competing between 1920 and 1970, 'third force psychology' (the humanistic approaches), pluralism and eclecticism appearing largely after 1970, and the 'return of professional authority and its postmodern critics' after 1980.

The competing nature of the differing theoretical paradigms is still very much present in the delivery of counselling in Britain today although cognitive behavioural approaches have gained the upper hand in the last decade.

Recent initiatives by lead organisations, for example, the National Institute for Clinical Excellence (NICE) and the National Occupational Standards for Counselling have developed core competencies (*see* Appendices 1 and 2) which outline the necessary competencies that practitioners must develop in their training in order to be eligible for professional recognition. Such initiatives have contributed significantly to the ongoing regulatory framework of the practice of counselling and psychotherapy in the UK by the Health Professions Council (HPC).

The application of counselling skills has developed considerably over this period to encompass a wide variety of roles and settings including educational, public sector, voluntary and charitable organisations. In more recent years, counselling activity has been developed to support employees in many private sector organisations, either in-house or outsourced, to promote employee well-being. The term counselling is used in a variety of ways, both informally and formally, and hence it is of paramount importance that students studying health and social care gain a clear understanding of the meaning of the term, and are able to clearly differentiate between formal and informal usage.

A good starting point at the commencement of studying the breadth and diversity of counselling application is to focus on preconceived ideas about the term 'counselling' with a view to clarifying your understanding and definition.

MOMENT OF REFLECTION

Activity One: Your understanding of the term counselling

Write down what your understanding of counselling is. Write freely allowing any-thing that comes to mind immediately. Try not to censor your thoughts and feelings. Your responses will have been shaped by previous education, media coverage, per-sonal experiences, wider reading, etc. Discuss your understanding with peers to see how your understanding differs.

Activity Two: Clarifying your understanding of counselling

Table 18.1 lists several definitions of counselling from leading authors and organi-sations in the field. Read these and consider your response to each one. Make notes if necessary. Which definition appeals to you – which do you think offers the closest definition to your own understanding outlined in Activity 1 above?

Table 19.1 Definitions of counselling

Burkes and Stefflre (1979: 14)	'Counselling denotes a professional relationship between a trained counsellor and a client. This relationship is usually person-to-person, although it may sometimes involve more than two people. It is designed to help clients to understand and clarify their views of their life space, and to learn to reach their self-determined goals through meaningful, well-informed choices and through resolution of problems of an emotional or interpersonal nature.'
British Association for Counselling and Psychotherapy (1984)	'The task of counselling is to give the client the opportunity to explore, discover and clarify ways of living more satisfyingly and resourcefully.'
Feltham and Dryden (1993: 6)	'A principled relationship characterised by the application of one or more psychological theories and a recognised set of communication skills ...'
Russell et al. (1998)	'Counselling is an activity freely entered into by the person seeking help, it offers the opportunity to identify things for the client themselves that are troubling or perplexing. It is clearly and explicitly contracted, and the boundaries of the relationship identified. The activity itself is designed to help self-exploration and understanding. The process should help to identify thoughts, emotions and behaviours that, once accessed, may offer the client a greater sense of personal resources and self determined change.'
Adams, R. (2007: 411)	'Counselling is an approach to human interaction that enables people to reflect on their situation and empowers them to deal with it themselves.'

The two activities above should now help you to begin to clarify your understand-ing of how the term 'counselling' is used. You are likely to notice in future weeks and months how the term is used by both yourself and other people. You will undoubtedly notice a wide variation in usage and may feel the urge to challenge views which you think offer either a false impression or misrepresentation of the term as you understand it.

COUNSELLING SETTINGS

Counselling as an activity has application in a wide range of settings and has developed to meet the needs of particular client groups and presenting concerns. From primary health care provision supporting clients with anxiety and depression (for example, counselling in GP surgeries) to psychological support for clients experiencing more severe mental health issues (for example, NHS provision in mental health units), counselling has grown both as a profession and method of mental health provision. Similarly, in the private sector, organisations have begun to see the benefits of supporting employees in the workplace, and counselling services (usually outsourced to external employee assistance providers (EAPs)) have developed to support employee health and well-being. McLeod (2008: 5) makes the economic case for counselling in the workplace by commenting that all published studies of the economic costs and benefits of workplace counselling have reported that counselling/ EAP provision at least covers its costs and that some studies have found substantial cost/benefit ratios.

THE APPLICATION OF COUNSELLING

The term 'arena' is used by Palmer and McMahon (1997) to differentiate the settings of individual, couple, family or group counselling. These arenas, or modes of practice, offer practitioners, clients and organisations considerable choice in the manner in which counselling is delivered as a professional activity although cost-effectiveness and budgetary restraint are likely to be the main determinants of the chosen mode of delivery by an organisation. The move towards practice-based commissioning of differing forms of psychological support means that organisations are required to minimise per capita costs for delivery of services and there is a move to incorporate more innovate forms of self-help such as online support, guidance and information systems. Delivery of counselling can vary widely and can include either individual counselling, couples work, group work, family therapy, telephone or online counselling provision.

Individual counselling

The majority of counselling activity in the UK is delivered as individual (or one-to-one) counselling. The benefits of individual counselling are considerable although this mode of practice is the most expensive to deliver on a per capita basis. Confidentiality is paramount in the delivery of any therapeutic activity but individual counselling offers the client the greatest opportunity to explore issues in a one-to-one confidential setting and this mode is hence more popular with clients who wish to discuss sensitive and emotive issues. The possibility of establishing a therapeutic relationship offers the client the opportunity to explore delicate material whilst the individual practitioner is able to focus very closely on these presenting concerns without any distraction from any external factors. Another significant benefit offered by individual counselling is that the practitioner is able to closely track the pace of the client's progress and consequently the therapeutic response can be shaped to meet the client's particular needs. For example, a client who finds it difficult to form relationships will be faced with the very real situation of a 'potential' therapeutic relationship with the practitioner. Although this is likely to result in considerable challenge, the opportunities offered for personal growth can be considerable.

Individual counselling activity, however, faces considerable criticism and it is important for health and social care professionals to be fully aware of the arguments. Apart from the resource intensive nature of the activity and consequently the cost implications, the social exclusion argument, expressed widely in academic texts, posits the view that individual counselling separates the client from their wider environment and hence limits the possibilities for growth. However, Kearney (1996) expresses the view that counselling does have the potential to radically transform external political structures as well as individual people. This raises the issue of whether counselling is a politically neutral activity and authors and practitioners are divided on this issue. This viewpoint will also be shaped by the theoretical orientation of a practitioner or organisation. Further criticisms of counselling include the possibility of a client becoming too reliant on the practitioner, which in turn could be viewed as inhibiting personal development and growth. This criticism could be angled at most health and social care professional roles and appears to come with the territory. Rather than seeing these as weaknesses of individual practice, practitioners and professional bodies argue that these obstacles represent a challenge to practice with the eventual aim of integrating the disparate parts of a client's presenting concerns in order that she/he may move towards greater self-reliance.

Couples counselling

Couples counselling developed considerably in the UK after the Second World War. The National Marriage Guidance Council (now Relate) was established in 1947 in order to support couples facing emotional difficulties. Rising divorce rates in the second half of the twentieth century fuelled the demand for couples counselling and in recent years with the advent of civil partnerships for lesbian and gay relationships, couples counselling has now been developed to support partners of any sexual orientation. The major difference of couples counselling, compared to individual counselling, is that the strongest initial relationship in the therapeutic encounter is pre-established and independent of the counsellor, albeit not at a strong point when seeking external support. This allows for the possibility for the counsellor to disengage and observe the patterns that a couple may present. Most couples work is offered in agency settings predominantly in the voluntary sector. The decision to approach couples counselling usually means that previous support networks (for example, family and friends) have been fully exhausted. Counsellors engaged in couples work follow specialist training to work with relationship issues. The role of counselling in couples work involves exploring communication, facilitating negotiation and in some cases dealing with the end of a relationship. In the event of separation or divorce, legal counsel is often sought and during this difficult period clients may consider the possibility of individual counselling.

MOMENT OF REFLECTION

Activity Three

How do you decide which mode of counselling is best for a client? List the factors you think a health and social care professional may need to consider when referring a client for counselling.

Group counselling

The use of group work in counselling and psychotherapy again developed in the years following the Second World War. One of the major reasons for this development was the need to support large numbers of people who were injured or bereaved during or after the war years and group work was seen as a cost-effective approach to supporting clients with similar concerns. This has continued to be the case in the interim period and groups tend to operate best around a single focus, for example, groups for clients with eating disorders. Other examples of group work include personal therapy or 'encounter' groups, addiction and bereavement issues. Community development, social care, religious groups and health care services have all used group approaches and there is a wide body of theory, mostly US led, that explores the application of counselling in groups. Group work is a very different experience for clients compared to individual counselling and care needs to be taken in considering referral of a client by health and social care professionals. The use of needs-based assessment tools can assist in determining suitability although ultimately the decision rests with the client. Group work has a history of application across all major theoretical paradigms, for example, using either a psychodynamic or humanistic approach to personal development. Group work is also used to support families in crisis (usually termed family therapy) and again is applied quite widely in health and social care provision in the UK.

INNOVATIVE APPROACHES TO COUNSELLING

In more recent years counselling has evolved to respond to the range of differing media available to support clients. There has been the development by service providers of a wide range of online resources, for example, highlighting local and national support networks, and there is a leaning towards encouraging self-help by accessing online resources. Some service providers have introduced an online counselling provision which offers the opportunity for counsellor and client to communicate in real time. There are also chat-specific forums for clients to talk around a particular topic. These innovative approaches are bringing counselling to a much wider audience. The Samaritans, for example, in 2002 reported that the provision of online support meant that it was reaching larger numbers of young Asian men, who were keener to approach services anonymously. In more recent initiatives, for example, Improving Access to Psychological Therapies (IAPT), the UK government has suggested the use of online self-help resources as an initial point of contact for clients suffering with anxiety and depression. Rather than replacing face-to-face practice, these innovative approaches are seen as supplementing existing provision.

MULTICULTURAL COUNSELLING

Multicultural (other terms used in academic studies also include transcultural or inter-cultural) approaches to counselling practice are central to the training, professional development and delivery of counselling practice in the UK. The specific cultural and ethnic needs of client populations require the practice of counselling to develop and evolve to respond appropriately and sensitively to differing cultural and ethnic requirements. There are many definitions of these terms, and a wide range of theories about the process and delivery of multicultural counselling (for wider discussion *see* Chapter 12). Naturally within the context of a multicultural society, practitioner train-ing, service development and the delivery of counselling requires significant focus on working with diversity and difference. Counselling training programmes in the UK lay great emphasis on the development of practitioner skills so that counsellors are trained to respond to a wide range of cultural and ethnic issues. The responsibility, how-ever, lies with the practitioner and professional guidelines, for example, the National Occupational Standards discussed above require that practitioners demonstrate equal-ity and diversity awareness when working in a counselling role. Rawson *et al.* (1999: 6) discuss this responsibility and make reference to Wrenn's (1962) concept of cultural encapsulation, requiring the practitioner to move to a point of transcultural compe-tence in order to be effective when working in a diverse multicultural society.

The considerable demographic changes in post-war years in Western cultures have resulted in transcultural communication being a necessity for practitioners using counselling and psychotherapy in professional settings. Terminology in this area of study has evolved considerably and multiculturalism has become a significant force impacting on the policy, culture and language used in professional practice. Pedersen (1991) describes the nature of the development of multicultural theory as a 'bottom-up' social movement rather than the 'top-down' traditional theories directed by specific leaders such as Freud, Skinner or Rogers.

The development of transcultural counselling practice has clear links with envi-ronment and society, particularly from a demographic point of view, and leads to a questioning of the philosophical assumptions underlying traditional Western theoreti-cal approaches to counselling training and practice. The practice of counselling offers the greatest challenge when the transcultural dynamic is fully considered and requires individual practice, policy issues and service delivery implications to be fully consid-ered by training institutions, professional bodies and service providers.

SIGNIFICANT ASPECTS OF COUNSELLING PRACTICE

Counselling practice requires consideration of the therapeutic relationship, ethi-cal approaches to therapeutic intervention, confidentiality, assessment, referral and management of the therapeutic relationship. Practitioners are required to review their work in professional supervision (or consultative support) although requirements here vary across professional bodies. Students of health and social care need to understand how these components contribute to the quality and standard of care that is provided from both an organisational and individual perspective.

1 The therapeutic relationship

Humanistic approaches to counselling lay great emphasis on the significance of the therapeutic relationship between counsellor and client. Mearns and Thorne (2007) describe the decision to become a counsellor as no task for the faint hearted and that those who accept the challenge of person-centred counselling are letting themselves in for a particularly rigorous discipline. The skills required to develop the person-centred orientation include self-awareness, genuineness, empathic understanding and the ability to focus on the therapeutic relationship. In contrast, those practitioners identifying as psychodynamic or psychoanalytic may pay less emphasis to the therapeutic relationship as such but would focus more on the aspects of the client's process such as transference or counter-transference which may have links with previous experiences, most likely from childhood and early adolescence. The common theme in generic practice, however, is for the counsellor to develop the ability to focus on the dynamics of the relationship between counsellor and client and to respond appropriately from a chosen theoretical model. The theoretical positions described earlier in this chapter give some indication of the range and breadth of differing theoretical positions that exist within the profession.

2 Ethical codes of conduct

Elsewhere in this book, discussion has focused on the significance for health and social care students to develop a personal system of ethics which will underpin the approach and manner in which they work with clients or patients. The ethical approach developed will relate to human conduct but will also reflect personal views of what is right or wrong in the approach to the delivery of health and social care interventions. Similarly, professional counselling bodies in the UK have been instrumental in developing ethical codes of conduct which relate to the professional practice. Sometimes an ethical conflict seems clear cut, for example, developing friendships outside the professional role with clients, but in other cases the issues are more challenging and at times unclear. Nelson-Jones (2008) identifies the legal duty of care that helpers have to their clients and usefully explains the importance of developing helper competence. Familiarisation with ethical codes of conduct of lead counselling organisations is recommended as one route to understanding the complex nature of ethical challenges faced in practice. See, for example, the BACP Ethical Framework listed in the reference list at the end of this chapter and the following discussion points.

MOMENT OF REFLECTION

Activity Four: Ethical challenges

Imagine you are working as a counsellor in primary health care. What ethical challenges do you imagine that you might face in your role? Make a list of these.

Discuss these challenges in a small group in order to highlight the dilemmas that counselling practice might pose to you as a health and social care professional.

3 Confidentiality

Confidentiality is central to ethical counselling practice, and where this is broken the impact will be apparent immediately on the professional relationship between counsellor and client. There are, however, limitations to confidentiality, many of which are dictated by law and it is important that clients are informed in advance of counselling of such exceptions to the confidentiality rule. Counselling organisations usually have a very clear policy statement on this issue in their introductory information, either in the form of written information or on their website. These limitations include a legal duty on the part of the counsellor to disclose information when:

- There is a clear risk to a third party disclosed by the client (for example, the Drug Trafficking Offences Act 1986).
- There is clear evidence of a risk to the client, for example where a client threatens suicide.
- There is evidence of a risk to children.
- There is evidence that information disclosed threatens national security (for example in contravention of the Prevention of Terrorism Act 2000).

Counsellors may also be forced to disclose sensitive personal client information in cases where refusal would make them liable to civil or criminal court proceedings. The general rule in any disclosure requires the counsellor or counselling organisation to discuss such circumstances with the client in advance before any disclosure to a third party, preferably gaining the client's consent, although clearly in some of the circumstances outlined above this may not be entirely possible.

4 Assessment or intake interview

Some approaches to counselling require a detailed assessment of client psychological needs at commencement of counselling, usually referred to as an assessment or intake interview, although the view of humanistic approaches is that this process medicalises the process of therapy. A counselling service will make clear the position at intake. Where an assessment tool is used (*see* earlier discussion of assessment tools in Chapter 2,

Working with people), the aim will be to identify whether the client is at a point where a therapeutic intervention might be appropriate. In cases where a client has a history of mental health issues, or is on psychotropic medication, this decision may involve ethical considerations, the necessity for case discussion or in some cases referral (*see below*) to a more appropriate organisation or agency. Consultation with a client's GP might also be necessary although this should always involve the client's prior consent.

5 Referral

Referral to another organisation or agency may be the most appropriate route for a client, particularly where a specialised type of service or provision is required (for example, if the client identifies a need to see a counsellor of her own ethnicity and a service is unable to meet this request). Where the decision to make a referral is made, full consultation should take place with the client to inform him/her of the referral suggestion and to check how s/he feels about such an option. Where a referral is agreed, consensus needs to be reached about what information will be provided to the organisation or agency. It is usually best if the client approaches the referral organisation/agency but in circumstances where there is a long waiting list, an agency referral may accelerate the process.

6 Supervision

Supervision, or consultative support, is a professional requirement for those engaged in counselling activity. Lead counselling organisations specify the number of hours required linked to counselling practice. Talking client issues through with a clinical supervisor, either in individual or group supervision, requires the counsellor to identify significant client concerns and ethical issues which are faced in counselling practice. Counselling supervision is a distinct and separate activity and should not be confused with line management which has an entirely different role and purpose. The National Occupational Standards for Counselling (*see* Appendix 2) require counsellors to be aware of the professional requirements for supervision, models of supervision, be clear of the objectives of supervision (for example, an awareness of how events in your private life may impact on client work), and recognise the benefit that supervision is likely to have on therapeutic practice. For a full list of requirements *see* NOS Unit CLG3: Contract for and utilise supervision in counselling.

7 Managing the helping relationship

Consideration needs to be given throughout the counselling process to managing the helping relationship. This may be the primary concern of the counselling provider, or in the case of private practice, the responsibility of the practitioner. Issues to consider are wide, but these include:

- the duration of counselling (short/medium/longer term)
- the issue of challenge
- ethical considerations (linked to professional codes of conduct)

- accessibility issues for clients with disabilities
- provision of written information detailing the services offered
- complaints procedure
- confidentiality
- supervisory process
- whether there is a financial charge for the service
- advance requirements in the event of session cancellation
- resource implications
- health and safety regulations
- client and counsellor safety.

MOMENT OF REFLECTION

Activity Five

Research information about counselling agencies (either hard-copy leaflets or electronic) to identify how the helping relationship is managed. What additional factors to those listed above have you found? Discuss with a partner or small group.

TRAINING IN COUNSELLING

The training route for those interested in pursuing a career in counselling requires the student to commit to professional training, with most courses at either undergraduate or postgraduate level. The Health Professions Council (HPC) currently has the responsibility of developing the regulation of the training requirements for practising counsellors and psychotherapists in the UK and is overseeing the development of the requirements for the approval of counselling and psychotherapy training courses.

CONCLUSION

The practice of counselling has explored the application of counselling skills in contemporary Britain. The chapter includes discussion of the ethics, principles and purpose underpinning counselling practice; discusses practitioner development of counselling skills; explores the dynamics of the therapeutic relationship and encourages an active process of self-exploration and enquiry. Practice issues explored include discussion of counselling settings; boundaries and ethics; assessment and referral; supervision and support; and consideration of how to manage the helping relationship. Students are advised to familiarise themselves with the NICE guidelines about the treatment and care of people with depression and anxiety (NICE 2004) and for those students interested in further training, the National Occupational Standards for Counselling (NOS) and requirements of the Health Professions Council (HPC) – *see* Appendices 1 and 2.

SUMMARY OF MAIN POINTS

You should be able to:

*   Display a critical understanding of the principles, purpose and ethics underpinning effective practice.
*   Demonstrate insight into the interpersonal and intrapersonal processes involved in counselling.
*   Display a critical understanding of the nature of counselling work within differing practice settings.

MOMENT OF REFLECTION

Discussion points

*   What considerations need to be given to the delivery of counselling practice?
*   What are the limitations of counselling in health and social care settings?
*   What responsibility does a counselling organisation have in developing provision within a multicultural society?

CASE STUDIES

The following case studies are offered to focus your thinking on counselling from both a client and a practitioner point of view. Discuss these case studies in either small groups or with a peer on your course.

Case study One

You are a 69 year old widow living in Grantham. Recently there have been a spate of burglaries in the area and you are becoming anxious about your safety. Your only daughter, Maude, lives in London. She calls most nights to check how you are. You decide to speak with a counsellor at your GP surgery about your concerns.

*   What might you expect from counselling?
*   How might counselling support you to deal with your anxiety about the burglaries?
*   Can you think of other health and social care interventions that might be useful in this scenario?

Case study Two

You and your partner have been trying for a family for some time but have not been successful to date. The anxiety of this is really getting to you and you decide to explore your thoughts and feelings about this with a nurse at your local GP practice who offers counselling support to couples trying for a family.

- How do you think counselling might support you and your partner?
- What might the outcome of the meetings with the nurse be?
- What other primary health care services might be useful to support you and your partner in this scenario?

Case study Three

You have recently arrived in the UK from Congo. You have come to the UK to study but are feeling very homesick. You hate the food here, the British people have been rude to you and the weather is terrible!

You decide to go and discuss this with a counsellor at your college – you have heard that they are there to support international students so thought you would give it a try.

- What issues might be usefully addressed in counselling?
- How might the counsellor support you? What would you be looking for?
- What other types of support might help you to settle better into the UK?

BIBLIOGRAPHY

Adams, R. (2007) *Foundations in Health and Social Care*, Basingstoke: Palgrave Macmillan.

BAC (1984) *Code of Ethics and Practice for Counsellors*, Rugby: BAC (now BACP).

Burkes, H. M. and Stefflre, B. (1979) *Theories of Counselling* (3rd edition), New York: McGraw-Hill.

Feltham, C. (2007) Individual Therapy in Context, in Dryden, W. (Ed.) *Dryden's Handbook of Individual Therapy* (5th edition), London: Sage.

Feltham, C. and Dryden, W. (1993) *Dictionary of Counselling*, London: Whurr.

Kearney, A. (1996) *Counselling, Class and Politics*, Manchester: PCCS.

McLeod, J. (2003) *An Introduction to Counselling* (3rd edition), Maidenhead: Open University Press.

McLeod, J. (2008) *Counselling in the workplace: the facts* (2nd edition), Lutterworth: BACP.

Mearns, D. and Thorne, B. (2007) *Person-Centred Counselling in Action* (3rd edition), London: Sage.

National Institute for Clinical Excellence (2004) *Guidelines to improve the treatment and care of people with depression and anxiety* [online]. Available at: http://www.nice.org.uk/niceMedia/pdf/2004_50_launchdepressionanxiety.pdf (Accessed 5 May 2009).

National Occupational Standards for Counselling. Available at: http://www.ukstandards.org.uk/Find_Occupational_Standards.aspx?NosFindID=4&FormMode=ViewModeSuite&SuiteID=1292 (Accessed 5 May 2009).

Nelson-Jones, R. (2008) *Basic Counselling Skills: A Helper's Manual* (2nd edition), London: Sage.

Palmer, S. and McMahon, G. (Eds) (1997) *Handbook of Counselling* (2nd edition), London: Routledge.

Pedersen, P. (1991) Multiculturalism as a generic approach to counselling, *Journal of Counselling and Development*, 70: 6–12.

Rawson, D., Whitehead, G. and Luthra, M. (1999) The challenges of counselling in a multicultural society, in Palmer, S. and Laungani, P. (Eds) *Counselling in a Multicultural Society*, London: Sage.

Russell *et al.* (1998) in Sanders, P. (2003) *Step into Study Counselling* (3rd edition), Ross-on-Wye: PCCS.

Wrenn, C. G. (1962) The culturally encapsulated counsellor revisited, in Pedersen, P. (Ed.) (1985) *Handbook of cross-cultural counselling and therapy*, Westport, CT: Greenwood.

APPENDIX 1

NICE guidelines to improve the treatment and care of people with depression and anxiety

Source: http://www.nice.org.uk/niceMedia/pdf/2004_50_launchdepressionanxiety.pdf (Accessed 5 May 2009).

The National Institute for Clinical Excellence (NICE) has issued guidelines for the NHS on the treatment and care of people with depression and anxiety. The guidelines take account of the announcement by the Medicines and Healthcare products Regulatory Agency (MHRA) on the safety of antidepressant drug treatments and will support health professionals when implementing the MHRA's advice. The guidelines also recommend effective psychological treatments for people with depression and anxiety and will set national standards for care across England and Wales. Depression is characterised by a low mood and loss of interest, usually accompanied by one or more of the following – low energy; change in appetite, weight or sleep pattern; poor concentration; feelings of guilt or worthlessness; and suicidal ideas. The guideline on depression recommends that for mild and moderate depression, psychological treatments specifically focused on depression (such as problem-solving therapy, cognitive behaviour therapy (CBT) and counselling) can be as effective as drug treatments and should be offered as treatment options.

The guideline also recommends that:

- Antidepressants should not be used for the initial treatment of mild depression, because the risk–benefit ratio is poor.
- Where antidepressants are prescribed for moderate or severe depression it should be a selective serotonin reuptake inhibitor (SSRI), because SSRIs are as effective as tricyclic antidepressants and their use is less likely to be discontinued because of side effects.
- All patients prescribed antidepressants should be informed that, although the drugs are not associated with tolerance and craving, discontinuation/withdrawal symptoms may occur on stopping or missing doses or, occasionally, on reducing the dose of the drug.
- Screening to be undertaken for all high risk groups – for example, those with a past history of depression, significant physical illnesses causing disability, or other mental health problems such as dementia.
- For severe depression, psychological treatment (CBT) should be used in combination with antidepressant medication.

Anxiety is characterised by feelings of apprehension and worry, spontaneous panic attacks, irritability, poor sleeping, avoidance and poor concentration. The guideline on anxiety recommends that patients should be offered any of the following three types of intervention, taking into account patient preference. In descending order of long-term effectiveness, these interventions are:

- Psychological therapy, such as CBT.
- Medication, such as an SSRI licensed for generalised anxiety disorder.
- Self-help, such as bibliotherapy (the use of written materials) based on CBT principles.

The guideline also recommends that:

- Involving individuals in an effective partnership with health care professionals, with all decision making being shared, improves outcomes.
- Access to information, including support groups, is a valuable part of any package of care.
- There are positive advantages for people with anxiety of services being based in primary care rather than in a hospital setting.

APPENDIX 2

National Occupational Standards for Counselling

Source: http://www.ukstandards.org.uk/Find_Occupational_Standards.aspx?NosFind ID=4&FormMode=ViewModeSuite&SuiteID=1292 (Accessed 5 May 2009).

National Occupational Standards (NOS) define the competences which apply to job roles or occupations in the form of statements of performance, knowledge and the evidence required to confirm competence. This set of National Occupational Standards has been developed by ENTO to define the competencies and knowledge of those working as counselling practitioners. Not all units will be appropriate to all work settings, for example it is recognised that not all counsellors would have an opportunity to manage the counselling practice. All units within this suite of National Occupational Standards for Counselling are non-specific to any theoretical model and should be applied to your work in the context of your own chosen theoretical approach.

There are many uses of National Occupational Standards including those which:

- inform qualifications
- contribute to the design delivery and evaluation of training
- contribute to the development of job specifications
- inform skills assessment
- inform training needs analysis
- ensure best practice at work.

Occupational Standards for Counselling (September 2007)

Unit CLG1   Take responsibility for your own continuing personal development in counselling
Unit CLG2   Reflect upon your work with clients through supervision and manage your continuing
              professional development in counselling
Unit CLG3   Contract for and utilise supervision in counselling
Unit CLG4   Promote the counselling service
Unit CLG5   Manage the counselling practice
Unit CLG6   Use effective communication within the counselling environment
Unit CLG7   Manage the counselling assessment process
Unit CLG8   Demonstrate equality and diversity awareness when working in counselling
Unit CLG9   Identify the mental health needs of clients when counselling and refer in an appropriate manner
Unit CLG10 Support and/or refer clients suffering from symptoms of physical illness when counselling
Unit CLG16 Manage breaks and holidays in the context of therapeutic work
Unit CLG17 Demonstrate an understanding of the social and political context of counselling
Unit CLG18 Interpret and apply ethical and legal frameworks in the practice of counselling
Unit CLG19 Contract for provision of counselling
Unit CLG20 Take an active role in the wider professional community for counselling
Unit CLG21 Undertake routine evaluation of your own counselling practice
Unit CLG22 Undertake research and evaluation relevant to counselling

CHAPTER 20

SUBSTANCE MISUSE

MARTYN HARLING

O B J E C T I V E S

After reading this chapter you should be able to:

- Define the term 'drug' and some of the common terminology associated with substance misuse.

- Critically understand society's changing response to the substances which are now commonly misused.

- Describe current (UK) legislation linked to illicit drug use, particularly the current classification of substances in the Misuse of Drugs Act (Home Office 1971).

- Understand the common drugs of misuse, their effects and health risks.

- Apply some of the knowledge gained from reading the chapter to a case scenario.

- Consider substance misuse service provision in the UK.

After reading this chapter you will understand the key terms:
Ecstasy, LSD, cocaine, heroin, amphetamine, cannabis, anabolic steroids, alcohol, tobacco.

There are two Moments of Reflection to work on throughout the chapter.

INTRODUCTION

Behaviour linked to the use of both illegal and legal drugs is of growing concern to many areas of health and social care provision. The twentieth and early twenty-first centuries have seen substance misuse develop from a position of limited state control to a global issue requiring international legislation and consideration by the World Health Organisation.

The chapter starts by considering what we mean by a 'drug' and society's view of a 'problem drug taker'. An historical perspective of the concepts of 'addiction' and substance misuse is considered alongside how differing views have influenced social policy and legislation in the UK. Some of the common illegal and legal substances used in contemporary society are described in terms of their effects and potential consequences for the individual user. The chapter provides discussion points and directs the reader to reference material and suggestions for further study resources relating to substance misuse.

MOMENT OF REFLECTION

Activity One: What is a drug?

Defining what we mean by a 'drug' is by no means easy. Write a list of all the substances you would describe as a drug. Think about the similarities and differences between the substances you have written on your list. Your list may include some that are illegal to use, others given out by doctors or sold in pharmacies and others available from high street health food shops.

The effects of these substances on the human body and mind will also vary. Some drugs may result in predominantly physical reactions, others produce a more pronounced psychological effect and many result in both.

Often our view of a certain 'drug' will be influenced by who provided it to us, its purpose and whether it achieves its desired effect.

HOW DO WE DEFINE A PROBLEM DRUG TAKER?

The list you generated in Activity 1 may also help to illustrate society's complex relationship with drugs. On the one hand we rely on drugs as a major aspect of medical care, but on the other hand revile certain drugs for causing social problems. Sometimes, as is the case with heroin or to use its medical name diamorphine, some substances fit into both categories. Added to such contradictory views around the substance itself, individuals use drugs in different ways. Some individuals may 'experiment' with the physical or psychological effects of certain drugs. Others use drugs as part of their 'recreational' activities (for example, drinking alcohol when socialising in pubs or clubs). Some individuals use legal and/or illegal substances at a problematic level which can result in psychological or physical dependency, commonly called 'addiction'. The term 'addiction' raises many stereotypical images within the general public and is a hotly contested issue amongst workers within the substance misuse field (*see* Davies 1997, for a detailed discussion about this). The term is often used to imply some form of illness, which is difficult to apply to drug use, where an individual has some level of choice around their behaviour. Rather than using the term 'addiction' it is perhaps more useful to talk about the potential for problematic drug use. The Advisory Council on the Misuse of Drugs (the official advisory body to the British Government) defined a problematic drug user as someone:

> who experiences social, psychological, physical or legal problems related to intoxication and/or regular excessive consumption and or dependence as a consequence of his/her own use of drugs or other chemical substances.
>
> (ACMD 1982: 34)

This definition can equally apply to the legally controlled drugs such as alcohol and tobacco, and to the illegal drugs controlled under the Misuse of Drugs Act (Home Office 1971).

The focus of this chapter is on the substances commonly available in modern society which are not taken under medical guidance and can be used at a problematic level.

A BRIEF HISTORY OF THE UK'S VIEW ON DRUGS

Before talking about specific substances it is worth noting that society's view on what are now illegal substances has changed over the course of British history. During the last few decades, much debate has centred on the health risks of various illegal drugs (notably cannabis and ecstasy), and their status within legislation. Whilst it is not possible to cover such debates within this chapter, it is important to note that the UK's response to certain substances has not necessarily emerged from considerations about their potential health risks.

Prior to the First World War substances which are now controlled by the Misuse of Drugs Act (Home Office 1971) (for example, heroin and cocaine) were available to the general public with few restrictions. During the First World War concerns were raised that prostitutes were selling cocaine to soldiers, compromising their ability and inclination to fight. This led to the introduction of the Defence of the Realm Act [DORA] Regulation 40B in 1916, effectively criminalising cocaine and opiate use. This law was extended into civilian legislation in the form of the Dangerous Drugs Act in 1920. Up to this significant point in history the use of opiates, cannabis and cocaine had all proved fashionable, at different times and within different sections of UK society. Drug misuse was considered acceptable within society but excessive use was viewed as a moral issue, linked to the willpower of the individual user (McMurran 1994). Since freedom of choice was considered to be a key element in an individual's decision to use alcohol or drugs to excess, those who chose to use excessively were deemed to be morally at fault, requiring punishment rather than treatment interventions. Moves toward a manufacturing based urban society, fears that drug use could damage the efficacy of the war effort during the First World War, increases in the power of medicine as a science and the rise of the USA as a world power, have all been identified as factors in establishing certain psychoactive substances as targets for national and international legislation (Kohn 1992; Davenport-Hines 2001; Walton 2001). The USA has consistently pioneered national responses to the perceived threat from certain drugs and since the First World War has proved to be a key figure in international responses (Davenport-Hines 2001).

Increases in the power of medical science in the late nineteenth and early twentieth centuries led to the excessive use of psychoactive substances being viewed in medical terms and categorised as a disease process rather than a moral failing (McMurran 1994). However, international controls placed on the availability of opiates and cocaine after the First World War meant that such substances were also effectively banned for medical purposes. This situation was challenged in 1926 by the Rolleston Committee Report which established the right of medics to prescribe such substances to those patients who had developed a dependency, usually after medical treatment (Berridge 1988; Ashton 1989). The Rolleston Committee Report firmly placed the treatment of those with problematic substance misuse within the realms of medicine. The resulting system, where individuals were administered their drug of addiction by their GP, has since been called the 'British system' of prescribing (Gossop 2000). Although, as Gossop (2000) points out, its application was limited to a small number of respectable individuals who had developed drug problems via medical treatment or as a result of injuries sustained through war.

Increases in the use of illegal drugs amongst young people after the Second World War led to public concern on both sides of the Atlantic during the 1960s. The USA increased its legislative response which was aimed at curbing the use of hallucinogens and marijuana which was, at the time, linked to social unrest and increasing levels of dissention over the war in Vietnam. Concern in the UK centred on heroin use with two medics, Lady Frankau and John Petro, receiving a great deal of media attention over high levels of prescribed heroin given to young dependent users. In 1965, the Brain Committee Report recommended overturning the Rolleston Committee Report, which resulted in the treatment of heroin use being removed from general medicine and placed within psychiatry (Davenport-Hines 2001). Legislation was also tightened in the UK in the form of the Misuse of Drugs Act (Home Office 1971) which introduced the current system of classifying drugs into three bands and the associated charges for possession and dealing.

CURRENT UK DRUG LAWS

The UK drug laws are rather complicated and at times confusing. However, there are two main laws restricting the availability of drugs: the Misuse of Drugs Act (Home Office 1971) and the Medicines Act (1968). The Misuse of Drugs Act is designed to prevent the use of certain drugs outside legitimate medical treatment and classifies substances as A, B or C, with class A considered the most serious and class C the least. Since the classifications of controlled drugs are periodically changed it is worth consulting reputable websites (see for example, www.drugscope.org.uk) in order to verify the current situation. Relying on the media for information is problematic as, whilst the declassification and subsequent reclassification of cannabis received a great deal of attention, the classification of fresh psilocybe mushrooms to a class A drug received little attention.

Table 20.1 Maximum penalties under the Misuse of Drugs Act (Adapted from the Misuse of Drugs Act 1971)

Class of drug	Maximum penalty for possession	Maximum penalty for supply
A	7 years prison and/or a fine	Life imprisonment and/or a fine
B	5 years prison and/or a fine	14 years prison and/or a fine
C	2 years prison and/or a fine	14 years prison and/or a fine

At the time of writing, class A drugs include ecstasy, LSD, cocaine, crack, heroin, magic mushrooms (containing the compound psilocin) and any class B if prepared for injection. Class B drugs include amphetamine and cannabis. Class C drugs include anabolic steroids and minor tranquillisers.

The Misuse of Drugs Act (Home Office 1971) outlines several offences connected with the supply and possession of a controlled substance (*see* Release 2009). Charges relating to supply do not require an individual to profit during the transfer of a controlled drug to another person (Release 2009). Hence a charge of supply could be made where an individual gives a quantity of a controlled drug to a friend (for example, buying two ecstasy tablets for a night out and giving one to a friend counts as supply of a class A drug). Potential sentences under the Misuse of Drugs Act are shown in Table 20.1.

As previously noted, drugs such as diamorphine (heroin) have legitimate uses in Western medicine and the Misuse of Drugs Act (Home Office 1971) allows certain drugs to be legally used during medical care. Substances are scheduled 1–5, with schedule 1 drugs being the most stringently controlled. Therefore, it is not possible for a medic in the UK to prescribe cannabis, a class B and schedule 1 drug, but it is possible to prescribe diamorphine (heroin), a class A and schedule 2 drug (*see* Release 2009, for more details).

The second piece of legislation, the Medicines Act 1968, controls the manufacture and supply of medicines to the general public (Release 2009). Medical drugs are divided into three categories. The first category can only be supplied by a pharmacist upon receipt of a prescription from a medic. The second can be sold 'over the counter' but only by a pharmacist. The third category, which includes aspirin and paracetamol, can be sold in any shop (with restrictions on the amount sold in any one sale).

SOME OF THE COMMON SUBSTANCES OF MISUSE AVAILABLE IN THE UK

The drugs which are used/misused in our society can be loosely categorised into five main groups: stimulants, depressants, narcotic analgesics, hallucinogens and anabolic steroids.

Stimulant drugs can act on the individual in physical and psychological ways. Users often describe physical excitement and increased energy levels along with heightened sensations and feelings. Examples of this group of drugs span the legal range including cocaine (class A), amphetamine (class B, unless prepared for injection in which case it becomes class A), nicotine (a legal but controlled drug) and caffeine (a freely available substance with no legal controls).

Depressants are a group of drugs which slow down various physical functions of the body and also dull the individual's feelings. The term 'depressant' relates to a slowing down of the central nervous system and not depression in the mental health sense. Whilst the use of depressant drugs, such as alcohol and solvents, can lead to depression in terms of a mental health diagnosis, this is not an automatic effect of such drugs.

Narcotic analgesics have a great deal in common with depressant drugs, but have some specific effects. Opiates fall into this category and are drugs made from the opium poppy, such as opium, morphine, heroin and codeine. Opiates have been used for thousands of years for their pain relieving properties and alongside their depressant effects they induce a sense of euphoria and a general feeling of well-being in the user.

Hallucinogens such as LSD (lysergic acid diethylamide), magic mushrooms and stronger forms of cannabis disrupt the sensory perceptions of the user. Changes in mood and the senses (for example, distortions of colours) are common, and intense hallucinatory visions are possible with more powerful hallucinogens such as LSD. Individuals can experience a very different world to those around them which may result in psychological disturbance.

Steroids are synthetic copies of naturally occurring hormones mainly based on testosterone, the 'male' hormone. Their effect is mainly physical, increasing muscle mass, thus to some extent increasing muscle strength. They may also promote aggressiveness in the person using them. They have been used by individuals in connection with intensive physical sports, occupations which require rapid responses to physical situations (for example, nightclub doorpersons) or for body building but may cause problems in the user's interpersonal relationships.

Many drugs used in modern society could be placed into more than one of these five categories. For example, ecstasy could be categorised as a stimulant and a hallucinogen or cannabis could be classified into the depressant or hallucinogen category.

The following section gives a basic outline of some of the major legal and illegal drugs used in the UK, placed in order of their categorisation under the Misuse of Drugs Act (Home Office 1971).

ECSTASY

Ecstasy is a synthetic range of substances which loosely combine some of the effects of amphetamine and LSD. It is illicitly supplied in a variety of tablets and capsules, and is also increasingly available in powder form. Ecstasy tablets are often stamped with logos in order to identify a particular batch. However, it is not unusual for a producer to change the strength or content of subsequent batches of the drug and sell them on the basis of the reputation of a previously supplied product. This means that a user should be wary of relying on previous experience in order to judge the effects and dose of a tablet that resembles one previously taken. Many tablets and capsules sold as ecstasy contain amphetamine or even the legal substance caffeine.

What does it do to the user?

Effects are experienced after 20 to 60 minutes and can last several hours. Users may experience mild euphoria, feelings of serenity and calmness, stimulation of empathy with others and heightened perception. Side effects can include dilated pupils, jaw tightness, sweating, dry mouth, some rise in blood pressure and heart rate, loss of appetite and difficulty with coordination.

What are the possible consequences of using the drug?

There are recorded fatalities linked to the use of ecstasy in the UK, although these are far less numerous than legal drugs such as alcohol and tobacco. Heat stroke, an individual's susceptibility and drinking too much water (without eliminating the excess) appear to be the main causes of death following ecstasy use. Most of the adverse psychological consequences of ecstasy use have been reported by long term, heavy users. These can include anxiety, panic, confusion, insomnia and visual and auditory hallucinations, although these effects often remit once use stops.

LSD (LYSERGIC ACID DIETHYLAMIDE)

LSD is a powerful hallucinogenic drug which was synthesised from a naturally occurring fungus (Ergot) by the chemist Albert Hofmann (1906–2008) around the time of the Second World War. Pure LSD is a clear liquid which is very powerful, requiring only a tiny dose to produce the desired effects. It is usually available within small squares of blotting paper, slivers of gelatine or small tablets (called microdots) which are swallowed.

What does it do to the user?

Effects are usually experienced after 30 minutes to one hour and can last up to 12 hours. Users report visual hallucinations often consisting of intensified colours, distorted shapes and sizes and the movement of stationary objects. They can experience changes in their perceptions of time and place, auditory hallucinations and heightened emotional states including heightened self awareness.

What are the possible consequences of using the drug?

Physical addiction does not develop with LSD as regular use of the drug ceases to provide the desired effect. However, adverse long-term psychological effects are possible. Such effects can include anxiety, depression, panic and paranoia. The risks of such symptoms developing may increase when there is an existing or latent mental health problem. Unpleasant reactions can occur whilst using the drug, commonly referred to as a 'bad trip'. These may include increasing levels of panic and fear, and uncertainty about how long the effects of the drug will last.

COCAINE

Cocaine is a stimulant drug which comes in the form of a white powder derived from the leaves of the coca plant of South America. Because it is imported into Europe from South America by organised crime syndicates it is considerably more expensive than the synthetically made amphetamine sulphate (*see below*) and its use is often associated with rich and famous members of society. Cocaine may be injected, snorted (sniffed into the nasal passages through a straw, rolled up bank note or such like) or smoked (in the form of crack), but cannot be swallowed due to its local anaesthetic properties. Crack is the alkaloid, smokable form of cocaine which is produced from cocaine powder often by local dealers. It comes in the form of small white lumps which are smoked in a pipe, often improvised by the user. When crack is heated in such a pipe it makes a crackling noise, hence its name.

What does it do to the user?

When snorted or injected the effects of cocaine start quickly but only last for between 20 to 30 minutes. Cocaine gives the user a feeling of confidence, stamina and euphoria and may result in an indifference to physical pain. When smoked in the form of crack, the effects are more rapid and intense, but only last for around 5–10 minutes.

What are the possible consequences of using the drug?

Psychologically, cocaine can make you feel anxious and the stimulant effect can leave you feeling run down and depressed afterwards, particularly after large doses or prolonged use. It can cause restlessness, insomnia and paranoia and may lead to nasal damage if sniffed. Injecting cocaine can lead to severe injection site injuries, due to its local anaesthetic properties. Injectors can miss a vein without realising, leading to the development of an abscess.

Cocaine does not cause physical dependence, but can lead to psychological dependence where an individual attempts to maintain the positive feelings they first experienced. It is not unusual for cocaine users to binge for several days, not use for several days and then use again. This pattern of usage leads the individual into the belief that they are controlling their cocaine use.

It is possible to overdose on cocaine which can result in heart failure and respiratory arrest, and lead to death.

HEROIN

Heroin belongs to the family of drugs called the opiates that also includes substances such as morphine and codeine which are commonly used in medicine for the relief of moderate and severe pain. They are derived from the opium poppy which grows in most areas of the world, but produces the best yield of opiates in certain climatic conditions. Much of the world's production of opium has traditionally centred on Northern India, Pakistan, Afghanistan and some areas of China.

Pharmaceutical grade heroin (called diamorphine) comes in the form of a white, water soluble powder. However, illegally sourced heroin comes in the form of a brown powder which is designed to be smoked. Unlike cannabis, which is often mixed with tobacco, rolled into a cigarette (spliff) and smoked, heroin is heated on a strip of aluminium foil and the resultant smoke inhaled through a tube held in the user's mouth. The smoke emitted from the heated heroin is said to resemble the shape of a Chinese dragon, hence the term 'chasing the dragon'. Illicit heroin can be injected, but unlike the pharmaceutical product needs to be mixed with an acid such as vitamin C (ascorbic acid) or acetic acid in order to break it down, prior to injection.

What does it do to the user?

The effects of heroin start quickly and can last several hours, but these do vary between individual users, depending on the amount used and the purity of the supply. It acts as a depressant drug, slowing down bodily functions whilst at the same time giving the user a sense of detachment and feelings of contentment. Pupils may become constricted and users report that the drug removes feelings of anxiety, blocking physical and emotional pain. Higher doses result in sedation and drowsiness often called 'gauching' by users.

What are the possible consequences of using the drug?

Tolerance to the drug can develop relatively quickly and physical dependence can result. The drug is then required in increasing doses in order to stave off potentially unpleasant withdrawal effects. Regular use decreases appetite, resulting in ailments caused by poor nutrition, and a general sense of apathy can lead to social problems such as homelessness and unemployment.

The strength of illegal heroin supplies varies considerably, increasing the risk of potential overdose, particularly if injected. Overdose can result in coma and death when the depressant properties of the drug close down the body's nervous system.

If dependency does develop a user may experience a wide range of withdrawal symptoms if they stop using the drug including muscle cramps, inability to sleep, gastrointestinal disturbances, oversensitivity of touch and smell and a range of other symptoms resembling influenza. These symptoms last for approximately 7–10 days and often result in the user seeking medical assistance or relapsing into using the drug again.

AMPHETAMINE

Amphetamine is a synthetic stimulant which is most usually available as an illegally manufactured compound. It comes in powder form and is usually white or slightly yellow in colour, although it is sometimes coloured pink by suppliers who claim this to be the sign of increased potency.

Amphetamine was widely prescribed by GPs in the 1960s as an appetite suppressant and general antidepressant. Its use soon spread amongst young people who used the drug at all-night clubs and social events. It fell out of favour as a prescribed substance during the late 1960s being replaced by other medications such as benzodiazepines. An illicit market subsequently developed in illegally manufactured amphetamine which is relatively cheap (in comparison with cocaine) and fairly easy to manufacture, given unrestricted access to certain chemicals.

It has few medical uses today, although derivatives of the compound are used in the treatment of attention deficit disorder in children and (rarely) for the treatment of individuals who are considered dependent on illegal amphetamine. Amphetamine powder can be sniffed, swallowed or injected.

What does it do to the user?

Amphetamine is a powerful stimulant and depending on the mode of ingestion effects occur within a few minutes and last for several hours. It provides the user with feelings of exhilaration, increased energy, and a sense of power and confidence. Users report an enhanced ability to concentrate and a marked reduction in appetite and the need for sleep. Heart rate can increase, along with blood pressure and pupils tend to dilate. Individuals may experience a dry mouth, and develop the urge to chew or grind their teeth.

What are the possible consequences of using the drug?

Regular use of amphetamine can lead to tolerance, where an increasingly larger dose is required to achieve the desired effect. The drug can place a strain on the heart and there have been cases where death has occurred due to heart failure.

Periods of extended use can lead to lack of sleep and poor nutrition. Psychological ill effects include pronounced mood swings, which can be aggressive or violent, paranoia and there is a suggestion of the possibility of developing psychosis.

CANNABIS

Cannabis is currently the most commonly used illicit drug in the UK according to the British Crime Survey (Murphy and Roe 2007). It is a product of the bushy cannabis sativa plant and comes in various forms including the leaves and buds of the plant, and more refined extracts such as resins, oils and powders. The plant is native to the Indian subcontinent but grows readily in warmer climates around the world. With modern advances in hydroponics (growing plants under artificial conditions indoors) cannabis can be grown in any area of the world. However, the cost of running such growing systems and risks from enforcement agencies tend to limit this method of commercial production to more organised criminal gangs.

Cannabis is often smoked in a pipe or cigarette mixed with tobacco (commonly called a spliff) but can be eaten on its own, drunk in a tea or added to foods such as cakes, cookies or chocolate. There is increasing interest in the use of cannabis as a medication for a range of illnesses including conditions of the central nervous system such as multiple sclerosis and for the relief of chronic pain. Research is currently being conducted into potential medical uses for some of the compounds found in the cannabis plant.

What does it do to the user?

The physical effects from smoking cannabis occur relatively quickly, although if eaten or drunk the effects can take longer to fully emerge. Psychological effects can include a feeling of relaxation, increased sociability, talkativeness, hilarity or introspective reflection. Users often report effects such as bloodshot eyes, dryness of the mouth, increased appetite (commonly called the 'munchies') and impaired coordination and movement.

What are the possible consequences of using the drug?

There is no conclusive evidence that regular use causes any lasting physical damage, but smoking the drug with tobacco will increase a user's risk of developing cancers and respiratory diseases.

Potential psychological problems can include increased anxiety, risk of panic attacks and even paranoia. Impaired memory functioning has also been reported and chronic use can result in lethargy and apathy thereby resulting in poor performance at work or in education. Commonly cited research has indicated that increasingly potent strains of cannabis may be linked to the development of psychosis in adolescents (Van Os *et al.* 2002). The UK government recently reclassified cannabis from a class C to a class B drug (26 January 2009) despite recommendations from the Advisory Council on the Misuse of Drugs (ACMD) that it should remain as a class C. This research was mentioned as one of the reasons for the reclassification of cannabis in the UK.

Cannabis is often seen as a 'gateway' drug, where users move from cannabis to other more dangerous substances. However, evidence around this progression is inconclusive.

ANABOLIC STEROIDS

Anabolic steroids are a group of synthetic drugs which mimic the effects of the male hormone testosterone. They should not be confused with the commonly prescribed corticosteroids that are used to reduce inflammation and swellings. There are many different preparations that can be categorised as anabolic steroids and some legitimate medical uses for these substances, such as for certain illnesses which lead to muscle wastage and for delayed puberty. However, pharmaceutical products are extremely rare within the illicit market, with the majority of steroids traditionally being obtained from abroad or veterinary sources (Tyler 1995). Illicitly sourced steroids may be forgeries or contain an increased dose of the substance they are packaged as. They are available as tablets or injectable solutions that are injected via an intramuscular injection rather than intravenously.

Anabolic steroids are often used in conjunction with other drugs; some are used for their body building properties, for example insulin or human growth hormone; some are used to reduce the side effects of the steroids, for example Tamoxifen and human chorionic gonadotrophin; and others used to maintain the motivation to body build, for example amphetamine or cocaine.

Most anabolic steroid users take the drug for a fixed time period, usually a few weeks and then stop using for a period of time (this is known as a cycle). Often users will mix various amounts of different anabolic steroids, orally and by injection (known as stacking). Anabolic steroid users tend to see themselves as interested in improving their physique and stamina and feel that this sets them aside from other, pleasure seeking drug users.

What do they do to the user?

This group of drugs has two main effects on the body, the anabolic effect, which improves muscle mass of the user, and the androgenic effect, which produces masculine characteristics, such as male pattern baldness, facial hair and a deeper voice. Some preparations have more anabolic property than androgenic and vice versa. The steroid user is generally interested in the anabolic potential of the drugs in gaining increasing muscle mass and perceived improvements in physique.

What are the possible consequences of using these drugs?

There are many potential problems with the use of anabolic steroids, particularly in relation to the comparatively large doses taken by many users. The masculinising effect of the drug can result in male pattern baldness, the development of facial hair and a deepening of the voice (in male and female users). Anabolic steroids can lead to a reduction in the body's own testosterone production, impotence, infertility, testicular atrophy and a reduced sperm count in men. Male steroid users may try to counteract such effects during the off-cycle (where the individual stops using anabolic steroids) by the use of human chorionic gonadotrophin, a substance found in the urine of pregnant women. Due to the synthesis of testosterone in the body, breast tissue may develop in men (gynaecomastia) and Tamoxifen (a drug used in the treatment of breast cancer) is often taken to combat this. Women can experience a reduction in breast size, an enlarged clitoris and changes in their menstrual cycle, and such effects in women appear to be irreversible.

Anabolic steroids can seriously affect the liver of the user causing damage and possibly cancer. Since the heart is also a muscle, and the thickening of this muscle is a disease process, heart problems may develop along with circulatory disease.

Research into the psychological effects of anabolic steroid use indicate that it may be associated with increased levels of aggression (Beaver *et al.* 2008) and increase the risk of domestic violence (Choi and Pope 1994).

ALCOHOL

Alcohol use is relatively common in Western societies and has been a traditional feature in religious and recreational activities for thousands of years. Alcohol is produced by the fermentation of fruit juices, solutions made from grain or vegetable materials. Fermentation occurs when yeasts break down the sugar over a period of time, resulting in the production of alcohol. Distillation is the process where water is removed from the fermented product in order to raise the concentration of alcohol. It is commercially available in the form of a range of different beverages varying in strength and flavour, commonly consumed in the form of wines, beers and spirits.

The law around alcohol use is rather complex and reflects the UK's longstanding relationship with the production and consumption of this drug. Currently children under the age of five years can only be given alcohol in an emergency under medical supervision. Alcohol is legal to consume over the age of five away from licensed premises. Under 16s can go anywhere in a public house if supervised (unless the pub has licensing conditions imposed), but may not consume alcohol. A 16 or 17 year old can consume beer, wine or cider (but not spirits) with a meal, in a pub, if bought by an adult accompanying them. Alcohol is legal to buy over the age of 18 years and is readily available in many other retail outlets, pubs and restaurants.

What does it do to the user?

The effects of alcohol consumption increase with dose and are dependent upon such factors as individual physiology, stomach contents and the mood of the user. Many individuals use alcohol as a relaxant and to lessen inhibitions in social settings, which in smaller doses is a possible effect of the drug. Increased doses result in impaired judgement and slower reactions, lack of fine motor coordination, blurred vision and slurred speech. Further increases in dose result in loss of gross motor coordination (such as loss of balance) and possible unconsciousness or even death.

What are the possible consequences of using the drug?

The use of alcohol is a growing concern in the UK in terms of individuals exceeding their recommended maximum intake and alcohol-related criminal activity. The Government currently views excessive alcohol use as having a major impact on public health with considerable financial implications for NHS resources (The Information Centre 2008).

In the short term users may suffer from a 'hangover', where they may feel nauseous, headachy and generally unwell as the effects of the alcohol wear off. They may be involved in accidents, be the victim (or perpetrator) of violence or become involved in other forms of crime.

In the longer term physical and psychological dependence may develop. There are a wide range of physical problems which may result from the use of alcohol. Liver diseases such as cirrhosis, heart disease, stomach problems and impotence are all possible with varying amounts of consumption. Alcohol prevents the uptake of important vitamins and long-term use may result in thiamine (vitamin B1) deficiency. Deficiency in thiamine and the presence of alcohol in the body can lead to brain damage in the form of Wernicke's encephalopathy or Korsakoff's syndrome. These conditions affect the memory and cognitive functioning. Sudden withdrawal from alcohol dependency can result in seizures and death, and it is therefore important to seek medical advice when considering detoxification from the drug.

Women appear to be particularly susceptible to the ill effects of alcohol use, requiring less alcohol than men to develop long-term damage. The Department of Health recommendations reflect this. They suggest that women should not drink more than two to three units of alcohol per day and men should not drink more than three to four units of alcohol per day (NHS 2008). Individuals often underestimate their alcohol intake, particularly when talking to health and social care workers. In order to calculate the number of UK units in a particular beverage it is necessary to know the percentage of alcohol present. The number of UK units equates to the percentage of alcohol by volume (usually indicated on packaging) multiplied by the volume consumed (in ml) divided by 1,000, hence 500 ml of strong lager at nine per cent alcohol by volume would equate to 4.5 units ($500 \times 9 \div 1,000 = 4.5$).

TOBACCO

Tobacco is the dried leaves of a plant native to the Americas which is most often smoked in the form of cigarettes or cigars although it can also be inhaled (snuff) or chewed. Whilst tobacco contains thousands of different chemicals, the main constituents noted in the substance are tar and nicotine. Tar is the dark, sticky substance which condenses as the tobacco smoke cools and contains the flavour sought by the smoker. It contains chemicals which are carcinogenic and others which inhibit the correct functioning of the lungs, thus contributing to diseases such as emphysema and bronchitis. Nicotine is a poison fatal to humans in relatively small doses. However, smoking does not deliver a significantly large dose of nicotine rapidly enough to cause death.

It is illegal to sell tobacco to anyone under the age of 18 years. Its use is also banned in confined public spaces due to the risks posed to others through passive smoking.

What does it do to the user?

Tolerance to tobacco use develops quickly. In the small doses received during smoking, nicotine is a mild stimulant. It is absorbed rapidly via the lungs causing an increase in pulse rate and blood pressure, reduced appetite and lowered skin temperature. Users report that it can produce symptoms of stimulation and arousal, and paradoxically, relaxation and calmness. This appears to be due to the drug's effect on the release of naturally occurring brain chemicals such as dopamine (Rassool 2009).

What are the possible consequences of using the drug?

There are clear risks to the circulatory system, increasing susceptibility to blood clots resulting in heart disease, heart attacks or strokes. The risk of cancer of the lung, mouth and throat are all well documented.

FURTHER RISKS ASSOCIATED WITH DRUG USE

In addition to the specific risks posed by each of the drugs discussed there are other consequences to consider in connection with drug use.

For the individual user the possession and supply of many of the substances discussed are controlled under the Misuse of Drugs Act (Home Office 1971), carrying the risk of extensive prison sentences and/or fines. Many employers require potential employees to undergo criminal record checks which may preclude an individual from employment options. From a financial perspective, maintaining a drug dependency has a monetary implication leading to the possibility of increased deprivation and social problems such as theft perpetrated in order to fund such use. Because the production of illegal drugs is not controlled and often originates from criminal sources they can be mixed with dangerous adulterants which can result in systemic illnesses such as tetanus and other health complications depending on the nature of the specific adulterant. If injecting equipment is shared, users are at risk of blood borne infections such as HIV and hepatitis.

The cost of legal drugs in terms of treating smoking and drinking related diseases has been recognised as a major drain on NHS resources. The UK government appears keen to focus on preventing rather than simply treating subsequent illnesses (Department of Health 2004). Treatment and counselling for smokers is currently available from the NHS and an extensive health promotion campaign has been used to encourage individuals to engage in such services. Health promotion activities have also targeted the public's awareness of alcohol use, focusing on the UK's binge drinking culture, where large numbers of individuals drink excessive amounts of alcohol over short periods of time, and the increasing numbers of women who drink over the recommended limit of alcohol.

The production of illegal drugs has also been noted for its potential in generating profits for organised crime and funding terrorist organisations across the globe. This issue has focused an international effort, aimed at controlling certain drugs, orchestrated by the United Nations (United Nations Office on Drugs and Crime (UNODC) 2009).

Drug use and pregnancy

Drug use during pregnancy carries additional risks for the unborn child and mother. Babies born to heroin dependent mothers may require medical attention to detoxify them from the drug once delivered. The lack of attention to nutrition and self care associated with heroin use may also increase the risk of harm to a baby. Cocaine use during pregnancy can damage the unborn child due to the drug's effect of constricting blood vessels. Smoking can result in a reduction in nutrients reaching the developing foetus, lowering birth weight and increasing the risk of miscarriage (NHS 2007). Alcohol use should be avoided as 'foetal alcohol syndrome' can develop causing brain damage and deformities in the baby (NHS 2008). In general, pregnant women may be reluctant to engage in health care services for fear of judgemental attitudes from professionals or the involvement of social workers.

MOMENT OF REFLECTION

Activity Two

Andy is 17 years of age and is currently attending a local college, studying for his 'A' levels and hopes to go on to be a teacher. He has obtained good grades in his assignments, but his attendance has recently deteriorated and his grades have fallen.

He has been smoking cannabis for around six months since meeting some new friends at college who supply him with the drug.

He has a long-term girlfriend who is very much against the use of all drugs, legal or illegal. Andy has so far managed to keep his cannabis use from her.

He lives at home with his mother and younger sister (aged 15), his father having left home some years ago. His mother struggles to support the family on a limited income from part-time work.

You work as an adviser at the college and Andy has asked to see you about his cannabis use.

- What advice would you give?
- What legal, health and social issues might be relevant to Andy?
- How would you help him to address any problems you think he may have?

SUMMARY OF MAIN POINTS

You should be able to:

- Appreciate the historical factors which have influenced society's response to substances of misuse.
- Demonstrate increased knowledge around the common drugs of misuse and know how to develop this knowledge base.
- Present a more measured view on why individuals use/misuse substances.
- Consider how current national legislation seeks to influence the supply and demand for drugs.

FURTHER STUDY

More detailed information on specific drugs can be found in books such as Rassool (2009), and Tyler (1995) provides an interesting and extensive history of drug use.

Drugscope, is the UK's leading independent source of information on drugs, providing a searchable index of drugs in the resources section of its website (www.drugscope.org.uk). Alcohol Concern provides a range of information relating to alcohol use on its website (www.alcoholconcern.org.uk). Both of these organisations are a good source of up-to-date information on issues which have emerged from the latest research and policy on drugs and alcohol.

Addiction and the *Journal of Substance Use* are the two leading academic journals in the field.

REFERENCES

Advisory Council on the Misuse of Drugs (1982) *Treatment and Rehabilitation,* London: The Stationery Office.

Ashton, M. (1989) Rolleston: The Defence of the Right to Prescribe, *Druglink,* January/February, 12–14.

Beaver, K. M., Vaughn, M. G., DeLisi, M. and Wright, J. P. (2008) Anabolic-Androgenic Steroid Use and Involvement in Violent Behavior in a Nationally Representative Sample of Young Adult Males in the United States, *American Journal of Public Health,* 98 (12), 2185–7.

Berridge, V. (1988) The origins of the English drug 'scene' 1890–1930, *Medical History,* 32, 51–64.

Choi, P. Y. L. and Pope, H. G. (1994) Violence Toward Women and Illicit Androgenic-Anabolic Steroid Use, *Annals of Clinical Psychiatry*, 6 (1), 21–5.

Davenport-Hines, R. (2001) *The Pursuit of Oblivion: A Social History of Drugs,* London: Pheonix Press.

Davies, J. B. (1997) *The Myth of Addiction,* Amsterdam: Harwood Academic Publishers.

Department of Health (2004) *Choosing health: Making healthy choices easier,* London: HMSO.

Gossop, M. (2000) *Living with Drugs* (5th edition), Aldershot: Ashgate Publishing Ltd.

Home Office (1971) *Misuse of Drugs Act,* London: HMSO.

Information Centre (NHS) (2008) *Statistics on Alcohol: England 2008* [online]. Available at: http://www.ic.nhs.uk/webfiles/publications/alcoholeng2008/Statistics%20on%20Alcohol-%20England%202008%20final%20format%20v7.pdf

Kohn, M. (1992) *Dope Girls: The Birth of the British Drug Underground,* London: Granta Books.

McMurran, M. (1994) *The Psychology of Addiction,* London: Taylor and Francis.

Murphy, R. and Roe, S. (2007) *Drug Misuse Declared: Findings from the 2006/07 British Crime Survey*, London: HMSO.

NHS (2007) *NHS Choices: Smoking and Pregnancy* [Online]. Available at: http://smokefree.nhs.uk/smoking-and-pregnancy/

NHS (2008) *NHS Choices* [online]. Available at: http://units.nhs.uk/index.php

Rassool, G. H. (2009) *Alcohol and Drug Misuse: A handbook for Students and Health Professionals,* Abingdon: Routledge.

Release (2009) *UK Law* [online]. Available at: http://www.release.org.uk/information/uk-law

Tyler, A. (1995) *Street Drugs* (2nd edition), London: Hodder and Stoughton.

United Nations Office on Drugs and Crime (2009) Home Page [online]. Available at: http://www.unodc.org/unodc/index.html

Van Os, J., Bak, M., Hanssen, M., Bijl, R., de Graaf, R. and Verdoux, H. (2002) Cannabis use and psychosis: a longitudinal population-based study, *American Journal of Epidemiology,* 156 (4), 319–27.

Walton, S. (2001) *Out of It,* London: Penguin Books.

CHAPTER 21

WORKING WITH CHILDREN

HELEN BURROWS, JILL BERRISFORD AND JO WARD

OBJECTIVES

After reading this chapter you should be able to:

▪ Understand the historical development of the context of working with children.

▪ Be aware of current themes in child development.

▪ Understand transitions, communication and participation.

▪ Be aware of values that underpin working with children.

After reading this chapter you will understand the key terms: 'Rights', 'paternalism', attachment, resilience, transition, communication, participation.

There are three Moments of Reflection to work on throughout the chapter.

INTRODUCTION

In whatever setting we work with children and young people, whether it is in health care, early years, education, social care, statutory safeguarding, youth justice, community development, guidance and mentoring – we need a range of skills, knowledge and values in order to work effectively. Whilst an earlier chapter, *The individual in society*, has outlined themes and theories in wider human development, we will look at specific understanding of some areas of child development in more detail. An understanding of child development enables us to put children's behaviour and abilities into better context, and points us in the direction of the skills we need to work with them at an appropriate level and in an appropriate way.

CHILDREN AND YOUNG PEOPLE AND OUR VALUES

As discussed earlier, for anyone working with children and young people in any setting, helping them to express their views, to manage transitions, to develop resilience and overcome difficulties is a vital role. However, it is not just important to understand how to do this, and to learn the skills to do this effectively, it is also important for us to understand *why* we do it.

The role of the state in shaping child care policy and practice is crucial in this respect and as Colton *et al.* (2001) suggest, has changed considerably over time. The emphasis on residential care for children moved to developing foster care provision and by the 1970s the focus became achieving permanence for children in a family. During the 1980s, the aim was to maintain children in their biological families if at all possible. The final stage Colton *et al.* identify is one in which the extended family are viewed as part of an important network for children. Horner (2003) suggests a further phase of integrated contributions by birth, extended and substitute families.

Behind policy and practice various ideological positions can be identified. Fox Harding (1997) identifies four:

1   **Laissez faire/patriarchy** – the role of intervention by the state is kept to a minimum, preservation of family privacy highly valued.
2   **The society as parent/state paternalism** – the state is seen as having a moral and legal obligation to protect children. The emphasis is on the importance of providing care for children in trouble, rather than punishment. If parents are unable to provide adequate care and protection for their children then they do not deserve to look after them and ties may be severed.
3   **The kinship defender** – state intervention is seen as important but it must be done by supporting and helping families to overcome their difficulties in caring for their children. Intervention is viewed as oppressive by the political left and right but often for different reasons.
4   **Children's rights** – the capacity of children and young people to be involved in decisions about their lives is acknowledged and encouraged. Their perspective needs to be included in the development of policy, practice and legislation.

Being aware of the context of our work helps us to reflect on and develop our values and understanding, and to explore the different approaches that we might take to tackling different situations. We might want to think about what we want to achieve in working with children – do we want to help them to learn, to protect them from harm, to help them to achieve their best potential, or to give them a healthy and safe environment to grow up in? And we might want to think about our motives – do we want to give them the sort of life experiences that we had ourselves, or conversely, help them to avoid the sort of experiences we had?

When we think about why and how we are going to work with children, it is also helpful to think about how we view them. Children and young people can be seen in many lights, often reflected in the language we use. For example, babies and very young children are often seen as sweet and adorable – 'poppet' (which originally meant a toy or doll), 'angel', 'sweetie' ('I could eat you up'). Whereas older children and young people can at the other extreme be demonised – 'hoodies', 'gangstas', etc. Popular media in particular feed this view of young people. Neither of these views shows respect for children and young people as individuals with their own differences, needs and views, and both extremes see them as basically alien to adult society. Taking either of these views might be described as paternalistic – as adults we think we know what is best for society, and whether we welcome, tolerate, dislike or fear children, we do not give them a say in how the world is run. Taking a different view, however, might lead us to see children and young people as valued individuals who have rights of their own. Whether we take a 'rights' or 'paternalistic' perspective will impact on how we try to work with children and young people.

CURRENT THEMES IN CHILD DEVELOPMENT

One of the most interesting current debates (which has in many ways been an ongoing debate for generations) is the convergence of nature and nurture – developments in genetics resulting from the sequencing of the human genome are proving illuminating, sometimes confirming existing ideas and sometimes challenging them. Genetic factors have been found to strongly influence some diseases and mental disorders, such as schizophrenia or autism, where the genetic component is strong, but the effect of environmental influences on the development of genetic traits is still open to much debate. Adverse experiences can make people either more resistant or more susceptible to particular conditions, and the interplay between genetic and environmental factors is as yet uncertain, despite the regular announcements in the press that 'the gene for ... has been identified' (debate summarised in Rutter 2002). This is closely linked to questions about the impact of non-shared environments – how people with similar genetic makeup develop similar characteristics or not. Criticisms of twin studies have pointed out that research on twins often looks for similarities, whereas there are also many differences, and no firm conclusions about the strength of genetic influences should be drawn (for example, Stoolmiller 1999; Baumrind 1993; Joseph 1998).

A further idea is that of continuity of development over the whole lifespan rather than 'stages' – this gives a much more positive and holistic view of the human condition. The availability of developmental pathways gives the opportunity to make choices and influence outcomes (Rutter 1999; Sroufe 1997).

Two areas in which the influences of environmental factors are felt to be particularly important are traits and behaviours related to attachment, and a child's levels of resilience. These areas of understanding explore how parenting affects child development for good or ill – the 'nurture' effects on typical and atypical development. Acute adversity has been found to be less damaging than long-term deprivation. This is particularly important when looking at children suffering abuse and neglect (Rutter 2002).

Attachment

In order to work effectively with children it is important that we have a basic understanding of attachment theory and the concepts of separation and loss as we understand them thus far.

John Bowlby (1951, 1969, 1973, 1988) is seen as the founding father of the concept of attachment. From the 1940s onwards, over a number of decades, he undertook numerous studies. As a result of these, he suggested that there is a human 'instinct' to form an attachment between the mother and child. Prolonged separation between mother and child, especially during the first few years of their life, was seen as a major cause of 'delinquent' behaviour and mental health difficulties. However, as research progressed, it is important to note that he became convinced that children can make significant attachment relationships with other people not just their mothers. Further research (Rutter 1981) has shown that children can develop a number of attachments and that developing relationships with fathers, siblings, extended family and friends is also important. Put simply, children thrive when they experience reliable, stable and loving relationships throughout their childhood with whomever it is that looks after them.

It now seems clear, that the nature of a child/young person's attachments is likely to have an effect on their emotional, behavioural and social development. In his studies, Bowlby highlighted three themes in his attempts to understand disturbed and upset behaviour. First, the failure of the attachment figure to provide a reliable and secure base as well as to help the child deal with feelings of anger in response to loss. Second, the loss of a close relationship and disruption of affectionate bonds. Third, the development of defensive strategies, particularly emotional withdrawal, to cope with the pain of loss and the associated feelings of anxiety. The combined effect of these experiences seems often to be linked to difficult behaviour and disturbed relationships.

David Howe suggests that what appear to be difficult behaviour and disturbed relationships to the outsider are in fact a rational and understandable response by children who are insecurely attached to their caregivers. Their behaviour is seen as an adaptive response to a situation in which anxiety and emotions are running high (Howe 1995: 95).

Bowlby's concept of 'internal working models' helps us understand the potential for the long-term impact of early attachment experiences. It is argued that these models form the basis for organisation and affective experience (Bretherton 1991; Main *et al.* 1985) helping us to make sense of new experiences and shaping subjective reality. Internal working models, whilst resistant to change, can be reformatted. Kate Cairns (2002) talks with passion and great insight about her experiences of doing just this with the 12 children she fostered over a period of 25 years.

Ainsworth *et al.* (1978) identified three patterns of attachment – secure, ambivalent and avoidant. An additional category was identified by Main *et al.* (1985) – disorganised/disorientated:

- *Secure* – the secure pattern provides the *optimal* context for development. It provides the child with a foundation from which to explore the world. The primary attachment figure facilitates the development of an internal working model in which the self is perceived as worthy, others are perceived to be reliable and available and the environment can be experienced as challenging but manageable with support.
- *Avoidant* – this pattern develops in the context of an unresponsive and rejecting relationship with the attachment figure. The self is perceived as unworthy and others are seen to be unavailable and hurtful. Due to lack of consistent support in stressful situations, the environment is experienced as threatening.
- *Ambivalent/resistant* – this pattern develops in response to inconsistent, unreliable and at times intrusive responses from the attachment figure. There is uncertainty about the worthiness of the self. Others are perceived to be unreliable, overbearing and insensitive, and the environment is experienced as unpredictable and chaotic.

- *Disorganised/disorientated* – this pattern develops when children have to respond to an attachment figure that they perceive as a source of threat. The primary caregivers are described as frightening *or* frightened. The self is perceived to be unworthy and others are perceived as frightening and dangerous. When the primary caregiver is frightened, the self is perceived to be unworthy and others are seen to be helpless. In both situations the environment is experienced as dangerous and chaotic.

Ainsworth *et al.* tested these theories experimentally through the 'Strange situation test' whereby infants' reactions to brief separations from their caregivers were observed and categorised (Ainsworth *et al.* 1978).

It is worth noting that many of us *are not* the benefactors of secure attachment patterns. Indeed, it is likely that probably half of the population of Great Britain will have experienced an avoidant attachment pattern during childhood (Howe 1995).

More recently, research undertaken by Schore (2001) focuses on the link between attachment and brain development, emphasising the link between attachment and the development of self regulation. He argues that when severe difficulties arise in the relationship to the attachment figure, the brain becomes inefficient at regulating affective states and coping with stress and that sustained stress hinders development.

Attachment theory can be criticised in several respects. First, for children living in difficult environments such as war or, in a less extreme example, children living away from their families for whatever reason, a secure attachment is not only likely to be unachievable, it may also be emotionally damaging. An avoidant attachment may be the best way of ensuring psychological survival.

Attachment can be seen as a Western concept based on the model of a single carer (usually the mother) being responsible for the upbringing of a child, whereas in many societies the extended family is the basis of child rearing. While attachment is in essence a fundamental biological impulse, different care giving methods will provoke different attachment styles (Rogoff 2003). Some of the tests to validate attachment theory, particularly the strange situation experiment, are very culturally specific to a US/UK context. For example, in societies where independence is encouraged from an early age, or conversely where babies are rarely separated from their mothers, the child may not respond in the expected way to the return of their parent in the test (Rutter 1995; Miyake *et al.* 1985). Finally, it has been argued from a feminist perspective that attachment theory was politically promoted by the government at the time. This was in order to help achieve their aim of getting women back into the home from the workplace, following the necessity of them working during the Second World War (Cleary 1999). However, these criticisms do not mean that attachment is meaningless or useless as a concept, but rather that we must be wary of making broad assumptions about what is or is not a 'good' attachment.

Resilience

We have been considering how lack of attachments can have a detrimental impact on our behaviour and impede our ability to form and sustain caring and loving relationships. However, despite the importance and validity of this theory there is an increasing body of knowledge and research, some of which will be referred to later, into the concept of resilience. On the surface, this may appear to contradict the theory of attachment. However, they offer different perspectives on why children and later adults behave the way they do.

Resilience stems from the question: why is it that despite spending their childhood in what would be deemed emotionally and physically adverse environments for well-being, some people are nevertheless able to function and thrive?

MOMENT OF REFLECTION

Activity One

Before going on to read about what research has to show us about this question, think for yourself: what might promote resilience in children?

Consider what you have already read and also your own experiences of childhood.

COMMENTARY

You may have considered the following factors when thinking about what promotes resilience: having significant and caring relationships with parents/carers and siblings; having positive and nurturing friendships; gaining a good education and school experience; being capable and/or very interested in a particular sport or activity; belonging to a club/group where a sense of belonging and identity was developed, etc.

In the UK, the resilience of children and young people from very disadvantaged family backgrounds has been found to be associated with: a redeeming and warm relationship with at least one person in the family or secure attachment to at least one unconditionally supportive parent or carer; positive school experiences; feeling able to plan and be in control; being given the chance of a 'turning point' such as a new opportunity or break from a high-risk area; higher childhood IQ scores; lower rates of temperamental risk; and having positive peer influences (Rutter *et al.* 1998).

A research review by Newman and Blackburn (2002) of the international literature on resilience factors in relation to the key transitions made by children and young people during their lives has added to this picture. As well as the first three factors identified above, the authors conclude that children and young people who are best equipped to overcome adversities will have: strong social support networks; a committed mentor or person from outside the family; a range of extra-curricular activities that promote the learning of competencies and emotional maturity; the capacity to reframe adversities so that the beneficial as well as the damaging effects are recognised; the ability, or opportunity, to make a difference, for example, by helping others through volunteering, or undertaking part-time work; and exposure to challenging situations that provide opportunities to develop both problem-solving abilities and emotional coping skills.

The definitions of resilience can vary considerably, but while diverse, within all of them are concerns with development; the ability to adapt and the nature of various outcomes for young people. In addition, most refer to the ability to cope with threats and adversity, how the individual and environment interact, and supportive and undermining factors.

In their critical overview of resilience research, Harvey and Delfabbro (2004) cite how a series of studies, among them Garmezy *et al.* (1984), Werner (1984) and Rutter (1981), demonstrated the achievement of 'normal psychosocial development' and 'life success' by young people in the face of multiple risks in their lives. These early studies were subsequently followed by others demonstrating similar findings and further developing the concept of resilience (Harvey and Delfabbro 2004). We can be excited by this research for the simple reason that it offers hope in the face of the often intractable difficulties children and families face in their lives.

As already alluded to, central to the concept of resilience is the idea of risk and protective factors. In simple terms, risk factors are those characteristics of a person or their environment that increase the chances of their having impaired development. For example, research by Parrot *et al.* (2008) indicates loss through bereavement, marital/relationship breakdown or illness, acting as a carer, being bullied at school, homelessness and poverty, or loss of control at work and long working hours might be risk factors. Other ones may include child abuse, significant childhood illness, parental drug or alcohol abuse, mental health problems and significant offending behaviour.

Protective factors are characteristics that reduce such chances 'either directly or by mediating or moderating the effect of exposure to risk factors' (Arthur *et al.* 2002: 576). For example, a secure attachment, outgoing temperament, a good school experience, one supportive adult, community network support, skilled help with behavioural problems, social support networks and problem solving skills are protective factors.

Another key idea within resilience is that of *positive* turning points in developmental pathways. A turning point can be viewed as a new opportunity, for example, leaving school, leaving home, finding a new skill or interest, beginning a new friendship/relationship.

Vignette of Terry

Terry is nearly 18 and of black African-Caribbean heritage. He has recently moved to live in a flat with Kate his girlfriend.

Terry has three younger siblings who all live at home with his parents, Sophia and Michael. The family are poor as Sophia and Michael have always found work hard to come by. When Terry was seven years old, Sophia got a cleaning job in the evenings and Michael found work away from home. Terry looked after his siblings in the evenings. There was often little or no food in the house and conditions in the home were poor. Urine and faeces from the family's three dogs was found around the home by social workers when they visited.

Terry was first arrested when he was 10 and had committed criminal damage, car theft and burglary by the time he was 13. He spent some months in secure accommodation before being released back to his family. He committed further offences and was placed in foster care at age 14. During his secondary school years he missed about half his schooling before going into foster care.

Terry spent a settled two years in foster care, finishing his secondary schooling with some achievements. He became a popular student with teachers, being well known for his sharp wit. He got a weekend job and showed a flair for business.

He decided he wanted to move to semi-independent accommodation from foster care when he was 16. After a small blip of reoffending soon after he left the foster carers, he met Kate and they have been in a positive relationship for the last two years, during which time he has not reoffended.

MOMENT OF REFLECTION

Activity Two

Identify what you consider to be the potential risk factors and protective factors in Terry's life and highlight what you consider to be any positive turning points.

COMMENTARY

You may have considered the following as positive turning points for Terry:

*   Meeting his girlfriend Kate and eventually moving into a flat with her.
*   Moving to a foster placement where he was able to settle.
*   Weekend job that highlighted his flair for business.

TRANSITIONS

In a previous chapter, *The individual in society*, we talked about the various transitions that we all go through during our lifetime. In this chapter we will be concentrating on the transitions experienced during childhood which may be either universal or inflicted upon us by the vagaries of our life circumstances.

For those working with children it is essential to manage such transitions well. Understanding the effects of transitions and endings can give us an insight into why these times may be so difficult. It can help children, parents and carers to manage their own feelings of loss and grief, and give them the knowledge to successfully come through the changes facing them. Good attachments and resilience are likely to be key contributors to successful transitions being made. To help somebody through a time of transition is an opportunity to help them develop and learn from the experience.

We all go through various transitions during our lives and the perception and impact of this will almost certainly be different for each person. For example, we all leave school at some point but our reaction is likely to vary depending upon, amongst other things, our experience and achievements whilst there.

Transitions inevitably involve a degree of loss which may be viewed positively or negatively. For example, leaving an abusive relationship involves loss but the benefits outweigh the loss. The loss may be of dreams and aspirations as well as physical losses. Understanding the negative feelings that often adjoin separation and loss can be key to the successful movement through a transition.

Jewett (1984) identifies three stages of grieving:

- Early grief – characterised by denial, disbelief, shock, numbness and alarm.
- Acute grief – characterised by yearning, protest and 'searching'.
- Integration – 'I have got through it', begin to move into reorganisation of their life.

These stages may not be sequential and may be revisited over a period of time.

In order to minimise the trauma of moving, it is important to realise that different cultures have different desires and expectations in regard to how to deal with loss and grief. Acknowledging and researching this will certainly be advantageous to the process.

Unaccompanied asylum-seeking children and young people who come into the UK have been through difficult and sometimes horrific experiences in their home countries and during their journeys. In addition to the difference in culture and ethnicity, they are often unable to communicate in English. Given the disruption and trauma they will have suffered, the transition is likely to be a mammoth task requiring compassion and skilled help.

Rituals and customs at a time of transition are important to people in most societies and generally the significant occasions in life are marked by some kind of ritual or custom, for example, birthdays, leaving school/university or marriage. In our experience, working with children and young people who are fostered and adopted, it is appreciated when rituals and celebrations are included in these transitions. An absence of rituals may hinder the process of moving on (Currer 2007), and the creation of new rituals and ceremonies is an important part of knitting together the new family. For example, in regard to children in public care, it may be appropriate to have a leaving party when a child moves from foster carers to adopters, and subsequently for the adopters to mark the adoption day. This probably works best if they are of an age to appreciate and understand what is happening and are involved in the process. Another example would be if the child is being adopted by their foster carers. It may be important to mark this significant change and transition by a yearly celebration.

Transitions are of particular importance to children and young people who become looked after by the local authority as they may have to endure a number of different placements involving considerable disruption. Damage may be minimised by handling these disruptions as sensitively and honestly as possible. In addition, over the years there has been a plethora of initiatives in order to try and improve placement stability. This has culminated in the Children and Young Persons Act 2008, and one of the key areas for improvement in the Act is stability of placements and consistency for children in care.

Children and young people growing up and leaving care or moving from a children's service to adult service in the case of a young person with a learning disability need to be sure their transition will be well planned and successful. The Children (Leaving Care) Act 2000 and the associated regulations and guidance seek to improve the life chances of care leavers and provide important new entitlements. It is too early to say how much this has impacted upon the experience of care leavers as yet, but the service and resources available have improved as a result of the Act.

COMMUNICATION WITH CHILDREN

> When [we are] observing, talking to, listening to or playing with children, [we] need to have the knowledge and skills to take into account the developmental processes of children, and specifically children's own changing perspective on the world. The child must be seen as an actor in his or her own life rather than just a passive recipient of parenting or other experiences ... [We] need to be constantly asking, What is the child's experience of this situation?
>
> (Brandon *et al.* in Thompson 2002)

Although written for social workers, this quote is fundamental for anyone working with children. Working directly with children through play is a task many workers can (and indeed should) carry out. It is not the same as play therapy but is based on the same principles.

Communication with children depends on entering the child's world. We so often fall into the trap of needing to tell the child something, or teach her something, without waiting to listen to or understand what the child wants to communicate to us. 'In every child there is a story that needs to be told – a story that no one else has yet had time to listen to' (Winnicott 1984). When working therapeutically with children, the worker needs to take into account *both* the child's experience of the past, *and* his/her hopes for the future.

MOMENT OF REFLECTION

Activity Three

Try and think of a situation when, as a child, you were desperately trying to tell someone something. What would have helped?

What techniques do you have in your personal set of skills to aid communication? If the child has a disability or communication problem, think about what would help – pre-prepared picture cards are often very helpful; ask the school or carer what communication method the child usually uses. There are now many computer programmes which you can use, either designed for the purpose or other mainstream ones.

Think of the child's chronological age but also their developmental age – give older children the opportunity to express themselves through play that may be more appropriate for a younger child, while at the same time respecting that they may find this 'babyish'.

Respecting and encouraging the child are key factors; giving the child enough time is another. Understand that the child may not want to tell you what you want to know at this time – he/she may have other things on his/her mind. It is crucial to build rapport and you might have to wait. If the child is talking about painful or difficult feelings, before finishing make sure you help the child to 'close down' the session and return to his/her usual way of coping – therapeutic containment.

Filial therapy is a means of working directly with children where the parents/carers act directly as the main agents of change; the parents undergo training which equips them to work therapeutically with their child in designated play sessions (described in Stringer 2009; Van Fleet 2000).

Many young people are not used to having their voices heard, and may have been misinterpreted and misunderstood. They may never have learnt to express their feelings and emotions. They may not have English as their first language, or it may not be the first language of their family, therefore cultural traditions of how to express themselves may come into play. In some languages there are not the words to describe elements of sexual abuse and sexual behaviour (Chand 2005).

You need to be able to create an atmosphere of privacy and trust for the child. Confidentiality needs to be explored – think about what does it mean to the child? It is important that the concept is explained to them in a way that they can understand.

PARTICIPATION

Participation is now a key part of the agenda in working with children. Looking back historically, children were widely viewed as far less important than adults. In Roman times, the law of *patria potestas* gave fathers absolute power (including the power of life and death) over their children (Archard 1993), and more recently, children were still widely seen in Western cultures as possessions of their parents. Now the concept of children's participation is discussed throughout the world (International Save the Children Alliance), it is influenced by the ideas of children as consumers, as active contributors to their own lives, and children's rights.

The United Nations Convention on the Rights of the Child, to which the UK is a signatory, states that:

> State parties shall assure to the child who is capable of forming his or her own views the right to express those views freely in all matters affecting the child, the views of the child being given due weight in accordance with the age and maturity of the child.
>
> (United Nations Convention on the Rights of the Child)

These are complex ideas, however.

Look at the ideas below. Try and think of examples where these might apply. How can conflicting principles be resolved?

- Rights versus rescue.
- Subjects or objects?
- Competent or incompetent?
- Making decisions or involved in decision making?
- Rights of children/rights of parents.

Shier (2001) argues that there are five levels of children's participation, based on the classic 'ladder of participation' described by Roger Hart (1992):

1   children are listened to
2   children are supported in expressing their views

3   children's views are taken into account
4   children are involved in decision-making processes
5   children share power and responsibility.

Meaningful participation is beneficial for children in many ways, but for Shier's model to operate at any level requires openings, opportunities and obligations.

- An opening occurs when a worker is willing to involve children in participation and decision making.
- An opportunity happens when the worker has the resources, skills and knowledge to make it happen.
- Obligations are when the organisation is committed to participation and builds it into its processes.

Organisations enter into different levels of participation, but for children to fully participate (at level 5) would mean adults having to relinquish some of their own power. Many people would invoke some of the arguments outlined above and feel this is not appropriate.

However, it is now largely accepted that participation is a beneficial development for both the children themselves and for society as a whole, despite the challenges involved in implementing it in a really meaningful way.

CONCLUSION

To work with children and young people successfully in any setting, it is important we help them to express their views, manage transitions, develop resilience and overcome difficulties. In order to help us understand *how* to do this, we have outlined contemporary theories of child development, particularly focusing on attachment, resilience and transitions. We have also examined the key themes of working in partnership with children and young people to safeguard and promote their development and needs. Lastly, but certainly not least, we believe it is crucial to understand *why* we do this work by looking at the values that underpin it.

SUMMARY OF MAIN POINTS

You should be able to:

- Understand the historical development of the context of working with children.
- Be aware of current themes in child development.
- Understand transitions, communication and participation.
- Be aware of values that underpin working with children.

REFERENCES

Ainsworth, M. D., Blehar, M. C., Waters, E. and Wall, S. (1978) *Patterns of Attachment, A Psychological Study of the Strange Situation*, New Jersey: Erlbaum.
Archard, D. (1993) *Children – rights and childhood*, London: Routledge.

Arthur, M. W., Hawkins, J. D., Pollard, J., Catalano, R. F. and Baglioni, A. J. (2002) Measuring risk and protective factors for substance use, delinquency and other adolescent behaviours: The Community that Care youth survey, *Evaluation Review*, 26 (6), 575–601.

Baumrind, D. (1993) The average expectable environment is not enough: a response to Scarr, *Child Development*, 64, 1299–317.

Benard, B. (2006) Using strengths-based practice to tap the resilience of families, in D. Saleeby (Ed.), *Strengths perspective in social work practice* (4th edition), Boston: Allyn and Bacon, pp. 197–220.

Bowlby, J. (1951) *Maternal Care and Mental Health*, Geneva: World Health Organisation.

Bowlby, J. (1969) *Attachment and Loss, Volume I: Attachment*, London: Hogarth Press.

Bowlby, J. (1973) *Attachment and Loss, Volume II: Separation, Anxiety and Anger*, London: Hogarth Press.

Bowlby, J. (1988) *A Secure Base: Clinical Applications of Attachment Theory*, London: Routledge.

Brandon, M., Schofield, G. and Trinder L. (1998) *Social Work with Children*, Basingstoke: Palgrave Macmillan.

Bretherton, I. (1991) The roots and growing points of attachment theory, in Parkes, C. M., Stevenson-Hinde, J. and Marris, P. (1991) *Attachment across the Life-Cycle*, London: Routledge, pp. 9–32.

Cairns, K. (2002) *Attachment, trauma and resilience: therapeutic caring for children*, London: BAAF.

Chand, A. (2005) 'Do you speak English? Language barriers in child protection wok with minority ethnic families', *British Journal of Social Work*. 35 (6), 807–21.

Cleary, R. (1999) Bowlby's theory of attachment and loss: a feminist critique, *Feminism Psychology*, 9, 32.

Colton, M., Sanders, R. and Williams, M. (2001) *An Introduction to Working with Children: A Guide for Social Workers*, London: Palgrave.

Currer, C. (2007) *Loss and Social Work*, Poole: Learning Matters.

Fox Harding, L. (1997) *Perspectives in Child Care Policy* (2nd edition), London: Longman.

Garmezy, N., Masten, A. S. and Tellegen, A. (1984) The study of stress and competence in children: A building block for developmental psychopathology, *Child Development*, 55 (1), 97–111.

Hart, R. (1992) Children's Participation: From tokenism to citizenship. Innocenti essay no 4. Florence, Italy: Unicef International Child Development Centre.

Harvey, J. and Delfabbro, P. H. (2004) Psychological resilience in disadvantaged youth: A critical overview, *Australian Psychologist*, 39 (1), 3–13.

Horner, N. (2003) *What is Social Work? Contexts and Perspectives*, Exeter: Learning Matters.

Howe, D. (1995) *Attachment Theory for Social Work Practice*, Basingstoke: Palgrave.

International Save the Children Alliance [online]. Available at: http://www.savethechildren.net/alliance/index.html (Accessed 13 May 2009).

Jewett, C. L. (1984) *Helping Children Cope with Separation and Loss*, London: BAAF.

Joseph, J. (1998) The equal environments assumption of the classical twin method – a critical analysis, *Journal of Mind and Behaviour*, 19, 325–58.

Main, M., Kaplan, N. and Cassidy, J. (1985) Security in infancy, childhood and adulthood, in I. Bretheron and E. Walters (Eds) *Growing Points of Attachment Theory and Research*, Monographs of the Society for Research in Child Development, 50 (209), 1–2.

Miyake, K., Chen, S. and Campos, J. (1985) Infant temperament and mother's mode of interaction and attachment in Japan: an interim report, in I. Bretherton and E. Waters (Eds), *Growing points of attachment theory and research*, Monographs of the Society for Research in Child Development, 50 (209), 276–97.

Newman, Tony and Blackburn, Sarah (2002) *Interchange 78: Transitions in the Lives of Children and Young People: Resilience Factors*, Scottish Executive Education Department/Barnardo's Policy, Research and Influencing Unit.

Parrot, L., Jacobs, G. and Roberts, D. (2008) Stress and Resilience Factors in parents with mental health problems and their children, *Briefing 23*, SCIE.

Rogoff, B. (2003) *The Cultural Nature of Human Development*. Oxford: Oxford University Press.

Rutter, M. (1981) *Maternal Deprivation Reassessed* (2nd edition), Harmondsworth: Penguin.

Rutter, M. (1995) Clinical implications of attachment concepts: Retrospect and prospect, *Journal of Child Psychology and Psychiatry and Allied Disciplines*, 36, 549–71.

Rutter, M. (1999) Resilience concepts and findings: implications for family therapy, *Journal of Family Therapy*, 21, 119–44.

Rutter, M. (2002) Nature, Nurture and Development: from Evangelism through Science towards policy and practice, *Child Development*, 73 (1), 1–21.

Rutter, M., Giller, H. and Hagell, A. (Eds) (1998) *Antisocial Behaviour by Young People*, Cambridge: Cambridge University Press.

Schore, A. N. (2001) The effects of a secure attachment relationship on right brain development, affect regulation, and infant mental health, *Infant Mental Health Journal*, 22, 7–66.

Shier, H. (2001) 'Pathways to Participation: openings, opportunities and obligations', *Children and Society*. 15, 107–17

Sroufe, L. A. (1997) Psychopathology as an outcome of development, *Development and Psychopathology*, 9 (2), 251–66.

Stoolmiller, M. (1999) Implications of the restricted range of family environments of heritability and nonshared environment in behaviour-genetic adoption studies, *Psychological Bulletin*, 125, 325–409.

Stringer, B. (2009) *Communicating Through Play*, London: BAAF.

Thompson, N. (2002) *Building the future – social work with children, young people and their families*. Lyme Regis: Russell House Publishing.

United Nations Convention on the Rights of the Child [online]. Available at: http://www.everychildmatters.gov.uk/uncrc/ (Accessed 13 May 2009).

Van Fleet, R. (2000) *A Parents' Handbook of Filial Play Therapy*, Boiling Springs, PA: Play Therapy Press.

Vygotsky, L. (1978) *Mind in Society*, Translated M.Cole, Harvard: Harvard University Press.

Werner, E.E. (1984) 'Resilient Children', *Young Children*, 1., 68–72.

Winnicott, D. W. (1984) *Delinquency and Deprivation*, London: Tavistock.

CHAPTER 22

USER INVOLVEMENT: USER LED APPROACHES IN ADULT CARE – WHO IS IN CHARGE?

MATTHEW GOUGH

OBJECTIVES

After reading this chapter you should be able to:

- Understand the drivers of service user involvement.

- Appreciate the different models of service user involvement.

- Understand personalization and tensions in service user involvement.

- Appreciate best practice in service user involvement.

After reading this chapter you will understand the key terms:
Consumerist, citizenship, empowerment, partnership, personalization, best practice.

There are two Moments of Reflection to work on throughout the chapter.

INTRODUCTION

The term 'service user' is not without its problems. However, in terms of maximizing respect, accuracy and having common currency it is an effective term currently available to describe people who have experience of disability and/or adult care services.

This chapter considers user involvement in adult care and finds at the heart of the discussion an issue of differing objectives and processes. There can be seen an emphasis on service effectiveness and quality of services (Fudge *et al.* 2008) as well as a political or philosophical commitment to user involvement as a means to increase power and control and promote empowering change for often marginalized people (Carr 2007; Harrison *et al*. 2002). With the different processes for user involvement, it can be seen that the two objectives inadvertently merge and synchronize, that is the processes used to improve the effectiveness of services, by involving service users, can create power transfers and challenges to institutional power bases (Carr 2007). Equally, this chapter finds that efforts to promote citizenship, that is a sharing of power, giving away control or involvement, can improve service outcomes.

The objectives and concepts become more blurred when the 'Personalization' agenda apparent within *Putting People First* (Department of Health 2007) and *Transforming Social Care* (Department of Health 2008a) is considered. Such an approach cedes significant market control to service users, with a devolving of power and budgets to consumers to promote control over services and support to live independent lives. In doing this, is the quest for political change in terms of the position of power for disabled people better served or does such a paradigm become less relevant?

This chapter focuses predominantly upon user involvement in an adult social care context. The debates that are generated by the personalization through personal individual budgets are yet to be realized in the National Health Service. However, with the advent of *High Quality Care for All* (Department of Health 2008b) and the proposals for direct payments for health care, many of this chapter's themes, which are currently specific to social care, will likely become even more relevant in health care settings.

PERSONALIZATION

With the advent and extension of direct payments and personalized budgets for all adults in social care, authentic power is arguably in the hands of people using services. Users are no longer grateful clients, but employers with the power to hire and fire personal assistants to meet their social care needs. If we take seriously the aims of *Putting People First* (Department of Health 2007), then service users have greater control over the assessment process, in terms of a greater degree of self assessment with an emphasis on outcomes based solutions to problems identified by the citizen. Direct payments passes direct responsibility to services users to manage their own support and become employers of personal assistants who may be involved in providing and support needs. Personalization and self directed support (or personalized budgets) are broader than direct payments, though direct payments may be the vehicle by which personalized budgets may be delivered. These initiatives are designed to give greater participation and direct involvement over the decisions governing a person's required services on an individual basis (Department of Health 2006a).

DEFINING PARTICIPATION

At animal farm, the hen and the pig were having a discussion. 'I have great difficulty,' said the pig, 'in fully understanding some of these language terms. For instance what is the difference between participation and being involved?' 'That's easy,' said the hen, 'you know the bacon and egg breakfast enjoyed by humans? Well, I participate and you are fully involved.'

(Anon.)

User involvement can mean different things in different contexts. It is quite legitimate to refer to user involvement whilst meaning the extent an individual is able to exert control and destiny of their own care. It is also acceptable to talk of user involvement at the collective level: that is, where people come together who have mutual interests and want to exert some control and influence over wider service provision. This may take the form of health or local authority partnership or implementation boards or committees.

It can be helpful to view user involvement as a continuum with regards to collective involvement or individual user involvement with varying levels of involvement and power. Arnstein (1969) conceptualized the idea of user/patient or citizen power as akin to rungs on a ladder (*see* Figure 22.1 below).

This ladder has been widely used and adapted to help us understand user involvement today. It can be simplified to five rungs and summarized differently to emphasize the more common stages which are apparent when discussing user involvement. Low level involvement can be *information sharing*, whereby service users are informed about decisions. A higher rung can be *consultation* which enables dialogue between service users and decision makers but does not fundamentally alter the location of power or decision making. *Partnership* and power sharing is the next stage whereby decisions are jointly made between service user and provider. *User decision making* is the penultimate stage with *user controlled services* as the top rung.

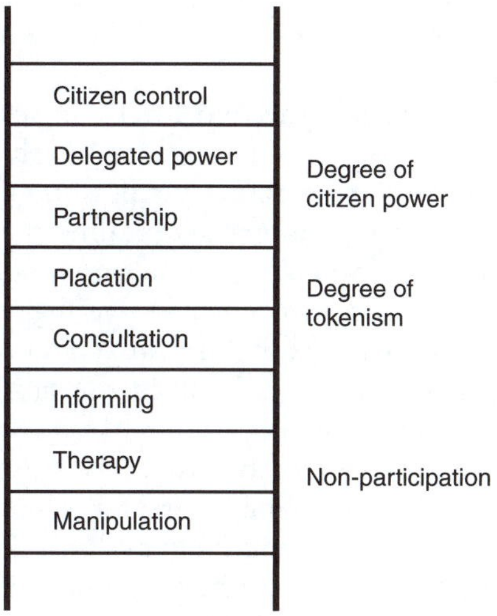

Citizen control	
Delegated power	Degree of
Partnership	citizen power
Placation	Degree of
Consultation	tokenism
Informing	
Therapy	Non-participation
Manipulation	

Figure 22.1 Arnstein's (1969) ladder of participation

MOMENT OF REFLECTION

Activity One

Think about when you may have been a patient or service user. How much control did you have over the experience? Where would you place your level of participation on Arnstein's ladder?

If we perceive user involvement as occupying any of the above rungs, we see that the nature and extent to which a service user has power and control will vary depending upon the processes position on the ladder. User involvement literature (Beresford and Croft 1993; Barnes and Walker 1997; Marsh and Fisher 1992) perceives that there are two different forces that impact upon involvement: the drivers of citizenship and consumerism.

Consumerism will tend to be characterized by being service centred, pursuing a managerialist agenda (Hambleton 1988). Traits within this model will likely include: the process is agency led, professionally dominated with the aim to improve the efficiency or effectiveness of services. Consumerist approaches would more likely sit comfortably at the lower rungs of the participation ladder.

Citizenship on the other hand has at its core a concern with the redistribution of power (Beresford and Croft 1993). The citizenship model of involvement seeks service users having control over their lives. The democratic power-sharing nature of citizenship will more likely be evident at the upper end of the ladder whereby control and power is with the service user.

An interesting metaphor to distinguish the two forces at play is shopping at a supermarket. Consumerism gives the shopper the choice of which beans are bought. Citizenship gives the shopper control of the running of the shop and whether beans are stocked at all. With supermarket shopping it is acceptable that the shopper does not manage the shop. However, having control over one's own personal care, which health and social care services directly affect, the stakes are higher. Personal health and social care services are by their nature personal, sensitive and often intimate. The things that matter most to people: our homes, our families, our health, our bodies, are at the heart of the health and social care industry.

Disappointment with care services for frustrating service user rights and aspirations is in part the rationale for users having a greater stake in those services (Wilson *et al.* 2008). 'Service users have been routinely and institutionally devalued, discriminated against, pauperized and denied their human and civil rights' (Beresford *et al.* 2007: 217). There is an obvious strong ethical argument for involving service users in the very services which they are affected by. Who better to influence, shape and control how services are planned and delivered than the person who is using them? User led/controlled services are vital to ensuring democratic sharing of citizen power. When services are led by service users they are more likely to be relevant and respectful to the people they are supporting as there is less distance between the people needing help and those running the service. There is much more likely to be a culture whereby equality and ownership is in evidence as the people have investment, meaningful stake and understanding. The culture of the environment is much less likely to be an 'us' and 'them' evident, insider and outsider, professional and (passive) client.

Hatton (2008) cites Foucault to help us understand the need for user involvement. We can understand the need for user led initiatives as a means for people's 'political imaginations' to be released (Hatton 2008: 76). Different alternative experiences are vitalized by users as active partners which envision the delivery of welfare and social care services. Services are bound to be more effective with the unique expertise afforded by the insight and contributions from people with lived experience (Beresford and Campbell 1994). Such inclusion fosters alternative models of how to view and work with people, challenging worker perceptions of users as passive stereotypes which in turn challenge practices and cultivate working differently with people (Beresford and Campbell 1994). If workers see users as equal citizens with political power and a voice, this is turn ought to promote better services as respect and more informed working practices follow.

One of the dangers with the argument that user involvement is most important for effective services is that it can become blurred with managerialist aspirations. Carr (2004) conceives that user involvement can merely become the 'technology of legitimation' (p. 18). That is, user involvement can be used to approve professional service planning rather than users being integral partners for the formulation of such service plans. This is more likely to be the case lower down the ladder of participation whereby the gains for citizenship are lesser, whereas consumerism may be fostered as political power exchanges are less fertile. Barnes and Walker (1997) argue that pursuing the consumerist agenda deflects attention away from the possibility of empowerment:

> the confusion between the models of consumerism and empowerment seriously inhibits progress towards empowering users because the limited goal of consumer consultation is sometimes mistaken for empowerment or regarded as sufficient expression of citizen participation.
>
> (Barnes and Walker 1997: 380)

Such rationale can perceive the establishment of user involvement as a counter-productive and reactionary step. Advocacy in Action *et al.* (2006) perceive that users being engaged in planning processes can cause them to be labelled and contained.

> 'Service-userism' is a classic creation of partnership to avoid power-sharing – the defensive response to challenging behaviours in those citizens previously stigmatized and oppressed within systems of health and social-welfare control.
>
> (Advocacy in Action *et al.* 2006: 336)

DRIVERS FOR USER INVOLVEMENT

There is both a grassroots and a top-down heritage to user involvement. Collective action, in terms of like minded people coming together, can be seen to have been organized in the 1970s and 1980s. Mental health system survivors as well disabled persons movements demanded respect and equality from a society that could be seen to be disablist with services that were stigmatizing and demeaning (Campbell 1996; Lindow 1995; Oliver 1996). The work of Beresford *et al.* (1993, 2005) and the Shaping Our

Lives (SOL) network has been influential in making clear the values and expectations regarding effective involvement. The national network of Centres for Independent Living has contributed much to facilitating user involvement (Department of Health 2009). Such work indicates the value and importance of user led initiatives in perpetuating greater user control and autonomy.

Braye (2000) identifies the two drivers for user involvement being principle and effectiveness. There is the moral/ethical rationale for user involvement, whereby services for the people ought to be shaped by the people. In addition to this, there is the business case: whereby services will be more efficient if responding directly to the needs of those citizens who will consume those services. Research by Nilsen *et al.* (2000, cited in Fudge *et al.* 2008), found that leaflets and patient information produced by service users was more readable, accessible, understandable and relevant than those materials designed without user input. Another way of classifying the drivers is as political or philosophical commitments to user involvement, in terms of the process being about power sharing and also quality of service provision: ensuring accountable, inclusive practice helps to ensure better informed and user relevant outputs.

User involvement literature (Beresford and Croft 1993; Barnes and Walker 1997; Carr 2007) place emphasis upon the emancipatory element of user involvement. This equates participation with engagement in the process of citizenship: people being seen and heard and challenging status quo approaches. Advocacy in Action *et al.* (2006) assert that the driving force of the user involvement agenda has to be understood as very much being owned by users, and the Government is responding to that rather than the response being the other way round:

> We know however that service-user involvement is not merely a response to guidance from above. Far from it! The voices of people fighting for justice have insisted on a hearing on their own terms for a very, very long time. Government legislation is a response to community grass-roots energy, passion, commitment and innovation.
> Advocacy in Action *et al.* (2006: 336)

So just what is that legislation and policy?

POLICY AND LEGISLATION

In the 1990s and 2000s, various pieces of policy and legislation have facilitated an expectation amongst service providers and commissioners that user involvement is an integral part of care. The NHS and Community Care Act 1990 requires local authorities to consult with people in receipt of services about such services. Indeed 'the first aim' of the community care legislation is to 'empower the consumers of community care' (Audit Commission 1992). This duty is further consolidated with the first direct payments legislation (Community Care (Direct Payments) Act 1996), practice guidance explicitly expecting local authorities to consult when planning services. Direct payments themselves are intended to give users more control as consumers of their direct personal care. Later policy and legislative drivers such as Valuing People (Department of Health 2001), the Health and Social Care Act (2001) and White Paper: Our health, our care, our say (Department of Health 2006a) all have at their heart an emphasis on user empowerment with requirements on health and local authorities to involve and consult people directly affected by service planning.

The growth of user involvement in the training of health and social care professionals is expected as mandatory as enabled by, for example, General Social Care Council requirements that for social work courses to be accredited, they must have involvement in both the planning and governance of programmes as well as the teaching (GSCC 2005).

EMPOWERMENT

Much emphasis is placed upon the individual benefits for service users being involved (Carr 2004). Personal and therapeutic benefits that may be cited to justify involvement emphasize the intrinsic and sometimes therapeutic benefits (Harding 2005). Being gainfully 'employed', or being able to use one's experiences to be heard can be powerfully healthy as Harding (2005) evidences:

> First, there is overwhelming evidence that working in any capacity can help you to maintain your mental health, and that unemployment is decidedly unhealthy, both physically and psychologically. I feel NHS user employment is particularly important as it enables people to consolidate and make use of what is to the rest of society misconstrued as a dirty secret or even a menace. For the individual themselves, the experience of distress is often a series of life-changing events; being able to make use of the revelations these bring is a natural panacea.
>
> (Hardy 2005: 269)

Carr argues that it is not just the intrinsic value for the individual of involvement processes, rather the changes which are achieved, that are key (Carr 2004). User involvement can be seen not just as an end, but rather as a means to an end. The process of user involvement itself may be empowering, but the ultimate goal of service users having control over services is more to do with improving people's lives by people determining their own destinies; that is more likely to happen if service users are shaping the factors (vital services) which shape that destiny. 'Participation is not simply an end in itself but a means to change' (Danso et al. 2002, cited in Warren 2007: 26). Such changes and improved outcomes are the purposes of involvement (Warren 2007). Exercising user involvement results not just in change for the individual service user and collective service users, but rather organizations, and institutions embedding a culture of user involvement, themselves experience significant change (Shaping Our Lives 2007). As user involvement is itself a cultural change for organizations, sharing power with people not traditionally holding power within services, then that in itself drives forward and perpetuates change (Shaping Our Lives 2007).

By service users either being involved in the planning of services or managing a service, they can be seen to change organizational culture on different levels. Beresford and Campbell (1994) argue that users provide unique expertise, in which, by them being in a visible influential position, traditional working practices are challenged. Perceptions are changed and new working models must be embraced as perceptions of users as passive stereotypes are challenged, thus providers have to work differently (Beresford and Campbell 1994). However, much of organizational prioritizing of user involvement over the last couple of decades can be seen to satisfy a consumerist agenda: ensuring that the care market efficiently serves its consumers rather than a real interest in citizenship power shifts.

The interesting paradigm we currently entertain is that the advance of direct payments, personalization, personalized budgets and its accompanying policy emphasis (Department of Health 2005, 2006a, 2007, 2008a, 2009), and the Government's efforts to tackle social exclusion through 'day service modernization' (Social Exclusion Unit 2004) and focus on 'job brokerage' and 'welfare to work' measures (Layard 2004) have emphasized the importance of these measures to promote active citizenship. As people are seen and heard more and have more power and control there is an impact upon the wider society beyond the social care market place. Thereby individual consumerist concern can perpetuate active citizenship and empowerment.

Carr (2007) argues that, from her review of service user involvement, a paradox has been created by the independence, well-being and consumerist choice agenda. By maximizing direct payments and personalized budgets an 'unparalleled degree of control over social care budgets' for service users is being created (Carr 2007: 268). Such control invariably leads to a change in culture whereby users inevitably have become more involved in training and organizational governance. However, Carr (2007) finds that the difficulties that mainstream organizations have in reconciling their duties and meaningfully sharing power with users creates tension. The tension itself forces change. The very fact that policy and legislation requirements are changing to foster consumerist requirements means that the decision making cultures within organizations find the requirements challenging. Such structures and cultures need to change to accommodate the tension, which in itself leads to changes in power. The paradox of being led by policy and legislation primarily concerned with individualistic consumerist changes in the market has therefore required collective voices to be incorporated. However, it is in the process of this incorporation that the tensions of organizational political culture clashing with the collectivist voice of user involvement and the meaningful democratization of power can be seen. Because effective user involvement is difficult and yet still has to happen, it exposes problems at the political, structural and economic levels thereby unsettling tradition bases of power (Carr 2007). Political and cultural change may arguably be apparent in the organizations which are trying to involve service users but does this have a wider impact?

Beresford *et al.* (2007) argue that governmental drivers such as 'Our Health, our care, our say' (Department of Health 2006a) have created an expectation that user involvement and user led approaches should be mainstream and that a culture has developed where user controlled research, training and service have facilitated change both at the individual and collective level. User defined outcomes and self assessment in planning adult social care services are becoming integrated into routine social care practices (Beresford *et al.* 2007).

So what are the factors which enable user involvement to be effective in terms of citizenship and what are the barriers which need to be overcome?

TENSIONS

From transnational research across Europe, Heikkila Julkumen (2003, cited in Hatton 2008: 88) identifies five key areas which can inhibit or foster effective user involvement: political/legal, administrative, professional, language and personal. The importance of political will has been discussed above and it can be seen that with political and legal expectation, a culture is fostered which creates expectation whereby user involvement can occur. There are administrative legal matters that impact on the personal which are looked at later. Perhaps impinging on several of these areas is the attitude of the professional. Much literature emphasizes the importance of work support for involvement process to be effective (Myers and MacDonald 1996; Marsh and Fisher 1992; Ross 1995 and Stevenson and Parsloe 1993).

STAFF ATTITUDES

Fudge *et al.*'s (2008) research into user involvement in health settings emphasizes that professionals really control the agenda of user involvement with organizations and how user involvement can be interpreted. This can be about the relative value placed upon professional judgement over user perspectives (Marsh and Fisher 1992). However, it can also be about fear, where staff can feel their role or status and influence under threat from sharing power with service users (Ross 1995). Giving up control and sharing power is somewhat fundamental to user involvement and of course that can be uncomfortable for some workers as Ross's research uncovers:

> For many staff, the idea of power sharing is terrifying because it means they are no longer in total control, that their authority might be questioned and their practices scrutinized.
>
> (Ross 1995: 794)

Ross's (1995) research found that there was a direct relationship between staff commitment to user involvement and their own feeling of being valued and included by management in decision making processes. The findings of Stevenson and Parsloe (1993) support this research: staff's confidence in user involvement hinges on how involved staff are, 'staff are more likely to empower users if they feel empowered themselves' (p. 25). If power is shared with professionals within organizations then it is more likely that power sharing with the user will be enabled.

PROFESSIONAL AGENDA

The issue of workers' support for user involvement is not without its issues. The quality of involvement can be affected by the nature of professional engagement and in particular if it is led by professionals or facilitated by them. There is a significant difference. Fudge *et al.* (2008) found that in their research, user involvement was less sustainable; less understood by users and lacked depth when initiatives were led by professionals rather than user activists. Even worse than ineffective or weak user involvement is the issue of exploitative involvement. This can be in the form of tokenistic engagement to 'tick all the boxes', similar to Carr's (2004) 'technology of legitimation', or to gain professional kudos or reward at the expense of respecting the voice of user contribution. Professionalizing the relationship between worker and user can be viewed, as discussed between user led organizations and staff, as 'the colonization of the life experience and value systems of citizens into expert territory' (Cairney *et al.* 2006: 315). Advocacy in Action *et al.* (2006: 336) view such types of partnership as 'one sided' and jeopardizing citizenship, 'this one-sided partnership sucks up all the energy and activism out of civil protest, feeds on what it can ingest, compromise, dilute or distort, and spits out the gristle.'

CAN USERS BE WORKERS AND WORKERS USERS?

In considering the issue of workers and service users, the discussion can become a little removed from the reality of workers and users not being clearly demarcated groups. The divide between paid workers and service user workers is artificial. Can workers be users? When does a user cease to be a user and become a professional? Does a worker-user need to be open about their use of services to be a user? Many people working in social care and health have direct personal experience of disability, exclusion, mental health problems or being a carer. It can seem odd when organizations have to demonstrate effective user involvement when workers themselves employed in such projects may have user experiences. Paradoxically, 'service userism' can contribute to the cultivation of a division that is at odds with the, albeit unacknowledged, reality.

SERVICE USER VOICE VERSUS PROFESSIONAL RESPONSIBILITY

It is also important in elevating the voice of service users, that the voice of professionals must not be denigrated. In many circumstances, professionals will still have the power and will have to over-rule service user expectations. In working directly with people, workers have to 'balance what service users say about their experiences with information and levels of understanding derived from sources outside of knowledge that lie outside of their direct experience', (Wilson *et al.*, 2008: 416). Wilson *et al.* (2008) emphasizes the need to not override other considerations of the worker role, beyond being directed by service user expressions. Whilst, obviously true, perhaps because the user voice and position have been so 'devalued, discriminated against, and pauperized' (Beresford *et al.* 2007: 217) the developing political will of user involvement is not in a position whereby the power it yields puts it into equal position for a balance to naturally prevail. To emphasize the importance of user involvement is to get it beyond the passive and patronized position (Beresford *et al.* 2007) which tends to be apparent in the worker and user relationship in adult social care.

THE EMPLOYMENT–BENEFITS ISSUE

Within the traditional welfarist approach to adult care is the expectation of people with long-term health problems to be dependent on state benefits. Recent government backed initiatives such as 'Welfare to Work', 'Tackling Social Exclusion' and the Layard Report (Layard 2004) have sought to challenge this expectation. Within this thinking is an increasing of expectations for disabled people to be supported into work. User involvement in participative processes is promoted in some of these quarters for many of the reasons outlined above and possibly as a means to entering the employment market. However, in terms of the key barriers to effective user involvement (Heikkila Julkumen 2003, cited in Hatton 2008: 88), the legal administrative obstacles make lawful meaningful user involvement very problematic. The Government's policy guidance, *Reward and Recognition* (Department of Health 2006b) written in conjunction with 'Shaping Our Lives' very clearly raises the expectation of the need to remunerate and honour user time with payment if required. However, trying to reconcile this with the other legal requirements that it makes clear must be complied with, such as minimum wage (employment law) with disability benefit permitted work rules and income support maximum payments (Department of Work and Pensions), excludes the very people who need to be involved from maximizing their participation. The guidance recommends organizations and users negotiate with their local Job Centre Plus to ensure transparency in their operation. The Social Care Institute for Excellence (SCIE) (Turner and Beresford 2005) and the Commission for Social Care Inspection's (CSCI 2007) reports both recommend that significant changes need to be made to benefits rules for the requirements for service user involvement in public agencies to be realized.

PEOPLE ARE UNREPRESENTATIVE

When we think of users involved in public agencies, a common criticism is that the people are only representative of themselves or not typical service users (Ross 1995). Users can be seen to be in a no-win situation. If users are confident and articulate enough to be listened to, then they run the risk of being perceived as not 'real' users and thus unrepresentative (Bewley and Glendinning 1994). Often, users may be the only – however limited the process – elected individual present, and yet other people in the room do not have their legitimacy questioned (Beresford and Harding 1993). Beresford and Croft (1993) assert such questioning of users' representative function can be used to undermine what the person is saying and this can be effective at undermining user confidence.

Hopton (1997) is critical of practiced user involvement for leaving out the majority of 'apolitical' service users, 'service users are not a homogenous group. We must develop ways of consulting all service users, not simply organized groups' (p. 45). However, thinking about user involvement as being primarily about representation may be a red herring. It may be more helpful to redefine user involvement in participative processes as being about accountability. It is important to hold service providers to account by the people receiving those services (Ross 1995; Beresford et al. 2007). By opening up this process the traditional power structures have to accommodate challenge and democratic change (Carr 2007).

Bramwell and Williams (1993) argue that it is the responsibility of service providers to involve a plurality of service user perspectives. By having one perspective there is a risk of disempowering other constituents under one view (Bramwell and Williams 1993). Warren (2007) identifies that whilst barriers exist to promote effective user participation generally, there are many particularly marginalized service user groups which lead to under-representation of several groups: homeless people; travellers; institutional or residential care residents; people affected by poverty; people who have needs across service categories, for example young black disabled people; people with severe disabilities; children and young people; people from certain geographical/rural areas; people from minority ethnic communities; gay and lesbian people; and people with dementia (Warren 2007: 20). Added to this could be people with mental health problems and people seeking asylum. Such groups may be referred to as 'difficult to reach', though reasons can be varied, from stigma and discrimination to ill health and poor levels of resource commitment denying access. So when considering issues of user involvement it is vital to remember that we are not talking of a homogenous group and that despite user involvement facing barriers, some individuals from parts of society may have no voice in participative processes because of multiple socially excluding obstacles.

RESOURCES

Users who give their time ought to be valued for their time (Department of Health 2006b, Turner and Beresford 2005; CSCI 2007), which can take the form of remuneration. Supporting this process itself can mean taking resources, dedicated time and money to ensure accessibility, and thinking creatively about how to run meetings and events. Taxi fares, interpreters, policies, staffing and system management are all basic requirements to making user involvement work for health and social care organizations. Some of these costs are only the same as what it may be to employ a diverse work force which does not discriminate in terms of disability, sexuality or maternity, for example. Such a diverse workforce is protected by employment and disability discrimination legislation. The benefits of having a diverse workforce can be seen as similar to wanting to promote user participation in services. Despite the cost, the benefits and statutory expectations can be understood and complied with as the requirements of a healthy, inclusive, effective and safe working environment.

USER LED ORGANIZATIONS

Returning to Arnstein's ladder (1969), we are reminded that ultimate citizenship power flourishes where people have control over services. Personalized budgets offer care management responsibilities to users to individually manage their own services. User involvement initiatives are aimed at ensuring greater service effectiveness. User led organizations offer a collectivist approach that goes beyond being able to exercise market restricted choices of support to actually directly determining the nature and character of support by running the service. Technically speaking, an organization that is managed by or staffed by people with direct experience of disability or using care services may be considered a user led organization (Department of Health 2009). There any many examples throughout the country of user led training and development organizations that may run collective user involvement forums or training courses. What is less well understood are the numbers of effective user led services that provide valuable support to other service users. Advocacy projects, drop-in centres, arts projects, crisis houses, horticulture projects and rights based information services all exist as services directly controlled by service users.

Such services have been around for a long time. What differentiates them from self-help support groups? The latter may be concerned with alleviating the 'problem' addiction, condition, whereas user led groups will tend to have more of an emphasis on civil rights, empowerment and control. They may be involved in the political process, campaigning for equality and civil rights. Such organizations may do this outwardly as a collective or have an ethos of working internally with peers on an individual basis, perhaps promoting advocacy and self-empowerment for the person.

Service user led organizations challenge the status quo both on the political level, but also in terms of typical attitudes towards what constitutes a service provider and what constitutes a service user. If provider and user become blurred it can threaten the status of both. The professional power base and comfort zone of workers can be threatened when the people whom you have power over and 'do to' become peers and colleagues.

The Government and stakeholder document, *Putting People First: Working together with user led organizations* (Department of Health 2009) clearly supports the expansion of user led organizations to all local authority areas. It is known that where user led organizations such as the Centre for Integrated Living are strong, that the take up of direct payments is much higher (Department of Health 2009). With the Government commitment to the increase of personalization and direct payments being a 'key' component of this (Department of Health 2006a, 2007, 2009), it makes sense that user led organizations grow. It is considered a sign of a healthy inclusive community when user led organizations are supported by their local authorities to thrive (Department of Health 2009).

CONCLUSION

In terms of citizenship and empowerment, collective control may be less apparent vis-à-vis the personalization agenda. Individually, in terms of a consumerist approach, the power of the individual service user is maximized, is it not? Because of market forces, the user is paying the piper and can name the tune? However, the consumerist notion of empowerment relies on the concept that there has to be a power of exit for power to be realized (Beresford and Croft 1993). The power to access and relinquish services (whether directly commissioned or indeed commissioned by a local authority power) is in the hands of workers and management deciding upon eligibility for services. Users can be seen as 'captive consumers' (Marsh and Fisher 1992) whereby their need for services inhibits their true power of exit and that this is gatekeeping via local authority assessment. With the Government's expectation for local authorities to facilitate self assessment and outcome based assessment, there is arguably greater scope for user influence over eligibility decision making. At the very least, the process should allow for more informed assessment decision making.

Ultimately, the decision whether someone is entitled to the payment to purchase their own care is made by the authority who administers the public purse and not the individual service user. Whilst this power relationship remains, there remains a dependency. Whilst a dependency remains, autonomy is fundamentally restricted. The personalization approach may therefore be successful in improving service outcomes for individual users. In terms of empowering service users collectively and of democratizing control, the processes involved may incorporate power sharing, however, power to enter and exit the care system in the first instance relies fundamentally upon external professional judgement. User led organizations offer collective and diverse ways to challenge the framework by which care markets tend to operate and are alternatives to such a framework. Whether such organizations will take a substantial role as providers of services remains to be seen.

MOMENT OF REFLECTION

Activity Two

List *three* different characteristics of self directed support and personalized budgets under each heading which act as a) drivers for a managerialist consumerist agenda and b) drivers for a citizenship empowerment agenda.

Competing agendas within the 'personalization' adult care services

a Managerial/consumerist drivers	b Citizenship empowerment drivers
1	
2	
3	

SUMMARY OF MAIN POINTS

You should be able to:

- Understand the drivers of service user involvement.
- Appreciate the different models of service user involvement.
- Understand personalization and tensions in service user involvement.
- Appreciate best practice in service user involvement.

REFERENCES

Advocacy in Action, Nottingham Staff and Students from the University of Nottingham (2006) Making It Our Own Ball Game: Learning and Assessment in Social Work Education, *Social Work Education*, 25 (4), 332–46.

Arnstein, S. (1969) A Ladder of Citizen Participation, *Journal of the American Institute of Planners*, 35 (4), 216–24.

Audit Commission (1992) *Community Care: Managing the Cascade of Change*, London: HMSO.

Barnes, M. and Walker, A. (1997) Consumerism versus empowerment. A principled approach to the involvement of older service users, *Policy and Politics*, 24 (4), 375–93.

Beresford, P. (2007) User involvement, research and health inequalities: developing new directions, *Health Society Care Community*, 15, 306–12.

Beresford, P. and Campbell, J. (1994) Disabled People, Service Users, User Involvement and Representation, *Disability and Society*, 9 (3), 315–25.

Beresford, P. and Croft, S. (1993) *Citizen Involvement: A practical guide for change*, Basingstoke: Macmillan.

Beresford, P. and Harding, T. (1993) *A challenge to change: A practical guide for change*, Hampshire: Macmillan.

Beresford, P., Shamash, M., Forrest, V., Turner, M. and Branfield, F. (2005) *Developing social care: service users' vision for adult support*, Report 7, London: SCIE [online]. Available at: http://www.scie.org.uk/publications/reports/report07.asp (Accessed 20 May 2009).

Beresford, P., Branfield, F., Lalani, M., Maslen, B., Sartori, A., Jenny, Maggie and Manny (2007) Partnership working: service users and social work learning and working together, in M. Lymbery and K. Postle (Eds) *Social Work: A Companion for Learning*, London: Sage.

Bewley, C. and Glendinning, C. (1994) *Involving disabled people in community care planning*, York: Joseph Rowntree Foundation.

Bramwell, L. and Williams, K. (1993) How much do you value our experiences?, *Open Mind*, 62, April/May.

Braye, S. (2000) Participation and involvement in social care. An overview, in Kemshall, H. and Littlechild, R. (Eds) (2000) *User Involvement and Participation in Social Care: Research Informing Practice,* London: Jessica Kingsley Publishing.

Cairney, J., Chettle, K., Clark, M., Davis, A., Gosling, J., Harvey, R., Jephcote, S., Labana, L., Lymbery, M., Pendred, B. and Russell, L. (2006) Editorial, *Social Work Education*, 25 (4), 315–18.

Campbell, P. (1996) The history of the user movement in the United Kingdom, in Heller, T., Reynolds, J., Gomm, R., Muston, R. and Pattison, S. (Eds) *Mental health matters: a reader*, Basingtoke: Macmillan Press.

Carr, S. (2004) *Has Service User Participation Made a Difference to Social Care Services?*, SCIE Position Paper 3, London: SCIE/Policy Press.

Carr, S. (2007) Participation, power, conflict and change: Theorizing dynamics of service user participation in the social care system of England and Wales, *Critical Social Policy*, 27 (2), 91 [online]. Available at: http://csp.sagepub.com (Accessed 29 July 2008).

Commission for Social Care Inspection (CSCI) (2007) *Benefit Barriers to Involvement: Finding Solutions*, London: CSCI.

Department of Health (2001) *Valuing People*, London: HMSO.

Department of Health (2005) *Independence, Well-being and Choice: Our Vision for the Future of Social Care for Adults in England*, London: HMSO.

Department of Health (2006a) *Our health, our care, our say: a new direction for community services*, London: HMSO.

Department of Health (2006b) *Reward and Recognition: The principles and practice of service user payment and reimbursement in health and social care*, London: HMSO.

Department of Health (2007) *Putting people first: a shared vision and commitment to the transformation of adult social care*, London: HMSO.

Department of Health (2008a) *Transforming Adult Social Care*, LAC (DH)(2008)1, London: HMSO.

Department of Health (2008b) *High Quality Care for All*, London: HMSO.

Department of Health (2009) *Putting People First: Working together with user-led organizations*, London: HMSO.

Fudge, N., Wolfe, C. and McKevitt, C. (2008) *Assessing the promise of user involvement in health service development: ethnographic study* [online]. Available at: http://www.bmj.com (Accessed 6 April 2009).

GSCC (2005) *Working towards full participation* [online]. Available at: http://www.gscc.org. uk/publications (Accessed 20 May 2009).

Hambleton, R. (1988) Consumerism, decentralization and local democracy, *Public Administration*, 66 (Summer 1988), 125–47.

Harding, E. (2005) Partners in care: Service user employment in the NHS: a user's perspective, *Psychiatric Bulletin*, 29, 268–9.

Harding, T. and Beresford, P. (1996) *The Standards We Expect*, London: National Institute for Social Work.

Harrison, S., Dowswell, G., Milewa, T. (2002) Guest editorial: public and user 'involvement' in the UK National Health Service, *Health and Social Care in the Community*, 10, 63–6.

Hatton, K. (2008) *New Directions in Social Work Practice (Transforming Social Work Practice)*, Exeter: Learning Matters.

Hopton, J. (1997) Who are we listening to?, *Nursing Times*, 8 October, 93 (41).

Layard, R. (2004) *Mental Health: Britain's Biggest Social Problem?*, London: Cabinet Office [online]. Available at http://www.cabinetoffice.gov.uk/media/cabinetoffice/strategy/assets/mh_layard.pdf (Accessed 20 May 2009).

Lindow, V. (1995) Power and Rights: the psychiatric system survivor movement, in Jack, R. (Ed.) *Empowerment in Community Care*, London: Chapman and Hall.

Marsh, P. and Fisher, M. (1992) *Good Intentions: Developing Partnerships in Social Services*, York: Joseph Rowntree Trust.

Myers, F. and MacDonald, C. (1996) Power to the people? Involving service users and carers in needs assessments and care planning – views from the practitioner', *Health and Social Care in the Community*, 4 (2), 86–95.

Oliver, M. (1996) *Understanding disability: from theory to practice*, Basingstoke: Macmillan.

Ross, K. (1995) Speaking in tongues: involving users in day care services, *British Journal of Social Work*, 25, 791–804.

Shaping Our Lives (SOL) (2007) *Developing social care: service users driving culture change*, London: SCIE.

Social Exclusion Unit (2004) *Mental Health and Social Exclusion*, London: Office of the Deputy Prime Minister.

Stevenson, 0. and Parsloe, P. (1993) *Community Care and Empowerment*, York: Joseph Rowntree Foundation.

Turner, M. and Beresford, P. (2005) *Contributing on equal terms: Service user involvement and the benefits system*, London: SCIE.

Warren, J. (2007) *Service User and Carer Participation in Social Work (Transforming Social Work Practice)*, Exeter: Learning Matters.

Wilson, K., Ruch, Lymbery, M. and Cooper, P. (2008) *Social Work: An Introduction to Contemporary Practice*, Essex: Pearson Longman.

USEFUL WEBSITES

Shaping Our Lives – is an independent user-controlled organization, think-tank and network working with a wide and diverse range of service users.
www.shapingourlives.org.uk

National Centre for Independent Living (NCIL) – is a national support, advice and consultancy organization that aims to enable disabled people to be equal citizens with choice, control, rights and full economic, social and cultural lives.
www.ncil.org.uk

Disabled Parents Network (DPN) – is a national organization of, and for, disabled people who are parents or who hope to become parents, and their families, friends and supporters.
http://www.disabledparentsnetwork.org.uk/cgi-bin/site/site.cgi

National Self Harm Network – UK focused survivor-led organization, committed campaigners for the rights and understanding of people who self-harm.
http://www.nshn.co.uk/

People First – is an organization run by, and for, people with learning difficulties to raise awareness of and campaign for the rights of people with learning difficulties and to support self advocacy groups across the country.
http://www.peoplefirstltd.com/index.php

UK Coalition of People Living with HIV and AIDS – an organization committed to 'enabling the diverse voices of people living with HIV and AIDS to be heard with a view to influencing change'.
http://www.ukcoalition.org/

CHAPTER 23

YOUNG PEOPLE AND YOUTH JUSTICE

ROGER HOPKINS-BURKE

OBJECTIVES

After reading this chapter you should be able to:

- Critically examine the historical development and construction of notions of young people and crime.

- Critically examine the historical development of the juvenile justice system in Great Britain.

- Critically examine the nature of the contemporary juvenile justice system in Great Britain.

After reading this chapter you will understand the key terms:
Justice/punishment, welfare/treatment, excluded tutelage, reintegrated tutelage.

There is a Moment of Reflection at the end of the chapter.

INTRODUCTION

This chapter is about the offending behaviour of young people and the way in which the authorities have responded to their activities.[1] Critical criminological orthodoxy that informs much undergraduate teaching in this area correctly recognises that many young people have a difficult transition from childhood to adulthood, which involves some offending behaviour, and proposes that left alone – or provided with some health and social care support – they will invariably grow out of it. Intervention by the criminal justice system and criminalisation will invariably make the problem worse (*see* for example Muncie 2004). This chapter is sympathetic to that agenda but, at the same time, recognises that the persistent offending of a small minority of three to four per cent of young people is a real and significant problem both for their victims and the perpetrators themselves who, without some form of criminal justice system intervention that challenges their problematic behaviour, face a life of social exclusion, serious offending and lengthy periods of adult incarceration. It thus departs from the orthodox academic critical criminological account and adopts a left realist perspective (*see* Hopkins-Burke 2008, 2009) that recognises the need to deal with the problematic actions of young offenders *and* the conditions which encourage those behaviours, and can be clearly identified as providing the theoretical foundations for the contemporary youth justice system.

This chapter is divided into two parts: the first considers the problem of 'delinquent' young people and attempts to control and discipline this significant section of the population in an historical and theoretical context; the second considers the development of a specific juvenile/youth justice system charged with an invariably criminal justice intervention in the lives of young people who have transgressed.

YOUNG PEOPLE, DISCIPLINE, CONTROL

It is important to consider the issue of delinquent young people in an historical context because the way we view childhood and the misdemeanours of the young today is very much a product of the modern world. In the pre-modern era childhood had not been a distinct period of development in the way that it is now (Aries 1962; Hoyles and Evans 1989), with our contemporary conception having its origins in the emergence of a recognisable middle class in the sixteenth century and its escalating demand for a formalised education for its sons. This is an important recognition because it was to be these developing bourgeois attitudes to childhood over the following four centuries that were to provide the dominant template of acceptable – and increasingly enforceable – child socialisation.

Childhood came increasingly to be viewed as a time of innocence and dependence, with protection, training and appropriate socialisation paramount. Youth, in contrast, came to be seen as an age of deviance, disruption and wickedness (Brown 1998), and this perception was strongly linked to the discovery of the pseudo-scientific concept of adolescence during the Victorian era and which from that time onwards came to be identified as a significant cause of delinquency (Aries 1962; Gillis 1974; Hendricks 1990a, 1990b; Jenks 1996; Brown 1998; Hopkins-Burke 2008).

The term 'adolescence' itself was constructed by the professional middle classes in accordance with the work of the influential early US psychologist G. Stanley Hall (1906), who described this stage of development in biologically determinist terms as one of 'storm and stress', and in which instability and fluctuation were normal and to be expected. His notion of 'normal adolescent demeanour' was ominously based on the 'unspontaneous, conformist and confident' white middle class youths with whom he came into contact and this model was again soon prescribed as the desirable model for young people of all social classes (Griffin 1997). Significantly, the marginalisation of whole cross-sections of young people – especially, the working class, girls and ethnic minority groups – became implicit from that time on with the social construction of a notion of adolescence acceptable to middle-class sensibilities. Although theories of 'delinquency' were to broaden their approach during the twentieth century (*see* Hopkins-Burke 2008), the ways in which adolescence is perceived continues to be heavily influenced by the 'storm and stress' model (Newburn 2002).

An historical perspective on youth justice is thus essential in helping to understand contemporary perceptions of young offending. Throughout history we can find references to the escalating problems of youth crime (West 1967; Pearson 1983) and the debates, discourses and political solutions in the past are remarkably similar to those of today. Fears about rising youth crime are constantly repeated, with the present continuously compared unfavourably with the peaceful days of a halcyon non existent golden age (Humphries 1981; Pearson 1983).

The emphasis on appropriate parenting in the contemporary youth justice system is again nothing new and the notion that 'the family' is in 'crisis', and/or that parents are 'failing', comprises a 'cyclical phenomenon with a very long history' (Day-Sclater and Piper 2000: 135), while the 'parenting theme' (Gelsthorpe 1999) has enjoyed, and continues to enjoy, a certain prominence within debates surrounding young people and crime.

Contemporary notions of childhood and adolescence were therefore socially constructed at the outset of industrial modernity, and children and their families were subsequently disciplined and controlled not least in the interests of an industrial capitalism which required a fit, healthy, increasingly educated, trained and obedient workforce. Reality was nevertheless more complex than such neo-Marxist explanations, while the orthodox social progress perspective, which proposes these disciplinary strategies to be the actions of motivated entrepreneurial philanthropists with genuine concerns about poor urban children and young people, is also too simplistic. Many of these philanthropists – or 'moral entrepreneurs' (Becker 1963) – clearly had little idea of the actual or potential long-term consequences of their actions while, at the same time, there is an identifiable failure to recognise the complexities of power and the outcomes of strategies promoted by agencies that often enjoy autonomy from the political centre and front-line practitioners who often enjoy considerable discretion.

It is the carceral surveillance society thesis – devised by Michel Foucault (1980) and developed by Jacques Donzelot (1980), Stanley Cohen (1985) and David Garland (2001) – where strategies of power are seen to be pervasive throughout society, with the state only one of the points of control and resistance (Foucault 1971, 1976), that enables us to make sense of the situation. It is thus observed that there are numerous 'semi-autonomous' realms and relations – such as communities, occupations, organisations, families – in civil society where surveillance and control are present but where the state administration is technically absent and, moreover, these arenas are often negotiated and resisted by their participants in ways over which even now, the state has little jurisdiction.

Hopkins-Burke (2004a, 2004c, 2008) has developed a variation on the carceral surveillance society thesis which acknowledges the orthodox premise that disciplinary strategies are invariably implemented by moral entrepreneurs, professional agents and practitioners who have little idea how their often humble discourse contributes to the grand overall disciplinary control matrix, but, at the same time, proposes that there are other, further, interests involved and these are significantly *ours* and in this context those of *our* predecessors. The bourgeois child tutelage project of the nineteenth and early twentieth centuries can be clearly viewed in that context (Hopkins-Burke 2008).

This hybrid or left realist perspective accepts that all accounts – neo-Marxist or social progress – are to some extent legitimate for there were and *are* a multitude of motivations for both implementing and accepting the increasing surveillance and tutelage of young people. The moralising mission of the entrepreneurial philanthropists and the reforming zeal of the liberal politician and administrator thus corresponded conveniently with those of the mill and mine-owners and a government which wanted a fit healthy fighting force, but it also coincides with the ever increasing enthusiasm for self-betterment among the great majority of the working class that has been described from differing sociological perspectives as 'embourgeoisement' (Goldthorpe 1968–9) and 'the civilising process' (Elias 1978, 1982). Those who were resistant to that moralising and disciplinary mission – the 'rough working' class of the Victorian era – have subsequently been reinvented in academic and popular discourse as the socially excluded underclass of contemporary society, with the moral panics of today a reflection of those of the past, and demands for action remarkably similar. These observations should be considered in the context of the following brief history of the development of the juvenile – and latterly, youth justice system – in England and Wales.

THE DEVELOPMENT OF JUVENILE JUSTICE IN ENGLAND AND WALES

The story of the development of the juvenile justice system is – for the first three-quarters of the twentieth century – one of a transition from a predominantly justice/punishment to a welfare/treatment model response, and is told in the context of repeated concerns and panics from widespread groups in society about the extent of offending by young people, and demands that something should be done.

Before the nineteenth century there was no special provision for young offenders, who were dealt with in terms of a criminal justice intervention that was no different from that applied to adults. They were nevertheless gradually singled out as a distinctive category in relation to both criminal behaviour and legal control, with the nature of the response initially located predominantly in the context of the contemporary justice/punishment model orthodoxy.

The beginnings of a welfare/treatment model approach that prioritised health and social care intervention in the lives of problematic young people was nevertheless emerging. Voluntary reformatories were opened by the Philanthropic Society in the early part of the nineteenth century but the Youth Offenders Act 1854 introduced state recognised Reformatories and Certified Industrial Schools which came to replace prison terms for many young offenders and provide a basic education plus a trade. The Industrial Schools Act 1857 introduced better provision for the care and education of vagrant, destitute and disorderly children perceived to be in danger of becoming criminals (Newburn 1995), while the Education Act 1870 led to the establishment of industrial day schools and truant schools (Hopkins-Burke 2008).

Table 23.1 The justice/punishment model of youth justice

- Based on the rational actor model of criminal behaviour notions that young people have free will and choose to offend.
- Offenders should be held responsible for their actions and punished if they transgress.
- The level of punishment inflicted should be commensurate with the seriousness of the offence committed.
- Offenders should be punished for the offence committed and not on the basis of whom they are or the social conditions in which they live.

Source: Hopkins-Burke (2008: 49)

There were widespread motivations for change and in particular there was pressure from politically powerful religious, philanthropic and penal reform groups apprehensive about the brutality of conditions in adult prisons and their impact on young offenders, but by the end of the century these concerns had spread to the general public, not least because of media campaigns encouraged by perceptible widespread social disorganisation, drunkenness, and anxieties about declining standards of parenting and family socialisation (Davis 1990; Humphries 1981; Pearson 1983).

The Summary Jurisdiction Act 1879 reduced both the number of children in prison – who were now to be tried by magistrates – and the penalties available. The Gladstone and Lushington Committees subsequently introduced alternatives to custody and the Children Act 1908 established specialised juvenile courts which were given powers to deal with both the delinquent and destitute. These were to involve a mixture of welfare and punitive strategies but nevertheless remained essentially criminal courts and the idea that the child was a wrongdoer was to continue to be the dominant orthodoxy (Gelsthorpe and Morris 1994).

The Probation of Offenders Act 1907 introduced community supervision as an alternative to custody and the following year the use of imprisonment for children under the age of 14 was ended. The Prevention of Crime Act 1908 established specialised detention centres where rigid discipline and work training could be provided in a secure environment, with the first of these at Borstal in Kent, which gave its name to numerous similar establishments. There was a mixture of discipline and training, with some placing an emphasis on education, and later some were to adopt a therapeutic approach (Hood 1965).

The welfare/treatment model was becoming increasingly influential and this is demonstrated by the Children and Young Persons Act 1933, which increased the age of criminal responsibility from seven to eight years and directed magistrates to take primary account of the welfare of the child. This latter clause heralded an important victory for the welfare lobby but highlighted a fundamental contradiction in youth justice policy that has continued to the present day. The justice/punishment and welfare/treatment models inevitably appear to be incompatible, with the former emphasising full criminal responsibility and punishment, and the latter the needs of the individual child and welfare treatment.

Crime levels among young people increased throughout the 1930s and accelerated throughout the Second World War, where seismic social conditions were highly significant in the formative years of a whole generation (Newburn 2002). The 'blackout', evacuation, and the closure of schools and youth clubs, were all blamed for much delinquency and this notion of family disruption or dysfunction has remained a dominant approach to explaining criminality among young people (Bailey 1987).

Table 23.2 The welfare/treatment model of youth justice

- Based on the predestined actor model of criminal behaviour notions that young people are not fully responsible for their actions because of biological, psychological and social factors.
- Treatment and rehabilitation is advocated rather than punishment.
- Cases are to be dealt with by welfare professionals and experts, and not the criminal justice system.
- Later variants of the model recommend limited or non-intervention in accordance with the principles of the victimised actor model of criminal behaviour.

Source: Hopkins-Burke (2008: 51)

The Criminal Justice Act 1948 was introduced in the aftermath of the war and in the context of the post-war Labour Government and the creation of the welfare state. It placed a number of restrictions on the use of imprisonment but at the same time introduced detention centres and attendance centres which appeared to reflect a more punitive approach (Morris and Giller 1987), but concern about the 'welfare' of juveniles was also evident and the legislation sought to end the placement of neglected children in approved schools alongside offenders. Local authority children's departments were also established with their own resources for residential care and trained staff to oversee fostering and adoption (Harris and Webb 1987).

The argument between the proponents of two apparently incompatible models of intervention was to continue into a post-war period characterised by a constant rise in recorded youth crime and where it was increasingly suggested that the approved school system was unable to cope with some of the hardened young offenders that were appearing before the courts (Newburn 1995).

The Ingleby Report 1960 focused on the perceived conflict between the judicial and welfare functions of the juvenile court and proposed an immediate increase in the age of criminal responsibility from eight to 12 years with only welfare proceedings brought below that age (Morris and Giller 1987). The Children and Young Persons Act 1963 increased the age of criminal responsibility to 10 years as a compromise.

These debates were central to the introduction of the Children and Young Persons Act 1969 which advocated a rise in the age of criminal responsibility to 14 years and proposed alternatives to detention in the guise of treatment, non-criminal care proceedings and care orders. Diversion was emphasised and it was proposed that all offenders under 14 years should be dealt with via care and protection, rather than criminal justice proceedings. The police were encouraged to use cautions and only refer juveniles to court following consultation with the social services. The expanding role of the social worker was reflected in the provision for care orders and it was they rather than magistrates who would make the key decision as to whether the young person would be sent to a residential institution or left at home.

The Children and Young Persons Act 1969 was proclaimed by its supporters to be a decisive instance of 'decriminalising' penal policy, but was never fully implemented not least because of the election in 1970 of a Conservative government opposed to the social welfare philosophy of the legislation. Two central features of twentieth century juvenile justice policy nevertheless culminated in the Children and Young Persons Act 1969. First, increasing attention was given to assessing the suitability of the family situation of the offender. Second, the distinction between the offender and the neglected child was increasingly obscured. Moreover, the notion of the 'responsible individual' enshrined in the justice/punishment model of intervention was replaced by the concept of the 'responsible family', with the outcome being increasing state intervention in family life and socialisation under the guise of protecting children considered living in 'undesirable' surroundings.

Youth justice and the new Conservatism

The Conservative government elected in 1979 was prepared to take a vigorous stance against crime and the White Paper *Young Offenders* (Home Office 1980) and the subsequent legislation, the Criminal Justice Act 1982, attacked the welfare/treatment emphasis of the Children and Young Persons Act 1969, and instigated a significant return to the justice/punishment model and notions of individual *and* parental responsibility. Moreover, there was a significant move away from executive decision making (social workers) and a return to judicial decision making (courts), and away from the belief in the 'child in need' (welfare) to what Tutt (1981) has termed 'the rediscovery of the delinquent' (justice). Nevertheless, the Criminal Justice Act 1982 was 'not an unremittingly punitive statute' (Cavadino and Dignan 1997) for it was to introduce significant restrictions on the use of custody.

Conservative juvenile justice policy during the period 1979–97 appears ostensibly to be founded on contradictions and inconsistencies. Thus, the Criminal Justice Act 1991 espoused an 'anti-custody' ethos, while the government subsequently announced the introduction of 'new' secure training units in 1993 and the Criminal Justice and Public Order Act 1994 introduced new tougher sentences for young offenders. Some have proposed that these apparently contradictory measures were the response of a government who had lost confidence in the ability of the 'experts' to find solutions to the problem of youth offending and was merely reacting to crises as they arose.

Certainly during the 1980s, the 'welfare' approach to juvenile justice came under increasing attack and not just from a right-wing law-and-order lobby. The proponents of a 'progressive', 'back to justice' policy criticised discretionary social work judgements as a form of arbitrary power, with many young people the subject of apparently non-accountable state procedures, their liberty often unjustifiably denied and their right to natural justice undermined (Davies 1982). With the experience of the 1970s – where the numbers of custodial sentences increased dramatically in the aftermath of the implementation of a welfare/treatment system – the progressive new justice proponents argued for a return to notions of 'due process' and 'just deserts', along with moves to decriminalise certain offences and a general shift towards using alternatives to custody (Rutherford 1978).

A justice/punishment model solution was proposed with a return to the use of determinate sentences based on the seriousness of the offence rather than the profile of individual offenders. The Criminal Justice Act 1982 thus introduced criteria to restrict the use of both care proceedings and custodial orders while juveniles were now to be legally represented. Custodial orders were to be made only where it could be established that the offender had failed to respond to non-custodial measures, for the protection of the public, or where the offence was serious. There appeared to be little consistency but this was not necessarily the case. The legislation had been clearly introduced with the objective of helping to 'restore the rule of law' (Pitts 1996) but had placed restrictions on the use of custody. This apparent inconsistency can be explained with reference to a legislative strategy that Bottoms (1974) terms 'bifurcation' and which involves separating the response to serious offenders from that of minor offenders, with the outcome being that the former are dealt with punitively and the latter much more leniently.

The late 1980s was to be proclaimed by some a 'successful revolution' in juvenile justice policy not least because the numbers of young people and juveniles incarcerated during the period was significantly reduced (Hagell and Newburn 1994). A key factor in this reduction was the projects developed as alternatives to custody within the DHSS Intermediate Treatment Initiative, with local authority practitioners required to evolve a 'new style of working' with less focus on the emotional and social care needs of offenders and more on the nature of the offence. Magistrates were consequently persuaded that IT schemes were not 'soft options', but 'high tariff' criminal justice disposals implemented by inter-agency juvenile panels comprising of representatives from the welfare agencies, the youth service, police and education departments.

Perhaps the most notable development during this period was the repeatedly affirmed government commitment to community-based diversionary schemes. Diversion had increased in the years following the introduction of the Children and Young Persons Act 1969, but by the 1980s there was growing recognition that custody was extremely expensive with the vast majority of those released reoffending. Treatment in the community was no less effective and certainly far cheaper (Cavadino and Dignan 1997).

Pratt (1989) proposed that the justice/punishment and welfare/treatment models of juvenile justice intervention had now been superseded by a depoliticised 'corporatist model', in which a partnership of social workers, youth workers, health workers, police and magistrates cooperated to produce a cost-effective mechanism for the processing of adjudicated offenders. The process was furthered by the Criminal Justice Act 1991 which sought to provide a national consistency to local initiatives and expand the use of diversionary strategies for juveniles to include young adults. The anti-custody ethos was justified with the promise of more rigorous community disposals that were not alternatives to custody but disposals in their own right.

'Punishment in the community' was now the favoured option but this required a significant change in focus for the juvenile court and the practices of probation and social work agencies. For probation it meant a shift in emphasis away from the traditional approach of 'advise, assist and befriend' towards tightening up the conditions of community supervision and community service work. For the court system it meant the abolition of the juvenile court (which had previously dealt with criminal and care cases) and the creation of youth courts and family courts to deal with these issues separately.

The impact of these decarcerative measures was shown to be fragile when, in 1991, the Home Secretary hastily established a new offence of 'aggravated vehicle taking' carrying a maximum five-year sentence. Two years later, the establishment of 'new' secure training units was announced amidst a furore of media and political debate about a small group of 'persistent young offenders' and 'bail bandits', and to appease the public outcry following the James Bulger case where two 10-year-old children were found guilty of abducting and killing a two-year-old child. Prime Minister John Major insisted that 'we should understand a little less and condemn a little more' and comments from police, judges and MPs that official figures showing a decrease in juvenile offending were quite simply 'wrong' also signalled a renewed tough stance on the part of government and a repoliticisation of youth crime (Pitts 2003). Within weeks of becoming Home Secretary in 1993, Michael Howard commenced a process of revising juvenile justice policy, and secure training centres were to be rethought along the lines of US-style 'boot camps' to provide tougher and more physically demanding regimes aimed at knocking criminal tendencies out of young offenders.

The notion that Conservative juvenile justice policies had amounted to a 'successful revolution' is worthy of closer examination. There was certainly no lack of enthusiasm for the apprehension and incapacitation of offenders, and an acknowledgment that the latter need not mean imprisonment. Perhaps the most significant component was the policy and legislative strategy of 'bifurcation' (Bottoms 1977), where a twin-track approach to justice had sought to identify those young people who had briefly stumbled in the pursuit of an 'upward option' of increased commitment to education and training (Cohen 1972) and to provide them with the impetus and support to overcome their offending behaviour. The persistent and more serious offenders considered more worthy of a punitive intervention could easily be identified as primarily belonging to those sections of working class youth who had failed to take advantage of the economic changes that had transformed Britain during the previous twenty years. These had taken a 'downward option' of ignoring the need for improved education and training (Cohen 1972) and had drifted into a non-skilled, unemployable underclass location.

Excluded now from legitimate employment opportunities and presenting themselves as unattractive propositions to young women as long-term partners these young men found themselves 'frozen in a state of persistent adolescence' (Pitts 1996: 281) with important implications for their involvement in crime because the evidence suggests that 'growing up' means growing out of crime (Rutherford 1992). Stripped of legitimate access to adulthood these young men now found themselves trapped in a limbo world, somewhere between childhood and adulthood, long after the 'developmental tasks' of adolescence had been completed (Pitts 1996). Having failed to heed the warnings provided by the welfare and juvenile justice system, persistent young offenders were to be targeted with a much harsher intervention than those considered non problematic. The new multi-agency forum managerialism was simply about identifying the two categories of offender and setting in motion a twin-track response.

The notion of a new political consensus is more suspect. Conservatives and Labour were in agreement over the need for realism but there was a substantial difference in their interpretation of that reality (Hopkins-Burke 1999). Conservative juvenile justice policy had been for many young people particularly strong on 'the stick' but rather weak on 'the carrot'. There were many complexities and ambiguities to government policy during the period and the closely connected twin concerns of political expediency and pragmatism had led repeatedly to apparent changes in direction, but in summary the perceived solution to the problem of offending by children and young people was to catch more of them and send out a clear message that they would get caught and punished. Significantly, the latter did not have to mean incarceration or, indeed, serious punishment, nor did they all have to be treated the same.

The purpose of 'the stick' was to make young people take responsibility for their actions and become fully aware of the consequences of any illegal transgressions. The small group of persistent offenders were, nonetheless, seriously over-represented among the ranks of the new unemployable underclass, which had been an 'unintended' creation of the dominant laissez-faire economic policy during the period, and juvenile justice policies in particular, and welfare policies in general, had at best done nothing to alleviate that situation, and at worst managed to exacerbate the problem. This author has elsewhere termed this the 'excluded tutelage' model of youth justice (Hopkins-Burke 1999). See Table 23.3.

Table 23.3 The excluded tutelage model of youth justice

- The solution to the crime problem involves catching more offenders in order to deter others.
- Involves a twin-track approach to justice that differentiates between those who have briefly transgressed and can be provided with the support to overcome their offending behaviour and the more persistent and serious offenders considered more worthy of a punitive intervention.
- The latter group predominantly consists of members of those sections of working class youth who have drifted into a non-skilled, unemployable underclass location.
- A failure of government non-interventionist socio-economic policies to significantly address the social exclusion of this group of young people.

Source: Hopkins-Burke (2008: 78)

Vivian Stern of NACRO, writing in 1996, points out that while other European countries favoured the reintegration of offenders back into the community and saw this as central to social and criminal justice policy, Home Office press releases and Conservative government ministers 'use the language of conflict, contempt, and hatred ... doing good is a term of derision, and seeking to help offenders means that you do not care about the pain and suffering of victims' (Stern, cited in Brown 1998: 74). It was New Labour criminal justice and social policy to seek the reintegration of this socially excluded underclass back into mainstream inclusive society.

New Labour and the contemporary youth justice system

Central to New Labour political thought was the 'Third Way' (Giddens 1998) philosophy of communitarianism, which emerged in the USA during the 1980s in response to perceived limitations in liberal theory. From this perspective it argued that the individual rights vigorously promoted by traditional liberals should be balanced with social responsibilities not least because autonomous individual selves do not exist in isolation but are shaped by the values and cultures of communities in which they live (*see* Emanuel 1991; Glendon 1991; Etzioni 1993, 1995).

The New Labour Government was elected in 1997 and its communitarian credentials can be clearly identified in the Crime and Disorder Act 1998. This flagship criminal justice legislation established the Youth Justice Board (YJB) and the contemporary youth justice system, and brought together staff and wider resources from the police, social services, the probation service, education and health, in the delivery of youth justice services, with the principal statutory aim of preventing offending by young people.

Two major criminological theoretical influences on New Labour youth justice policy can be identified as left realism and reintegrative shaming. The former has its origins in the election of the populist Conservatives in 1979 and the subsequent response of a group of radical criminologists who were concerned that the debate on crime control had been lost to the political right. These 'new realists' argued for an approach to crime that recognised both the reality and impact of crime but which also addressed the socio-economic context in which it occurred (Lea and Young 1984). Inasmuch as the 'right realists' – who had provided at least a partial intellectual justification for the New Conservative criminal justice perspective – had focused their efforts on targeting the offender, 'left realists' emphasised the need for a 'balance of intervention'.

Left realism can be summarised briefly: first, there is recognition of the necessity and desirability of offenders taking responsibility for their actions, and second, it is acknowledged that account must be taken of the circumstances in which the crime took place. Since the beginning of a distinctive juvenile justice response in the mid-nineteenth century there had always been a tension between the apparently incompatible polar opposites of the justice/punishment and welfare/treatment models of intervention. The contemporary youth justice system provides a model of intervention that addresses both justice and welfare issues and it is an approach that had become popularised by the oft-quoted sound-bite of Tony Blair – made when he was Shadow Home Secretary in 1994 – 'tough on crime, tough on the causes of crime'.

John Braithwaite (1989) provides a radical reinterpretation and reworking of the labelling theory tradition with his notion of reintegrative shaming. He argues that

Table 23.4 The reintegrative tutelage model of youth justice

- Based on the left realist notion that crime requires a comprehensive solution and there must be a 'balance of intervention'.
- Young people who commit crime must face up to the consequences of their actions and take responsibility (rational actor model of criminal behaviour).
- An effective intervention needs to address the causes of offending as well as punishing the offender (predestined and rational actor model).
- Part of a wider set of educative and welfare strategies that seek to reintegrate socially and economically sections of society.

Source: Hopkins-Burke (2008: 79)

Western societies have a long established tradition of negative shaming, where young offenders become social outcasts, and consequently turn to others sharing their plight for succour and support, with the inevitable outcome being the creation of a criminally inclined underclass living outside of respectable society. In contrast, his notion of reintegrative shaming involves a closely linked two part strategy for the constructive intervention in the life of the offender. First, the offending activities of the individual are shamed with some form of reparation made to the victim and the community, and some form of punishment administered where this is felt to be appropriate but, second, rituals of reintegration are subsequently undertaken to restore the individual to an inclusive society which values their role and person.

Reintegrative strategies are usually termed restorative justice and are central to the contemporary youth justice system. These seek to balance the concerns and interests of victim and community with the need to reintegrate the young person into society and thus enable all parties with a stake in the justice process to participate (Marshall 1998). These interventions have been shown to be effective elsewhere in reducing reoffending by young people (Sherman and Strang 1997; Nugent *et al.* 1999; Street 2000), especially by violent young people (Strang 2000), and provide greater satisfaction for victims (Wynne and Brown 1998; Umbreit and Roberts 1996; Strang 2001).

It is this notion of reintegration back into the community that enables us to explain the approach to youth justice favoured by New Labour and which enables us to distinguish its policies from those of its populist Conservative predecessors, and this author has previously termed this the 'reintegrative tutelage' model of youth justice (Hopkins-Burke 1999, 2008).

CONTEMPORARY YOUTH CRIME

It is evident from self-report studies undertaken in recent years that most young people are not involved in criminality of any kind (Communities that Care 2001; Flood-Page *et al.* 2000; MORI 2001, 2002, 2003), while the great majority of those who do offend continue to 'grow out' of it (MORI 2003) regardless of the virtually continuous 'moral panics' that suggest the very opposite. The evidence we have of the relationship between young people and criminality in the contemporary world would thus seem to contradict popular perceptions. Indeed, the crime statistics show that young people are the group more likely to be victims of crime (Furlong and Cartmel 1997; Home Office 2002).

It is also significant that many young people do not appear to possess a liberal 'let them grow out of it' attitude to the criminal behaviour of their peers. The left realist variant of the carceral society thesis outlined above recognises our material interests in the creation of the social control matrix, and crucially among those who wish to see a rigorous intervention in the lives of those socially excluded young people who are over-represented among the numbers of persistent offenders are both *ourselves* as parents and perhaps more importantly *our children* themselves. It is the latter who want protection from what they widely perceive to be the dangerous threatening elements in their age group. Thus, a survey conducted by IPO-MORI for the Youth Justice Board showed that 60 per cent of young people between 10 and 17 years of age want to see more police on the beat as the best way to protect them from becoming a victim of crime at the hands of other young people, while 38 per cent called for harsher punishments for those in their age group who offend.

The decline in youth crime reflects a similar decrease in crime overall in society (Young 1999). The evidence suggests that these changes were in progress before the introduction of the contemporary youth justice system and while it is difficult to disentangle the possible causes and the impact of particular policies, Armstrong (2005) observes that there do appear to be some fairly sound grounds for optimism. Hopkins-Burke (2008) observes the real possibility that increasing numbers of young people have simply desisted from involvement in offending behaviour in recent years because it is simply no longer a rational or 'cool' choice in a changed socio-economic context where the only hope of legitimate material success is the adoption of an 'upward' strategy of educational attainment.

Improved education opportunities and provision are clearly a significant cornerstone of the New Labour 'reintegrative tutelage' project, but taking advantage of these opportunities is problematic for many young people and not necessarily those who are members of a socially excluded underclass. Fergusson *et al.* (2000) argue that current 'quasi-market' systems actively encourage instability in the trajectories of a substantial minority of young people in pursuit of post age 16 education and training. Powerful pressures are generated that force young people, who are often ill-informed and unable to identify or pursue a preferred option, to make particular rational choices while markets draw them into particular modes of participation. The outcome is often unsuitable options pursued with little commitment and which are short-lived. In reality, there is a significant blurring of boundaries between those who have taken a conscious 'upward solution' of education and career pursuit progression and those who have taken a 'downward solution' of laissez-faire non-participation albeit invariably by default (Hopkins-Burke 2008). There is a significant group in the middle who are sufficiently motivated to take an upward trajectory but unable to acquire sufficient cultural capital to obtain a stable, successful economic location. Such young people, with significantly weakened social bonds (*see* Hirschi 1969), are very much at risk of being absorbed into the readily available and invariably welcoming offending subcultures on the street (Hopkins-Burke 2008).

The reintegrative tutelage project thus appears to be established on fragile socio-economic foundations, with the economy unable to provide accessible legitimate *sustainable* opportunities for increasingly large sections of young people. In these circumstances, the notion of restorative justice, on which the contemporary youth justice strategy is based, is equally problematic. Supporters argue that the reinvigoration of community through restorative justice mechanisms can facilitate strong bonds of social control (Strang 1995), but as Crawford and Clear (2003) observe, alternative justice systems, through necessity, presuppose an existing degree of informal control upon which mutuality, reciprocity, and commitment can be reformed and, problematically, the appeal to revive or transform community has arisen at exactly the time when it appears most absent, when Durkheimian anomie or normlessness is the norm in society (*see* Durkheim 1933).

Young people are significant targets in the Government's battle against crime and disorder, social disorganisation, and most notably, antisocial behaviour (Squires and Stephen 2005). This zealous focus on antisocial behaviour 'signals exclusion and rejection' (Burney 2005: 2), instead of empowering and uniting the community; it ostracises certain families or individuals, whilst also pitting the community against the individual, as the former effectively has to police the latter to make sure they comply with the requirements of the anti-social behaviour order (ASBO). This allows for the development of resentment and division rather than the creation of a strong inclusive community.

When a young person becomes the subject of an ASBO, the community in which they live may be informed through the local newspapers – or through the distribution of leaflets – and this publicity includes information regarding the restrictions placed on the activities of the individual and a photographic image, so that the person is easily recognised. Not only is this contrary to the long-established principle in youth justice, established by the Children and Young Persons Act 1933, which places significant restrictions on the naming of a young person involved in criminal proceedings but it is also a classic example of 'disintegrative, rather than reintegrative, shaming because it does nothing constructive for the individual to ensure their reintegration into the community, but serves to alert a mistrusting community to their misbehaviour and places them under the surveillance of their neighbours' (Fionda 2005: 243).

Jamieson (2005) observes that the authoritarian penal populism of the 'respect' agenda – of which the ASBO agenda has such a central part – has a particular electoral appeal to contemporary society. The punitive emphasis of responses to 'antisocial' and criminal behaviour provides an opportunity to reassure the public that firm measures are in place to deal with such behaviours. She observes while such interventionist measures may well provide some respite from troublesome behaviour in the short term – and may even serve to deter involvement – the denigration inherent in the derogatory rhetoric and punitive emphasis of that agenda promotes profoundly negative portrayals of the parents, children and young people primarily targeted (Burney 2005; Squires and Stephen 2005). The danger of this contemporary approach is that it not only encourages intolerance and hostility, but also serves to obscure the often complex and diverse needs underlying 'parenting deficits' (Etzioni 1993; Dennis and Erdos 1992), 'anti-social' and 'criminal' behaviour, and is thus entirely incompatible with the aims and objectives of the reintegrative tutelage project.

THE FUTURE OF YOUTH JUSTICE

The contemporary youth justice system is very much a creation of the New Labour government first elected in 1997 and it is appropriate to briefly speculate on the future of youth justice in the eventuality of a change of government. Four possible scenarios have been outlined.

First, the system could remain relatively untouched albeit for some minor changes and amendments. Research certainly suggests that there has been a reduction in offending by young people in the intervening years although it is difficult to establish a direct causal link between system input and output. There has been some improvement in the life-chances (education and training) and general health (drug treatment programmes) of young people brought within the system remit although these positive changes are nevertheless ancillary to the central aim of reducing offending behaviour (Hopkins-Burke 2008). An incoming government could, however, recognise public money well spent and – with some justification – leave well alone.

Second, we could go further, with the system not just retained but radically revised along the lines suggested by John Pitts (2003). Thus, the YJB could be granted greater independence and autonomy from a controlling, however well-meaning, government, and which, it is argued, would provide it with greater widespread credibility, while, at the same time, it would be appropriately consistent with the requirements of the 'new liberal' moral communitarian agenda outlined by this author elsewhere (Hopkins-Burke 2008, 2009).

Third, it could be abolished altogether. We are living in the aftermath of the biggest economic downturn since the Second World War and all political parties recognise the necessity of making significant cuts in public spending and this is likely to be the case for some years. The contemporary youth justice system is expensive to administer and some will argue that it is insufficiently cost effective. This cost-cutting agenda would be supported by research which shows that more young offenders are incarcerated in England and Wales than anywhere else in Europe and this has become increasingly the case since the introduction of the present system (Goldson and Muncie 2006; Muncie 2008).

Fourth, there could be a less radical variant of the third scenario and the retention of a significantly curtailed system. Proponents could use the same justifications but with the additional observation that the increase in youth justice business can be attributed to the 'net-widening' propensities of the contemporary system (Cohen 1985; Hopkins-Burke 2008). The revised, significantly cheaper, system could use the risk assessment process fundamental to the contemporary system to ascertain those deserving of a rigorous criminal justice intervention while the others are simply siphoned out of the system at an early stage without any input. Welfare and heath concerns would thus not be dealt with in this scenario.

It will be left to the reader to speculate which political parties are likely to favour which strategies. This author is an unequivocal supporter of the contemporary youth justice system and thus favours its retention, albeit with the amendments suggested by the second scenario, while the issue of net-widening suggested by the fourth scenario should also be addressed. We will await the outcome with interest.

AN OVERVIEW

1   The concept of adolescence was socially constructed according to middle-class sensibilities which led to the marginalisation of significant sections of young people.
2   An historical perspective on youth justice helps to understand contemporary perceptions of young offending.
3   The bourgeois child tutelage project can be understood in the context of the left realist variant of the carceral surveillance society thesis.

4   The early story of the development of the juvenile justice system is one of a transition from a justice/punishment to a welfare/treatment model response.

5   The Children and Young Persons Act 1969 was heralded as a decisive instance of 'decriminalising' penal policy but was never fully implemented.

6   Conservative juvenile justice policy during the period 1979–97 can be best understood by the concept of 'bifurcation'.

7   The small group of persistent offenders were seriously over-represented among the ranks of the socially excluded underclass and this has been termed the 'excluded tutelage' model of youth justice.

8   The contemporary youth justice system was established by the Crime and Disorder Act 1998.

9   Left realism and reintegrative shaming are the two major criminological influences on New Labour youth justice policy.

10 The reintegration of the socially excluded underclass is central to New Labour social policy and has been termed the 'reintegrative tutelage' model of youth justice.

11 Most contemporary young people are not involved in criminality of any kind; most of those who do offend continue to 'grow out' of it, and they are the group most likely to be victims.

12 Most contemporary young people do not possess a liberal 'let them grow out of it' attitude to their offending peers.

13 Many young people have desisted from offending in recent years because it is no longer a rational or 'cool' choice.

14 The reintegrative tutelage project appears to be established on fragile socio-economic foundations with the economy unable to provide legitimate *sustainable* opportunities for many young people.

15 The battle against crime and disorder, social disorganisation and antisocial behaviour is incompatible with the reintegrative tutelage project.

16 The future of the contemporary youth justice system will depend on the outcome of the last General Election.

SUMMARY OF MAIN POINTS

You should be able to:

- Critically examine the historical development and construction of notions of young people and crime.
- Critically examine the historical development of the juvenile justice system in Great Britain.
- Critically examine the nature of the contemporary juvenile justice system in Great Britain.

MOMENT OF REFLECTION

Questions

1 The notions that the family is in 'crisis' and/or parents are 'failing' are nothing new but part of a 'cyclical phenomenon with a very long history'. Discuss.

2 Children and young people were disciplined and controlled throughout the nineteenth and first half of the twentieth centuries in a form that was functional and appropriate to the needs of industrial capitalism. Is this a simplistic account?

3 Discuss the view that youth offending is less likely to be a relatively non problematic part of a normal transition to legitimate adulthood for those who experience multiple factors of social exclusion.

4 Is the welfare/treatment model of youth justice progressive and humanitarian?

5 Can the New Labour youth justice agenda introduced in 1997 be legitimately considered merely a continuation of that introduced by their Conservative predecessors in the previous eighteen years?

6 Can New Labour youth justice policy be considered a success and if so in what ways?

NOTE

1 It is informed by the author's core text *Young People, Crime and Justice* published by Willan Publishing in 2008.

REFERENCES

Aries, P. (1962) *Centuries of Childhood: A Social History of Family,* (Trans. Robert Baldick) New York: Alfred A. Knopf.

Armstrong, D. (2005) A Risky Business? Research, Policy, Governmentality and Youth Offending, *Youth Justice,* 4 (2), 100–16.

Bailey, V. (1987) *Delinquency and Citizenship: Reclaiming the Young Offender 1914–48,* Oxford: Clarendon Press.

Becker, H. (1963) *Outsiders: Studies in the Sociology of Deviance,* New York: Free Press.

Bottoms, A. (1974) On the Decriminalization of the Juvenile Court, in R. Hood (Ed.) *Crime, Criminology and Public Policy,* London: Heinemann.

Bottoms, A. (1977) Reflections on the Renaissance of Dangerousness, *The Howard Journal,* 16 (2), 70–96.

Braithwaite, J. (1989) *Crime, Shame and Reintegration,* Cambridge: Cambridge University Press.

Brown, S. (1998) *Understanding Youth and Crime,* Buckingham: Open University Press.

Burney, E. (2005) *Making People Behave: Anti-social Behaviour, Politics and Policy,* Cullompton: Willan Publishing.

Cavadino, M. and Dignan, J. (1997) *The Penal System: An Introduction,* London: Sage.

Cohen, P. (1972) Sub-Cultural Conflict and Working Class Community, *Working Papers in Cultural Studies,* No.2, Birmingham: CCCS, University of Birmingham.

Cohen, S. (1985) *Visions of Social Control*, Cambridge: Polity Press.

Communities that Care UK (2001) Risk and Protective Factors Associated With Youth Crime and Effective Interventions to Prevent it, *Youth Justice Board Research No 5*, London: Youth Justice Board.

Crawford, A. and Clear, T. R. (2003) Community Justice: Transforming Communities through Restorative Justice?, in E. McLaughlin, R. Fergusson, G. Hughes and L. Westmarland (Eds), *Restorative Justice: Critical Issues*, London: Sage/Open University.

Davies, B. (1982) Juvenile Justice in Confusion, *Youth and Policy*, 1 (2).

Davis, J. (1990) *Youth and the Condition of Britain*, London: Athlone Press.

Day-Sclater, S. and Piper, C. (2000) Re-moralising the Family? Family Policy, Family Law and Youth Justice, *Child and Family Law Quarterly*, 12 (2), 135–51.

Dennis, N. and Erdos, G. (1992) *Families Without Fatherhood*, London: Institute of Economic Affairs.

Donzelot, J. (1980) *The Policing of Families: Welfare versus the State*, London: Hutchinson University Library, London.

Durkheim, E. (1933 originally 1893) *The Division of Labour in Society*, Glencoe: Free Press.

Elias, N. (1978) *The Civilising Process, Vol. 1: The History of Manners*, Oxford: Blackwell.

Elias, N. (1982) *The Civilising Process, Vol. 2: State-Formation and Civilisation*, Oxford: Blackwell.

Elliot, P. S. and Voss, H. L. (1974) *Delinquency and Drop-out*, Toronto: Lexington.

Emanuel, E. (1991) *The Ends of Human Life: Medical Ethics in a Liberal Polity*, Cambridge, MA: Harvard University Press.

Etzioni, A. (Ed.) (1991) *New Communitarian Thinking: Persons, Virtues, Institutions and Communities*, Charlottesville: University of Virginia Press.

Etzioni, A. (1993) *The Spirit of Community: The Reinvention of American Society*, New York: Touchstone.

Etzioni, A. (Ed.) (1995) *New Communitarian Thinking: Persons, Virtues, Institutions and Communities*. Charlottesville: University of Virginia Press.

Fergusson, R., Pye, D., Esland, G., McLaughlin, E. and Muncie, J. (2000) Normalised Dislocation and the New Subjectivities in Post-16 Markets for Education and Work, in *Critical Social Policy*, 20 (3), 283–305.

Fionda, J. (2005) *Devils and Angels*, Oxford: Hartley Publishing.

Flood-Page C., Campbell, S., Harington, V. and Miller, J. (2000) *Youth Crime Findings from the 1998/99 Youth Lifestyles Survey*, Home Office Research Study 209, London: Home Office.

Foucault, M. (1971) *Madness and Civilisation: A History of Insanity in the Age of Reason*, London: Tavistock.

Foucault, M. (1976) *The History of Sexuality*, London: Allen Lane.

Foucault, M. (1980) *Power/Knowledge: Selected Interviews and Other Writings 1972–77*, C. Gordon (Ed.), Brighton: Harvester Press.

Furlong, A. and Cartmel, F. (1997) *Young People and Social Change*, Buckingham: Open University Press.

Garland, D. (2001) *The Culture of Control*, Oxford: Oxford University Press.

Gelsthorpe, L. (1999) Parents and Criminal Children, in A. Bainham, S. Day Sclater and M. Richards (Eds) *What is a Parent? A Socio-legal Analysis*, Oxford: Hart.

Gelsthorpe, L. and Morris, A. (1994) Juvenile Justice 1945–1992, in M. Maguire, R. Morgan and R. Reiner (Eds), *The Oxford Handbook of Criminology*, Oxford: Clarendon Press.

Giddens, A. (1998) *The Third Way*, Cambridge: Polity Press.

Gillis, G. R. (1974) *Youth and History*, London: Academic Press.

Glendon, M. A. (1991) *Rights Talk: The Impoverishment of Political Discourse*, New York: Free Press.

Goldson, B. and Muncie, J. (2006) *Youth Crime and Justice*, London: Sage.

Goldthorpe, J. H. (1968–9) *The Affluent Worker in The Class Structure*, 3 Vols, Cambridge: Cambridge University Press.

Griffin, C. (1997) Representations of the Young, in J. Roache, S. Tucker (Eds) *Youth In Society*, London: Sage.

Hagell, A. and Newburn, T. (1994) *Persistent Young Offenders*, London: Policy Studies Institute.

Hall, G. S. (1906) *Youth: Its Regime and Hygiene*, New York: Appleton.

Harris, R. and Webb, D. (1987) *Welfare, Power and Juvenile Justice*, London: Tavistock.

Hendricks, H. (1990a) Constructions and Reconstructions of British Childhood: An Interpretive Study 1800 to the Present, in A. James and A. Prout (Eds) *Constructing and Reconstructing Childhood*, London: The Falmer Press.

Hendricks, H. (1990b) *Images of Youth: Age, Class and the Male Youth Problem 1880–1920*, Oxford: Clarendon.

Hirschi, T. (1969) *Causes of Delinquency*, Berkeley, CA: University of California Press.

Home Office (1980) *Young Offenders*, Cmnd 8045, London: HMSO.

Home Office (2002) *British Crime Survey*, London: HMSO.

Hood, R. (1965) *Borstal Re-Assessed*, London: Heinemann.

Hopkins-Burke, R. D. (1999) *Youth Justice and the Fragmentation of Modernity*, Scarman Centre for the Study of Public Order Occasional Paper Series, University of Leicester.

Hopkins-Burke, R. D. (Ed.) (2004a) *'Hard Cop/Soft Cop': Dilemmas and Debates in Contemporary Policing*, Cullompton: Willan Publishing.

Hopkins-Burke, R. D. (2004b) Policing Contemporary Society, in R. D. Hopkins-Burke, *'Hard Cop/Soft Cop': Dilemmas and Debates in Contemporary Policing*, Cullompton: Willan Publishing.

Hopkins-Burke, R. D. (2004c) Policing Contemporary Society Revisited, in R. D. Hopkins-Burke, *'Hard Cop/Soft Cop': Dilemmas and Debates in Contemporary Policing*, Cullompton: Willan Publishing.

Hopkins-Burke, R. D. (2008) *Young People, Crime and* Justice, Cullompton: Willan Publishing.

Hopkins-Burke, R. D. (2009) *An Introduction to Criminological Theory* (3rd edition), Cullompton: Willan Publishing.

Hoyles, M. and Evans, P. (1989) *The Politics of Childhood*, London: Journeyman Press.

Humphries, S. (1981) *Hooligans or Rebels?*, Oxford: Blackwell.

Jamieson, J. (2005) New Labour, Youth Justice and the Question of 'Respect, *Youth Justice*, 5 (3), 180–93.

Jenks, C. (1996) *Childhood*, London: Routledge.

Lea, J. and Young, J. (1984) What Is To Be Done About Law and Order?, London: Penguin.

Marshall, T. (1998) *Standards for Restorative Justice: An Overview*. London: Restorative Justice Consortium.

Marshall, T. F. (1997) Seeking the Whole Justice, in S. Hayman (Ed.) *Repairing the Damage: Restorative Justice in Action*, London: ISTD.

MORI (2000) *Youth Survey 2000*, Research conducted for the Youth Justice Board, London: Youth Justice Board.

MORI (2001) *Youth Survey 2001 for the Youth Justice Board for England and Wales*, London: Youth Justice Board.

MORI (2002) *Youth Survey 2002 for the Youth Justice Board for England and Wales*, London: Youth Justice Board.

MORI (2003) *Youth Survey 2003 for the Youth Justice Board for England and Wales*, London: Youth Justice Board.

Morris, A. and Giller, H. (1987) *Understanding Juvenile Justice*, London: Croom Helm.

Muncie, J. (2004) *Youth and Crime* (2nd edition), London: Sage Publications.

Muncie, J. (2008) The 'Punitive Turn' in Juvenile Justice: Cultures of Control and Rights Compliance in Western Europe and the USA, in *Youth Justice* 2008 (8), 107.

Newburn, T. (1995) *Crime and Criminal Justice Policy*, London: Longman.

Newburn, T. (2002) Young People, Crime, and Youth Justice in M. Maguire, R. Morgan and R. Reiner, *The Oxford Handbook of Youth Justice* (3rd edition), Oxford: Oxford University Press.

Nugent, W., Umbreit, M., Winnamaki L. and Paddock, J. (1999) Participation in Victim Offender Mediation Reduces Recidivism, *Connections* (VOM Association), 3, Summer.

Pearson, G. (1983) *Hooligan – A History of Respectable Fears*, London: Macmillan.

Pitts, J. (1996) The Politics and Practice of Youth Crime, in E. McLaughlin and J. Muncie (Eds) *Controlling Crime*, London: Sage in association with the Open University.

Pitts, J. (2003) Youth Justice in England and Wales, in R. Matthews and J. Young (Eds) *The New Politics of Crime and Punishment*, Cullompton: Willan.

Pratt, J. (1989) Corporatism: The Third Model of Juvenile Justice, *British Journal of Criminology*, 29, 236–54.

Rutherford, A. (1978) Decarceration of Young Offenders in Massachusetts, in N. Tutt (Ed.) *Alternative Strategies for Coping with Crime*, Oxford: Blackwell/Martin Robertson.

Rutherford, A. (1992) *Growing Out of Crime* (2nd edition), London: Waterside Press.

Sherman, L and Strang, H (1997) Restorative Justice and Deterring Crime, *RISE Working Papers*, Canberra: Australian National University.

Squires, P. and Stephen, D. E. (2005) *Rougher Justice: Anti-social Behaviour and Young People*, Cullompton: Willan Publishing.

Strang, H. (1995) Replacing Courts With Conferences, *Policing*, 11 (3), 20–21.

Strang, H. (2000) *Victim Participation in a Restorative Justice Process: The Canberra Reintegrative Shaming Experiments*, PhD Dissertation, Law Program, Research School of Social Sciences, Canberra: Australian National University.

Strang, H. (2001) *Repair or Revenge: Victim Participation in Restorative Justice*, Oxford: Oxford University Press.

Street, R. (2000) Restorative Justice Steering Group: Review of Existing Research, London: Home Office (unpublished).

Tutt, N. (1981) A Decade of Policy, *British Journal of Criminology*, 21 (4), 246–56.

Umbreit, M. and Roberts, A. (1996) *Mediation of Criminal Conflict in England: An Assessment of Services in Coventry and Leeds*, Rochester, Minnesota: Center for Restorative Justice and Mediation, University of Minnesota.

West, D. J. (1967) *The Young Offender*, New York: International Universities Press.

Wynne, J. and Brown, I. (1998) Can Mediation Cut Re-offending?, *Probation Journal*, 46 (1).

Young, J. (1999) *The Exclusive Society: Social Exclusion, Crime and Difference in Late Modernity*, London: Sage.

CHAPTER 24

THE PROFESSIONALIZATION OF THE YOUTH JUSTICE WORKFORCE

VICKY PALMER

OBJECTIVES

After reading this chapter you should be able to:

- Understand the historical emergence of the youth justice system.

- Understand 'professionalization' in youth justice.

- Understand the difficulties of youth justice.

- Appreciate the continuities with health and social care.

After reading this chapter you will understand the key terms:
Youth justice system, professionalization, modernization, case managers, agency, structure, managerialism, rights, responsibilities, Third Way, McDonaldization, effective practice, rehabilitation, crime prevention.

There are two Moments of Reflection to work through at the end of the chapter.

It is a terrible business to mark a man out for the vengeance of men. But it is a thing to which a man can grow accustomed, as he can to other terrible things; he can even grow accustomed to the sun. And the horrible thing about all legal officials, even the best, about all judges, magistrates, barristers, detectives and policemen, is not that they are wicked (some of them are good), not that they are stupid (several of them are quite intelligent), it is simply that they have got used to it. Strictly they do not see the prisoner in the dock; all they see is the usual man in the usual place. They do not see the awful court of judgement; they only see their own workshop.

(G. K. Chesterton, *The Twelve Men*, 1909: viii)

INTRODUCTION

The last decade has witnessed an unprecedented transition in youth justice practice in England and Wales following New Labour's fixation on modernization within a new, risk-averse society. To avoid past difficulties of young people 'falling through the net' and hence missing out on crucial forms of intervention to effect positive change in their behaviour, contemporary youth justice has embraced the benefits of partnership working. Here, key agencies are required to work together under one roof to form new methods of collaboration, which are also open to inspection by internal and external audits. These checks have been put in place to ensure that case managers – those who oversee the management of community orders and sentences of detention – are adhering to national standards laid down by the Youth Justice Board. These standards dictate such criteria as how often a young person should be seen by their case manager and the maximum number of days to be taken to prepare a court pre-sentence report. Workers are now obliged to utilize evidence based approaches to practice such as that advocated by Utting and Vennard's (2000) study of effective programmes. The rebranding of youth justice via the 1998 Crime and Disorder Act was a radical shift, which saw the label of the 'Local Authority Youth Justice Team' substituted with the title 'Youth Offending Team'; the subtlety of which heralded the launch of a novel epoch in the history of juvenile justice that has seen fundamental changes to both policy and practice.

This chapter focuses upon the 'professionalization' of practitioners who work within youth justice. It commences with an investigation of the disparate notions of the term 'professionalism', attempting to place this in perspective with the evolution of the modern youth justice system. In order to further contextualize the changes that have taken place in youth justice, it attempts to understand modernization in youth justice by illustrating some of the machinations of New Labour's neo-liberal, 'Third Way' policies. It then examines the impact that these policies have had, both in the training of youth justice practitioners and allied helping professions, and their impact upon modern practice.

There follows a brief overview of the literature pertinent to youth justice, both historical and contemporary, paying particular attention to areas that have perhaps been under-researched and investigated, such as the absence of the voice of both practitioners' views and those of the young offenders themselves. The literature findings also provide a critical analysis of what is presently taught to youth justice practitioners, and how this translates – or otherwise – in practice. Finally, this chapter raises some points for future reflection and consideration regarding the focus and content of curricula for students of health and social care, and concludes with an exercise focusing upon investigating the readers' knowledge of what constitutes criminal behaviour.

THE ELUSIVE NATURE OF PROFESSIONALISM

When one considers the concept of professionalism, it generally brings to mind connotations of competency and proficiency, yet any exploration beyond this veneer reveals a multiplicity of meaning. Professionalism, as explicated by Hoyle (1975: 315), refers to 'those strategies and rhetorics employed by members of an occupation in seeking to improve status, salary and conditions.' However, Hoyle's focus here seems more upon the material aspirations and the generation of symbolic capital, that is the accumulation of economic, social and cultural capital (Bourdieu 1986) of those employed within an organization, and overlooks that which defines adeptness and capability, including employers and their regulators. Clarke and Newman's (1997: 7) analysis of professionalism sees it functioning:

> both as an operational strategy, defining entry and negotiating the power and rewards due to expertise, and as an organizational strategy, shaping the patterns of power, place and relationships around which organizations are coordinated.

Although this synopsis incorporates the rules and regulations of employment and locates the importance of power, many attempts at definition seem to overlook the inexorable driver to those ends: the teaching of knowledge with which to achieve aspirations of professionality (Evans 2008). Whereas youth justice practitioners themselves would perhaps recognize expertise as a prerequisite to the development of a profession, Etzioni (1969) would locate the 'profession' of youth justice practice more as a 'semi-profession', maintaining that practitioners claim full professional status to which they are not entitled. This, Etzioni would suggest, is because they have not subjected themselves to five years or more of training and because within their instruction, knowledge is communicated to rather than created by its members (McMahon 2007). Etzioni argues that there are some hurdles that some groups are unable to overcome:

> the semi-professionals' efforts to change themselves, more fully to live up to the claim floated, generate a major source of tensions because there are several powerful societal limitations on the extent to which these occupations can be fully professionalized.
>
> (Etzioni 1969: vii)

Hence the notion of professionalism would appear to be both elusive and nebulous, holding different meanings to different individuals and stakeholders but seemingly something towards which individuals and organizations strive. As a qualified social worker, probation officer and youth justice practitioner, the author's own preferred definition requires there to be 'a number of key identifiable traits, one of which is autonomous decision making, underscored by a distinct, theoretical, expert knowledge base' (May and Buck 1998: 1). This is perhaps a result of the possibility that it most closely represents the ethos of professional training prior to the overload of bureaucratic practices, rather than any authoritative or definitive view.

THE ETHOS OF THE NEW YOUTH JUSTICE

Youth justice, as a 'profession' in its own right, has only truly surfaced over the last decade. Prior to this, it was incorporated into the remit of the local authority social services department with contributions made by the probation service for older young offenders. An initial review of related literature elucidates this perception with the earliest related narrative revealing itself in the *Probation Journal*'s 1930 Volume 1 edition with a commentary by Norman, entitled, 'Juvenile Courts' (Norman 1930). The *British Journal of Social Work* waits until 1974 to publish its own original article by Power *et al.* (1974), 'Delinquency and the Family'. The *Journal of Youth Justice* does not take root until 2001, following a raft of major legislative reforms designed to tackle youth crime, thus launching youth justice as a distinct discipline. The emergence of a discrete youth justice system sees its origins in the Crime and Disorder Act of 1998, which was passed during the currency of Tony Blair's leadership of the Labour Party.

Since the inception of the New Labour administration in 1997, youth justice policy has apparently witnessed an unprecedented transformation, closely allied to Tony Blair's intention of 'toughening up every aspect of the criminal justice system' (Blair 2004: 6). Revision of its function was to be complemented by the reconfiguration of key established professional relationships in order to ensure that agencies worked closely together under one roof in an attempt not only to promote inter-agency working, but also to ensure it. To this end, a variety of practitioners were assembled to make up the newly created Youth Offending Teams (Field 2007). Owing to their diverse backgrounds, the majority of these professionals required retraining in the ethos and ideology of contemporary youth justice, which strives towards the ultimate aim of the prevention of offending by children and young people via an approach that seeks to balance their rights with their responsibilities. The instruction of this novel agenda was invested in higher education and its context is embedded within the seminal piece of legislation that was enacted in 1998, effectively seeking a detachment from previous, allegedly ineffectual methods of working.

Through the Crime and Disorder Act 1998, the contemporary youth justice system statutorily draws its workforce from a range of key and ancillary health and social care professions, namely: health, probation, police, education and the local authority. This emphasis on multi-agency working has shifted the ethos of youth justice practice from its historic, secure location within social work and probation practice to a more relevant but potentially detached discourse propagated via the expansion of idiosyncratic training routes offering the provision of dedicated, youth justice orientated modules (Wilson *et al.* 2008). This sea change is clearly situated within New Labour's managerialist agenda of modernization, with its attendant target-driven features of transparency, accountability, monitoring, inspections and performance indicators (Batmanghelidjh 2008; Fergusson 2007; Muncie 2004). Work with both adult and young offenders has become increasingly subject to central government set parameters with heterogeneous approaches and appraisals of offenders rooted in actuarial risk-measurement tools, adroitly conceptualized by Fergusson (2007: 183) as 'a contentless tool-box which takes its ideological orders from above'.

It is clear then that youth justice practice has undergone an unprecedented reorganization in order to encourage crucial professionals to work together to prevent offending and reoffending by children and young people in England and Wales. The next section will look at how staff training and development has changed over the past 30 years, culminating in where we are at now in terms of the professionalization of the youth justice workforce.

YOUTH JUSTICE TRAINING IN CONTEXT

The Youth Offending Service attracts the preponderance of its case managers from social work trained professionals within the probation service and the social services department (Field 2007). Prior to the mid-1990s, the training for both professions was sited decisively within social work education where students strove originally towards the Certificate of Qualification in Social Work (CQSW) at undergraduate or post-graduate level, then in the early 1990s, the Diploma in Social Work (DipSW). The Conservative government insistence that the probation service should 'toughen up' effected a termination of this interrelationship and 1996 beheld the emergence of a distinct educative route for probation officers in the guise of the Diploma in Probation Studies (DipPS). This conspicuous cessation of the previous link with social work, with its attendant focus on a therapeutic alliance (Dowden and Andrews 2004), located probation officers' training 'within more of a legal/criminological/research frame-work, much more in line with the emergence of probation as a correctional service' (Annison *et al.* 2008: 261).

The gateway for social workers into their profession, since 2003, has been via the attainment of the social work degree (SWD) at either graduate or postgradu-ate level (General Social Care Council 2009) and this may have implications for the Youth Justice Board in its future consideration of appropriate qualification levels for its staff. This deliberation would not seem inappropriate given the Youth Justice Board's endeavour to offer parity to its practitioners, via its qualifications structure, with social workers (Youth Justice Board 2008).

For the Youth Offending Service workforce, 2003 saw the inception of a new qualification framework intended for practitioner training and retraining with the introduction of the Professional Certificate in Effective Practice (PCEP), followed in 2005 by the Foundation Degree in Youth Justice (FdYJ) (Youth Justice Board 2008). The Youth Justice Board originally prescribed curriculum content with three PCEP modules uninspiringly entitled, 'Aims, Values and Partnerships', 'Effective Practice' and 'Quality Assuring Effective Practice' (Youth Justice Board 2003a). After successful completion of PCEP, learners could opt to advance their academic credentials by com-mencing the FdYJ, whose itinerary offers a broader, more complementary knowledge base, including coverage of the history of the youth justice system, the evolving legal framework, child and adolescent development, contemporary youth crime in context and an examination of youth custodial provision.

Youth justice policy has been radically overhauled by New Labour over the last decade via the splicing together of the concept of 'agency' with its antithesis, 'struc-ture', in its management of young people who offend. 'Agency' stresses the importance of individual responsibility in their propensity to offend. A focus on this perception tends to attract 'justice' methods in dealing with offenders, that is, a matching of the levels of formal intervention to the seriousness of the offence, at the expense of attending to individuals' putative needs. 'Structural' approaches, on the other hand, see crime as the fault of societal influences and favour 'welfarism', which emphasizes that children should be dealt with in a different manner to adults and that their dis-tinct needs should be catered for. This could be seen however as a simplistic breaking down of a truly complex issue. For example, Giddens (1984) asserts that 'structure' and 'agency' is essentially inter-linked as individuals are inseparably concerned with society and dynamically enter into its constitution. People are not exterior to social structures and vice versa, hence there is the need to meld the two together.

The blending of both concepts has been conceived as the 'Third Way', which 'represents a quest to transcend social democracy ... which looks to the state for answers, and neo-liberalism ... which looks to the market for solutions' (Pitts 2001: 54). The policies intrinsic to the 'Third Way' tend to distinguish several overarching, central tenets, including the optimization of an organization's performance by the appliance of generic management skills, and the balancing of individual rights with the interests of the community. Each of these is then combined with an approach that sees partnership agencies working together in order to achieve more effective inter-agency cooperation (Pitts 2001). Giddens (2001) believes that there is no single version of the 'Third Way', yet essentially views it as a new form of social democracy. He indicates that this approach centres on modernization, involving government reform that employs a regulatory role in civil society rather than one that would seek to dominate it, alongside a linkage of rights and responsibilities and the pursuit of equality.

It may be the case that modern youth justice strategies aim to achieve their aims through an entwining of apposite, yet contradictory, aims and objectives. These involve the inducement of paternalistic welfarism through the utilization of early intervention provision and of court disposals such as parenting orders, referral orders and supervision orders. Such incentives, however, would be in exchange for responsibility by means of activities designed to make amends for the harm that has been done, victim and offender mediation sessions and offending behaviour programmes. All of this is ultimately underpinned by the sanction of punishment in the form of more stringent court orders including curfews, unpaid work and incarceration. However, it has been posited that:

> neither position offers a conclusive rationale on which to base the youth justice system. This is perhaps borne out by the evidence of practitioners reinserting welfare options into a structure which is increasingly dominated by notions of just deserts and correctionalism.
>
> (Smith 2005: 12)

In reality, this conflicting combination calls for a sensitive mode of discharge by practitioners of youth justice, the agency by which this is taught being higher education.

The Youth Justice Board, in its attempt to professionalize its increasingly discrete workforce, has fully embraced the philosophy of the 'Third Way', that intermingling of welfare and justice approaches, taking much of its lead from the National Offender Management Service (NOMS). However, it is clear that probation practitioners are becoming ever more uneasy with the maelstrom of change towards a more scientific and prescribed method of labour (Annison *et al.* 2008; Eadie and Canton 2002). These observations are epitomized by the compelling narrative of a newly qualified probation officer who contends that, 'The sheer volume of worthless, needless, repetitive paperwork and bureaucracy. It's like ivy – parasitic, and covers, obscures and strangles the true purpose of probation' (Annison *et al.* 2008: 266). Others posit that managerialism's unremitting surge has manifested in a faceless, routinized style of practice at the expense of professional prudence (Baker 2005). Indeed, it would seem that the proliferation of bureaucratic practices within the helping professions has led to a dilution of client-centred face-to-face casework (Burnett and Roberts 2004; Chui and Nellis 2003; Schön 1983; Worrall and Hoy 2005). This in turn has fed in to the notion that, 'Social care has tended to be re-orientated away from its commitment to holistic provision and social justice and towards homogenized and bureaucratic responses' (Ritzer and Barnard 2008: 48); a process axiomatically coined, 'McDonaldization' (ibid.: 46; Ritzer 2004). This potentially dehumanizing development and progression of bureaucratization within both adult and youth justice, with its intrinsic 'mind your back' obligation of credentialism, allied to its steady erasure of social work values and evisceration of practitioner autonomy, may have the effect of marginalizing the young people it was originally intended to work with (Howe 2008; Bryman 2008).

THE ASCENDANCY OF YOUTH JUSTICE

> To those who look at the rich material provided by history, and who are not intent on impoverishing it in order to please their lower instincts, their craving for intellectual security in the form of clarity, precision, objectivity, truth, it will become clear that there is only one principle that can be defended ... anything goes.
>
> (Feyerabend 1975: 27)

The justice versus welfare dichotomy has featured as an unyielding, controversial aspect of British juvenile/youth justice policy – particularly sentencing – for many years. We observe its concepts being wrestled with in Norman's musings on the founding of juvenile courts:

> There are ... two conceptions for the development of such courts, one being that the Juvenile Court should be a Juvenile Police Court and the other that such courts should be organized for the reformation of Juvenile Offenders.
>
> (Norman 1930: 67)

Norman's deliberations saw him reading from the fourth Report of the Children's Branch of the Home Office which expounded that, 'The qualities which are needed in every Magistrate who sits in a Juvenile Court are a love of young people, sympathy with their interests, and an imaginative insight into their difficulties. The rest is common sense' (Norman 1930: 68).

We may agree with Norman's list, with the addition of an in-depth knowledge of the body of theory surrounding child development. However, it would seem that these admirable values no longer stand up unaccompanied in modern times with the Youth Justice Board's drive towards the promotion of 'effective practice': methods of working that have been appraised and verified to reduce offending by our youth (Youth Justice Board 2008). We may also witness the irony of Weberian prophetic philosophy at play here, suggesting that:

> It is the destiny of our era, with its characteristic rationalization and intellectualization ... that precisely the ultimate and most sublime values have withdrawn from the public sphere.
>
> (Lowith 1982: 40)

Nowadays, some would say that administrative tasks befit the principal focus of youth justice, since tick-boxes relating to targets provide more uncomplicated techniques of measurement than any qualitative consideration of human misfortune (Argyris and Schön 1994; Batmanghelidjh 2008). Youth crime has apparently concerned itself with a more punitive discourse 'which talks of clamping down ... of zero tolerance of anti-social behaviour' (Bradley 2008: 1). This may be at odds with the ethics of workers who favour a mode of practice reflective of their individual and specialized values such as empathy, human dignity, respect and the establishment of a caring rapport (Argyris and Schön 1994; Eadie and Canton 2002).

To summarize, the training of youth justice practitioners has taken a fundamental new direction to that which previously existed, one that embraces New Labour's 'Third Way' politics. The risks inherent within such a radical shift are that workers become constrained within an ever-increasing bureaucratic system, leaving increasingly less time to devote to vulnerable and often misunderstood young people who are in trouble with the law. It has been noted by Annison *et al.* (2008) and Eadie and Canton (2002), that many practitioners resent the contamination of their work by the tick-box culture and that they would perhaps prefer a more responsive and age-specific approach towards their work with children.

The following sections will scrutinize the noticeable absence of the true feelings of both service users and practitioners, since it is possible that their views may assist to gradually nudge the system in a 'new' direction. Acknowledgement will be afforded to the notion that sometimes there is no solution to young people's propensity to offend and further critique of the present situation regarding the training of the contemporary youth justice workforce is presented together with a number of areas to be considered for improvement.

LOCATING THE GAPS IN PROVISION

> Across the board there was one bit lacking, which was service user input.
> (General Social Care Council 2009: 34)

There seems to be a conspicuous absence in the tendency towards the Youth Justice Board's sacrifice of social work values in order to embrace the paradigm of New Labour's managerialist agenda, in that the young offenders' views remain unspoken (Beresford 2008; GSCC 2009; Wilkes 2005). The quote above is from a newly qualified social worker reflecting on the social work degree, and the literature would suggest that this is nothing new and that their voices lay dormant from the paternalism of the eighteenth and early nineteenth centuries until the late 1960s when, 'The view of the other was sought and the client spoke' (Howe 2008: 3). The 'effective practice' equivalent of the golden years of social work could be seen to lie in cultivating the quality of rapport with and the bearing fruit of results for consumers (Davies 1985). It favoured a treatment model where quality over quantity and familiarity over computations of outputs were preferred. It aligned itself with the work of Rogerian[1] psychology, believing that the human being possesses the most compelling understanding of himself; rather than a peripheral self-professed authority (Howe 2008). The absence of the voice of the 'client' seems ironic when the machinations of the Youth Court itself even now tolerate the young person's right to be heard under the Criminal Procedure Rules 2005, rule 41 (Moore 2009). Although it is acknowledged that the two arenas are not the same, it remains interesting that the courts themselves are concerned with the views of young offenders but they are seemingly rendered silent elsewhere, yet young offenders' accountability to both agencies is on a similar footing.

Further omissions have been uncovered in terms of the stance of practitioners, a questionable omission given the depth and breadth of some professionals' experience. There are some notable exceptions in the literature such as that pertaining to probation officers, which has derivative applicability to youth justice practitioners as well as those working in health and social care. For example, in the National Association of Probation Officers' (NAPO) 2007 centenary publication, *Changing Lives: An Oral History of Probation,* retired officers' views are sought on the service's long history and their own reflections upon their careers. What emerges is a vast sense of grief at the loss of practitioner autonomy, characterized by ex-Assistant Chief Officer Sue Wade's condemnation of managerialism, 'I'm happy with the idea that everybody should come up to a certain standard, but it's killed off enterprise and innovation' (NAPO 2007: 43); and exemplified by an ex-probation officer's views of contemporary probation practice:

> It was only really in the end that I began to see that everything was going the wrong way, and now I am absolutely appalled at what we've got … I'm deeply concerned over the quality of training of probation officers.
>
> (NAPO 2007: 43)

The author would support this concern alongside further unease about the probation service's inability to retain qualified probation officers as this appears to be mirrored in the field of youth justice. Historically, a career in the probation service was viewed and accepted as a career for life, however the downside to the absorption of managerialism has been the movement towards the reality of the service becoming a parking lot for a more transient workforce. This is partly a result of high caseloads that are rife in the service, rendering quality work with offenders impossible. This fear is not unfounded given the recent, high profile cases of probation service failings regarding the brutal murder of the two French students, Gabriel Ferez and Laurent Bonomo in South London in 2008. One of the perpetrators of that crime was on non-parole licence and was being supervized by the probation service. The officer holding the case was newly qualified, yet held 127 cases at the time of the murder. The probation supervision took place in Lewisham, where no probation officers had more than two years' post-qualification experience (*NAPO News* 2009). This should be regarded as a warning sign for the youth justice system, where reductions in youth offending team funding have already begun in earnest (Puffett 2009).

ANSWERING THE UNANSWERABLE: IS IT POSSIBLE TO PREVENT YOUTH CRIME?

Contemporary youth justice practice retains little acknowledgement of the evident reality that certain human dilemmas have no answer (Bateman and Pitts 2005). This is evidenced to some extent by the fact that youth crime rates have remained constant from year to year across Europe (Hammarberg 2008). Youth justice policy in England and Wales seems to cling to the naïve and optimistic belief, typified by the words of Wilson *et al.*:

> If welfare interventions were not perceptibly helping young offenders, diverting them from crime, or preventing them from being incarcerated … then alternative strategies had to be sought.
>
> (2008: 517)

It appears then that there is a political requisite to know the problem of youth crime and hence the means by which to solve it (Haines and Case 2008). This does not automatically presume, however, that the old client-centred casework holds a nirvana, and it would be as well to mark Shaw's shrewd words, 'there is a danger in some quarters of replacing the rehabilitation myth with the myth of crime prevention' (Shaw 1983: 128). Furthermore, the treatment model itself has attracted criticism, with its clandestine, Foucauldian tendency towards control and utilization (Harding 1987; Hopkins-Burke 2008). Nevertheless, it is worth at least acknowledging that, 'Some human problems have no solution. Sympathy is more important than ideology: without compassion, social work is empty' (Howe 1987: 110). For we cannot always grasp precisely why somebody develops unlawful tendencies; we are dealing with complex constructs of reality in terms of the unique circumstances of offenders' lives. Moreover, it perhaps needs to be recognized that there are limitations in the capacity for measurement in interventions with young offenders as their behaviour is often remarkably individual. As Whyte (2004: 9) crucially indicates:

> Criminal behaviour in young people cannot simply be tackled as an episode of individual criminality dissociated from the social context or from the available child welfare, education and health, social and recreational provision.

This pivotal matter may require further consideration in the future development of training for youth justice professionals.

THE MOULDING AND SHAPING OF THE YOUTH JUSTICE WORKFORCE

> In the dominant twentieth-century model of the well-managed organization, the manager tries to achieve the task as he sees it by controlling his employees' behaviour. He does this by making the work so simple that anybody can do it.
>
> (Argyris and Schön 1994: 152)

It is possible that current youth justice discourse exemplifies this perception by means of the simplistic, repetitive, mantra-like vernacular that is omnipresent in its self-published literature. Phraseology such as, 'what works[2] ... what doesn't work ... what's promising ... what's unknown ... effective practice' (YJB 2003b) abound, shaping a more positivist, science-driven approach (Maclure 2003). Knowledge contained within the narrative, originating from the YJB, may be seen to hijack the domination of the truth, upholding it as a system of fact (Hall 1997). However this is not to suggest that this regime of truth is capable of dominating everyone working within the sphere of youth justice. This is illustrated by Rogowski's (2002) examination of a selection of youth court pre-sentence reports – documents prepared by social workers and probation officers for sentencing purposes – which revealed that:

> Despite the changes in the probation service and despite government attempts to push social workers in the same direction, it becomes clear that at the end of the twentieth century, the social workers of these young people were still firmly embedded in the welfare mode.
>
> (Rogowski 2002: 178)

He believed that this was largely the result of the persistence of a mode of working reminiscent of the social democratic era of the 1960s and 1970s. However, the implications of this are that these methods may in time be lost as those who benefited from welfare-orientated training retire or leave the youth offending service owing to a mismatch of ideologies. Contemporary students of youth justice receive minimal tuition concerning a welfare mode of delivery, particularly within the content of the PCEP programme.

The content of the PCEP course has already been scrutinized to some extent by Kubiak and Hester (2009), who wryly refer to it as the 'holy grail'. Expressing equal concern over the subject material and alluding to its dogma, they refer to the relentless, unquestioned presentation of the 'what works' agenda, the absence of any critique and the 'airbrushing' of history (Kubiak and Hester 2009).

Their views are reinforced by Bateman and Pitts' (2005: 253) informed take on PCEP, which they perceive, 'oversimplified understanding of the history of youth justice, which managed to ignore welfarism, corporatism and progressive minimalism without missing a beat'. This criticism, aimed directly at the Youth Justice Board, has gained further momentum via Stephenson *et al.*'s (2007) exceptionally balanced analysis of the redesigned youth justice system. Here, the authors acknowledge the accusation that the Youth Justice Board has 'adopted a "ground zero" approach denying the previous achievements in youth justice' (Stephenson *et al.* 2007: xv). By example, within one of the module contents of the Foundation Degree in Youth Justice entitled, 'Child and Adolescent Development', the seminal 1960s work of John Bowlby in this sphere was simplistically condensed into half a page of an 80-page workbook (YJB 2006). This may suggest that theories of attachment, separation and loss (Bowlby 1975) have less prominent significance in youth justice practice, since those that suffer profoundly from their effects are often those with whom little can be done to effect change.

With the exception of Hester (2008) and Kubiac and Hester (2009), there appears to be no specific study into the professionalization of youth justice practitioners. Professionalization in this context can be considered a transformation towards a workforce equipped to provide a controlled, quality service that is open to scrutiny, audit and accountability. One that is 'ready to match the pace of external change with internal dynamism' (Clarke and Newman 1997: 58). And one that is built around the indistinguishable assumptions of bureaucracy and professionalism to generate the notion put forward by Clarke and Newman (1997) of the 'bureau-professional'. Though more can be gleaned from the literature with respect to practitioner narrative (Annison *et al.* 2008; Baker 2005; Field 2006; Jamieson 2005; Matthews 2009; NAPO 2007), any correlation so far with higher education has leaned towards probation officer and social worker accredited professional training courses.

It would be useful to consider how the process of professionalization within youth justice training enables practitioners to 'internalize the norms and values that prevail within the social order' (Wanli 1998: 1). It would also be interesting to determine whether there has been a marginalization of the teaching of wider reflection, as advocated by Muncie (2004), lest we risk the manufacture of a Huxleyan workforce, contented in New Labour's brave new world, bearing, 'a more than superficial resemblance to blue-collar workers, deskilled by the numbing monotony of the assembly line' (Schön 1983: 337). This concern has been raised by others in relation to the youth justice workforce, with criticisms levelled at New Labour's approach that has 'zombified youth justice practitioners through its attempts to micromanage the system.' (Stephenson *et al.* 2007: xv). A new, obligatory, e-training programme that is presently being rolled out nationally to youth justice staff may exemplify this concern, one that has been described as shackling practitioners to their computers for 100 hours at the expense of face-to-face contact with youngsters (*Youth Justice News* 2009). Moreover, it would be pertinent to examine the course of managerialism and its conjunction to Foucauldian power–knowledge discourse, where individuals:

> are always in the position of simultaneously undergoing and exercising power. They are not only its inert or consenting target; they are also the elements of its articulation.
>
> (Foucault 1980: 98)

Any critique of education, however, should not involve a dismissal of the reality of managerialism, as protocols, goals and directives constitute a secure baseline for the negotiation of the multifaceted, intricate youth justice system. But a revision of the literature would intimate that a more humanistic approach should at least be considered for reincorporation into the equation. Although this may appear to represent a value statement, it is one that is commonly mentioned in the literature. For example, this view is embodied in the findings of Field's (2007) research of the views of YOT personnel on the matter of young offenders' welfare needs, with a salient remark that had been reiterated in a number of interviews:

> If you take the needs of the young person, if their basic needs aren't being met, their welfare needs, how on earth can they actually concentrate on not offending? If they are homeless, you are not going to address that offending behaviour because as far as they are concerned, they have got a priority need that they have to sort out before they are going to sit and listen to anything you have got to say.
>
> (Field 2007: 314)

This observation accords with that of one of the most renowned humanist psychologists, Abraham Maslow (1954). He believed that a hierarchy of human needs that comprise physiological needs, safety, love and belongingness and self-esteem are the drivers that stimulate the behaviour of individuals. He suggested moreover that people's behaviour is explained by their absence (Davies 2008); hence the homeless young person referred to above may be focused on offending due to the lack all four rudimentary needs.

It may be one thing to teach students the rudiments of the 'McGuire principles' (Youth Justice Board 2003a), such as the significance of 'risk assessment' and the 'structure' of ensuring that the objectives are clear, but quite another to impart to them how to diffuse a situation when they are met at the door of a home visit by a client wielding a shot gun, spitting expletives, accompanied by a dog trained to fight. Guidance on such scenarios appears to be absent in the Youth Justice Board's literature. This may well symbolize a stark contradiction between youth justice discourse and what happens in reality. For explanations of youth justice have frequently failed to address the manner in which the policy and practice dichotomy is often eclipsed by establishment realities. For example, some practitioners may believe that assisting young people to secure employment is more productive than mulling over the details of their offending and hence make this the primary focus of their work. Others may prefer to work independently within the family environment of the child, rather than refer parents to parenting courses. As Eadie and Canton (2002: 15) judiciously observe:

> The relationship is never straightforward, and among the influences at this level are occupational culture – by which we mean training, values and practice wisdom.

Ultimately, however, we need to take forward and be mindful of Hester's (2008: 1) observation:

> Understanding the central importance of reflective and knowledgeable practitioners is a step in the right direction and would ensure that children's rights are protected by developing 'know how' as a counter-balance to the asymmetry of forces that exist between the young person and their wider social environment. Addressing this asymmetry through the education of practitioners is, I believe, a step that we must take.

For, as a society, we should not wish to dissipate the creativity of youth justice professionals at the expense of the 'what works' agenda, since this could eventually jeopardize much of the authentically sound practice that remains in existence (Bateman and Pitts 2005).

CONCLUSION

Achieving the status of 'professional' within the youth justice workforce is no easy task owing to the variety of meanings that the term suggests. In addition, since youth justice as a discrete profession has only emerged since the passing of the 1998 Crime and Disorder Act, the notion of the youth justice professional remains in its infancy. Although no longer an arm of the local authority social services department, both social workers and probation officers remain integral players in youth offending teams. However, their pivotal role and professional status have tended to become submerged and undermined with the increasing reliance upon other key agencies, alongside volunteers and under-trained personnel (Pitts 2003). Owing to this, it has been argued that modern youth justice practitioners have become de-professionalized (Pitts 2001).

Running parallel to this, along with the experience of other health and social care professionals, has been a significant rise in the utilization of bureaucratic procedures together with formulaic methods of practice that seemingly bear scant resemblance to the type of complex and sensitive work which would ordinarily be called for when working with young offenders. In effect, social work values appear to be becoming marginalized to make way for a new rationalized and standardized managerialist agenda that epitomizes New Labour's policies. This change has seemingly occurred regardless of the longevity of experience and knowledge of previous juvenile justice practitioners and without consultation of representatives of the young offenders that this agenda seeks to manage.

The prevention of offending by children and young people has always been difficult to achieve (Hammarberg 2008; Shaw 1983), hence the problem can only apparently be contained by means of management, containment and control. These three approaches have not only been targeted at young offenders with progressively more punitive outcomes, but have also ostensibly been exercised with respect to practitioners via a proliferation of prescriptive practices which serve to dampen autonomy and creativity. As Orwell (1946: 383) reminds us, 'One of the aims of totalitarianism is not merely to make sure that people will think the right thoughts, but actually to make them less conscious'.

It would now seem timely to reverse the trend of 'intellectual purging' (Trevithick 2005: 58) that has taken place in all forms of practice within health and social care and this reversal is already showing signs of fruition. The social work profession has recently been tasked with introducing a new and advanced social work professional status, 'so the most highly skilled social work practitioners stay close to the frontline' (Balls and Johnson 2009: 2). It may be the case that this decision is eventually mirrored across the field of health and social care as well as in the youth justice arena, so that the more apposite, reflective and humanistic side of social care regains its primacy.

SUMMARY OF MAIN POINTS

You should be able to:

*   Understand the historical emergence of the youth justice system.
*   Understand 'professionalization' in youth justice.
*   Understand the difficulties of youth justice.
*   Appreciate the continuities with health and social care.

MOMENT OF REFLECTION

Activity One

1   To what extent and in what form is a managerialist agenda taught to health and social care practitioners?

2   What is the emphasis of teaching on welfare, justice, responsibility or an amalgam of these ideologies?

3   What emphasis is placed on professional autonomy and discretion?

4   To what extent are bureaucratic procedures instructed to youth justice staff and those in health and social care?

5   What association is retained to social work practice and values?

6   What do you believe the gaps in content are in health and social care education?

7   What is the correlation between knowledge that is taught and practice reality?

MOMENT OF REFLECTION

Activity Two

Which of the following scenarios would be defined as criminal?

1 Painting the outside of your own home with a colourful graffiti-style mural.

2 Brightening up the outside of a derelict youth club with a colourful graffiti-style mural.

3 A 13-year-old boy climbing a tree in his local park, snapping a branch in the process.

4 An 11-year-old girl chalking a hopscotch grid on the pavement outside her house for a game with her friends.

5 You are driving your two-year-old niece back home to her parents following a party on a hot day with your car windows open. She is securely in her car seat in the back of your car, clutching her party-bag. She takes one of her sweets out of the bag to eat, and in the process, the sweet wrapper blows out of the window.

6 Two 14-year-old boys are arguing in the school playground. The argument escalates into a fight and other pupils gather round to watch. One boy sustains a split lip and bruising, the other, cuts and scratches.

NOTES

1 Psychologist Carl Rogers (1902–1987)was concerned with the whole person. He believed that people are not simply motivated by internal compulsions or forced into actions by their environment, but are always dynamically attempting to make sense of their experiential understanding (Howe, 2008).

2 The 'what works' agenda advocates a number of 'principles' of effective practice primarily drawn from the work of James McGuire. He developed seven applicable principles from studies conducted in Canada and the USA. Programmes and services which work best possess the following features: 1) Theoretical soundness – based on an explicit model of the causes of crime; 2) Risk assessment – an assessment of the risk of reoffending; 3) Criminogenic needs assessments – made on risk factors, e.g. substance misuse; 4) Responsivity – workers adapt to individual differences and learning styles; 5) Structure – the objectives are clear; 6) Methods – the use of a cognitive behavioural approach; and 7) Programme integrity – delivery should be undertaken by appropriately trained staff (McGuire 2000).

REFERENCES

Annison, J. Eadie, T. and Knight, C. (2008) People First: Probation Officer Perspectives on Probation Work, *Probation Journal*, 55 (3), 259–71.

Argyris, C. and Schön, D. (1994) *Theory in Practice: Increasing Professional Effectiveness*, London: Jossey-Bass Ltd.

Baker, K. (2005) Assessment in Youth Justice: Professional Discretion and the Use of Asset, *Youth Justice*. 5 (2), 106–22.

Balls, E. and Johnson, A. (2009) *Joint Letter to Social Workers in England*, Department for Children, Schools and Families and the Department of Health [online]. Available at: www.dcsf.gov.uk/swtf/ (Accessed 24 September 2009).

Bateman, T. and Pitts, J. (2005) *The RHP Companion to Youth Justice*, Lyme Regis: Russell House Publishing.

Batmanghelidjh, C. (2008) in Barnard, A., Horner, N. and Wild, J. (Eds) (2008) *The Value Base of Social Work and Social Care*, Maidenhead: Open University Press.

Beresford, P. (2008) *Service User Values for Social Work and Social Care*, in Barnard, A., Horner, N. and Wild, J. (Eds) (2008) *The Value Base of Social Work and Social Care*, Maidenhead: Open University Press.

Blair, T. (2004) *Confident Communities in a Secure Britain: The Home Office Strategic Plan 2004–2008*, London: The Stationery Office.

Bourdieu, P. (1986) The Forms of Capital, in J. Richardson (Ed.) *Handbook of Theory and Research for the Sociology of Education*, New York: Greenwood, pp. 241–58.

Bowlby, J. (1975) *Attachment and Loss*, London: Penguin.

Bradley, K. (2008) *Juvenile Delinquency and the Evolution of the British Juvenile Courts, 1900–1950*, Kent: Institute of Historical Research.

Bryman, A. (2008) *Epistemological Considerations: Social Science Research Methods* (3rd edition), Oxford: Oxford University Press.

Burnett, R. and Roberts, C. (Eds) (2004) *What Works in Probation and Youth Justice: Developing Evidence-Based Practice*, Cullompton: Willan Publishing.

Chesterton, D.K. (1909) 'The Twelve Men' in Harding, J. (Ed.) (1987) *Probation and Community: A Practice and Policy Reader*. London: Tavistock Publications Ltd.

Chui, W. H. and Nellis, M. (Eds) (2003) *Moving Probation Forward: Evidence, Arguments and Practice*, Harlow: Pearson Education.

Clarke, J. and Newman, J. (1997) *The Managerial State: Power, Politics and Ideology in the Remaking of Social Welfare*, London: Sage.

Davies, M. (1985) *The Essential Social Worker: A Guide to Positive Practice* (2nd edition), Aldershot: Gower.

Davies, M. (2008) (Ed.) *The Blackwell Companion to Social Work* (3rd edition), Oxford: Blackwell.

Dowden, C. and Andrews, D. (2004) The Importance of Staff Practice in Delivering Correctional Treatment: A Meta-Analysis, *International Journal of Offender Therapy and Comparative Criminology*, 48, 203–14.

Eadie, T. and Canton, R. (2002) Practising in a Context of Ambivalence: The Challenge for Youth Justice Workers, *Youth Justice*, 2, 14–26.

Etzioni, A. (1969) *The Semi-Professions and their Organization: Teachers, Nurses, Social Workers*, New York: The Free Press.

Evans, L. (2008) Professionalism, Professionality and the Development of Education Professionals, *British Journal of Educational Studies*, 56 (1), 20–38.

Fergusson, R. (2007) Making Sense in the Melting Pot: Multiple Discourses in Youth Justice Policy, *Youth Justice*, 7 (3), 179–94.

Feyerabend, P. (1975) *Against Method*, London: New Left Books.

Field, S. (2007) Practice Cultures and the 'New' Youth Justice in (England and) Wales, *British Journal of Criminology*, 47: 311–330.

Foucault, M. (1980) *Power/Knowledge: Selected Interviews and Other Writings 1972–1977*, New York: Pantheon.

General Social Care Council (GSCC) (2009) *Raising Standards: Social Work Education in England 2007–2008*, London: General Social Care Council.

Giddens, A. (1984) *The Constitution of Society*, Cambridge: Polity Press.

Giddens, A. (Ed.) (2001) *The Global Third Way Debate*, Oxford: Wiley-Blackwell.

Haines, K. and Case, S. (2008) The Rhetoric and Reality of the 'Risk Factor Prevention Paradigm' Approach to Preventing and Reducing Youth Offending, *Youth Justice*, 8 (5), 5–20.

Hall, S. (Ed.) (1997) *Representations: Cultural Representations and Simplifying Practices*. London: Sage.

Hammarberg, T. (2008) A Juvenile Justice Approach Built on Human Rights, *Youth Justice*, 8, 193–6.

Harding, J. (Ed.) (1987) *Probation and the Community: A Practice and Policy Reader*, London: Tavistock Publications Ltd.

Hester, R. (2008) Power Knowledge and Children's Rights in the Teaching of Youth Justice Practice, *Inter-University Centre Journal of Social Work*, 17, Fall 2008 [online]. Available at: www.bemidjistate.edu/academics/publications/social_work_journals/issue17 (Accessed 12 April 2009).

Hopkins-Burke, R. (2008) *Young People, Crime and Justice*, London: Willan Publishing.

Howe, D. (1987) *An Introduction to Social Work Theory*, Aldershot: Wildwood House Ltd.

Howe, D. (2008) *An Introduction to Social Work Theory*, Aldershot: Ashgate Publishing Ltd.

Hoyle, E. (1975) *Professionality, Professionalism and Control in Teaching*, in Houghton, V. *et al.* (Eds) *Management in Education: The Management of Organisations and Individuals*. London: Open University Press.

Jamieson, J. (2005) New Labour, Youth Justice and the Question of 'Respect', *Youth Justice* 5, 180–93.

Kubiak, C. and Hester, R. (2009) Just Deserts? Developing Practice in Youth Justice, *Learning in Health and Social Care*, 8 (1), 47–57.

Lowith, K. (1982) *Controversies in Sociology: 12 – Max Weber and Karl Marx*, London: George Allen and Unwin.

Maclure, M. (2003) *Discourse in Educational and Social Research*, Buckingham: Open University Press.

Matthews, J. (2009) People First: Probation Officer Perspectives on Probation Work – A Practitioner's Response, *Probation Journal*, 56 (1), 61–7.

May, T. and Buck, M. (1998) Power, Professionalism and Organisational Transformation, *Sociological Research Online*, 3 (2), [online]. Available at: http://www.socresonline.org.uk/socresonline/3/2/5 (Accessed 24 August 2009).

Maslow, A. (1954) *Motivation and Personality*, New York: Harper.

McGuire, J. (2000) 'What Works in Reducing Criminality', Paper presented at the Conference, *Reducing Criminality: Partnerships and Best Practice*, [online]. Available at: www.stcloudstate.edu/mcguire-whatworksinreducingcriminality.pdf (Accessed 24 August 2009).

McMahon, E. (2007) *Professionalism in Teaching: An Individual Level Measure for a Structural Theory*, Ohio: Ohio State University.

Moore, T. (2009) *Youth Court Guide* (3rd edition), Haywards Heath: Tottel Publishing.

Muncie, J. (2004) *Youth and Crime* (2nd edition), London: Sage.

NAPO (2007) *Changing Lives: An Oral History of Probation*, London: National Association of Probation Officers.

NAPO News (2009) Probation in Context in the Aftermath of the Sonnex Verdict, *NAPO News*, 211, July/August 2009. London: The Trade Union and Professional Association for Family Court and Probation Staff.

Norman, H. E. (1930) Juvenile Courts, *Probation Journal*, 1 (5), 67–8.

Orwell, G. (1946) Politics and Literature, in *The Penguin Essays of George Orwell*, Harmondsworth: Penguin.

Pitts, J. (2001) *Crime, Disorder and Community Safety*, Oxford: Routledge.

Pitts, J. (2003) *The New Politics of Youth Crime: Discipline or Solidarity?*, Lyme Regis: Russell House Publishing.

Power, M. J., Ash, P. M., Shoenberg, E. and Sirey, E. C. (1974) Delinquency and the Family, *British Journal of Social Work*, 4 (1), 13–38.

Puffett, N. (2009) Youth Justice Board cuts Budget for Youth Offending Teams, *Children and Young People Now*, 16 June 2009.

Ritzer, G. (2004) *The McDonaldization of Society*, Revised New Century Edition, Thousand Oaks, CA: Pine Forge Press.

Ritzer, G. and Barnard, A. (2008) *Globalization Defined*, in Barnard, A., Horner, N. and Wild, J. (Eds) (2008) *The Value Base of Social Work and Social Care*, Maidenhead: Open University Press.

Rogowski, S. (2002) *Young Offenders: A Case Study of their Experience of Offending and the Youth Justice System and how this Relates to Policy and Practice Developments over the Post-War Period*, Manchester: Manchester Metropolitan University (Department of Applied Social Studies).

Schön, D. (1983) *The Reflective Practitioner*, Aldershot: Ashgate.

Shaw, S. (1983) Crime Prevention and the Future of the Probation Service, *Probation Journal*. 30 (4), 127–9.

Smith, R. (2005) Welfare Versus Justice – Again!, *Youth Justice*, 5 (3), 2–16.

Stephenson, M., Giller, H. and Brown, S. (2007) *Effective Practice in Youth Justice*, Cullompton: Willan Publishing.

Trevithick, P. (2005) *Social Work Skills: A Practice Handbook*, Maidenhead: Open University Press.

Utting, D. and Vennard, J. (2000) *What Works with Young Offenders in the Community?*, Essex: Barnardo's.

Wanli, L. (1998) *Power and Discourse: Michel Foucault and his Theories* [online]. Available at: www.eng.fju.edu.tw/crit.97/Foucault/Foucault.htm (Accessed 5 February 2009).

Whyte, B. (2004) Effectiveness, Research and Youth Justice, *Youth Justice*, 4 (3), 2–21.

Wilkes, T. (2005) Social Work and Narrative Ethics, *British Journal of Social Work*, 35 (1), 1249–64.

Wilson, K., Ruch, G., Lymbery, M. and Cooper, A. (2008) *Social Work: An Introduction to Contemporary Practice*, Harlow: Pearson Education Ltd.

Worrall, A. and Hoy, C. (2005) *Punishment in the Community: Managing Offenders, Making Choices*, Cullompton: Willan Publishing.

Youth Justice Board (2003a) *Professional Certificate in Effective Practice Tutor Pack*, Session 9, Module 1, Day 1, London: ECOTEC.

Youth Justice Board (2003b) *Assessment, Planning, Interventions and Supervision*, London: ECOTEC.

Youth Justice Board (2006) *Foundation Degree in Youth Justice: Child and Adolescent Development*, London: ECOTEC.

Youth Justice Board (2008) *Workforce Development Strategy*, London: YJB.

Youth Justice News (2009) YOT Staff Face 100 Hours of Computer Training, *Children and Young People Now*, 26 March 2009 [online]. Available at: www.cypnow.co.uk/Youth-Justice/news (Accessed 26 March 2009).

CHAPTER 25

CONCLUSION

ADAM BARNARD

PART 1

Skills for study and practice prepared you for study in health and social care. The chapter introduced you to the core skills necessary for study. Writing, reading and note-taking, and reading effectively were considered. Writing essays, literature reviews, essay plans, essay structure and written arguments and reflective learning allow you to gain the necessary knowledge and skills to succeed on a health and social care programme of study. The chapter also introduced you to the 'Moments of Reflection' that are used in subsequent chapters.

    Working with people discussed interpersonal communication and people skills in a professional health and social care context. Theories and concepts of interpersonal behaviour such as communication theory and practice, listening skills, assertiveness behaviour, teamwork, interviewing skills, the significance of feedback, assessment and how to use these skills in an applied setting were discussed. These skills are seen as transferable and relevant to study, work and social life.

    The individual in society provided an introduction to the developmental psychology and sociology necessary for health and social care by providing an understanding of how human beings grow and change over their lives. The introduction to physical, psychological, emotional and social changes that people experience during their lifespan and the factors that affect those changes was considered. External factors, such as the society in which individuals live, the opportunities they have and the difficulties specific groups may encounter have a massive impact on people's lives. The chapter argued for an understanding of human growth and development in its historical, cultural and sociological context. Key aspects of growth and development were discussed with a particular emphasis on life transitions and how individuals' experiences of these are influenced by factors such as gender, ethnicity and disability.

    Concepts of equality and diversity extended these aspects of diversity, and examined the concepts of equality and key mechanisms in relation to social differences that facilitate or inhibit the promotion of equality. The chapter then explored mechanisms that can operate to limit the promotion of equality such as prejudice, stereotyping, discrimination and oppression. The chapter then considered social differences such as class, gender, ethnicity, culture, age, sexuality and disability. The ways the mechanisms and social differences impact on each other were discussed. The chapter concluded with a discussion of the legislative framework that exists to address equality and diversity.

The final chapter of the first part of the book, *Introduction to social policy* addresses social policies that have the potential to affect the lives of the users and the providers of health and social care services. The chapter started with an exploration of what social policy actually is, and an attempt to locate the subject and to understand its relevance to people through the life course. The chapter explored the historical context in which welfare organizations have developed from the Poor Laws to the development of charities and the birth of the modern welfare state. Current social policy issues from immigration to an ageing population and from homelessness to work and welfare were illustrated by case studies.

PART 2

Studying at a higher level in health and social care examined how to construct written arguments at levels two and three of an undergraduate programme. The elements of a good argument, how to use chains of reasoning, and how to produce coherent and comprehensive arguments were discussed. The different levels of sophistication of arguments were discussed along with central processes for producing a good piece of written work. The chapter also addressed the idea that there are competing and multiple perspectives within health and social care and that a good argument is one that can entertain and critique different perspectives on a topic.

Health and health care in Britain discussed 'health', ways of thinking about health, and health services in Britain. It looked at the term 'health' and explored health inequalities in relation to socio-economic status, ethnicity and gender. The focus then shifted to look at issues relating to health care and examined the organization of the National Health Service, the issue of 'quality', and patient and public involvement in health as key themes shaping health services in Britain.

Key themes in health and social care examined how social policy and practice respond to emerging health and social needs, and the outcomes experienced by individuals and groups. The practical challenges associated with three key policy aims: providing individualized care; protecting adults and children from harm; and the promotion of well-being, were illustrated. Focusing on the service users' experience and observed outcomes in these settings, the contributions of the different professions, their organization and management were examined, and how they contribute to the quality of health and social care services.

Philosophical and political debate in health and social care examined political and philosophical issues that impact upon health and social care by introducing key philosophical, political, and ethical theories. The moral concepts of rights, responsibility, freedom, authority and power were introduced. The chapter started with a consideration of philosophy and the purpose of philosophical inquiry for health and social care. The discussion then considered key political philosophies and ethical theories. The chapter concluded by suggesting health and social care is centrally involved with philosophy, politics and ethics.

Research in health and social care distinguished between producers and consumers of research. The traditional dichotomy between quantitative and qualitative research methodologies and adoption of mixed methods and triangulation was discussed. Experiments, case studies, interviews, observation and surveys were explored along with the distinction between primary and secondary data sources. Statistical techniques and terms were explained in order to help the reader to become more research literate and a better consumer of research. The reader was finally introduced to the minefield of research ethics and their implications for research in general terms. Key issues were emphasized in relation to health and social care research and in particular issues related to access, law, informed consent and data protection.

Introduction to the criminal justice system used the broad definition of health and social care focused on the promotion of well-being of individuals, communities and society. As such, consideration of health and social care includes central areas such as criminal justice. This chapter focused on the contours of the criminal justice system and provided the reader with an introduction to definitions of criminal justice and the key areas of the police, prosecution, the courts, probation, prison, multi-agency working and victims. The chapter concluded with a discussion of the future direction and challenges of the criminal justice system.

Theories of counselling provided a broad introduction to the theory that underpins counselling activity. It started by exploring definitions of counselling and how counselling fits in with contemporary society. It identified the theoretical bases of major counselling paradigms, and put their development into a historical context. Key theorists in the major counselling approaches were examined alongside the explanations and assumptions about psychological development which underpin these. Consideration was also given as to how these explanations engender differing models of helping and the application of counselling skills. The discussion explored: the ethics, principles and purpose underpinning counselling practice; practitioner development of counselling skills; the dynamics of the therapeutic relationship; and an active process of self-exploration and enquiry. The relevance of developing the skills of the reflective practitioner was discussed. Practice issues explored included: discussion of counselling settings; boundaries and ethics; assessment and referral; supervision and support; and consideration of how to manage the helping relationship. Case studies were offered to give an understanding of the relevance of the theory and practice of counselling in studying health and social care.

Place, neighbourhood and health drew upon the wide ranging literature on neighbourhood in order to provide the reader with an understanding of place poverty and neighbourhood effects, and how this shapes the prevalence of, and responses to, social problems. The chapter argued for the need to adopt a holistic understanding of place and neighbourhood. The chapter provided a framework for evaluating the impact of place and neighbourhood upon the prevalence of health and social problems within specific localities, and explored contemporary policy approaches to measuring and mapping social problems. Overall, the aim of the chapter was to enable the reader to understand the factors that shape the quality of life and opportunities within different localities.

Health, housing and regeneration argued it is increasingly relevant to consider housing as a substantial element of public health and social welfare, and to integrate health aspects into strategies of sustainable housing construction and neighbourhood or urban planning. This chapter examined the relationship between health, housing and well-being to enable an understanding of how potential health impacts associated with the built environment can be addressed. The chapter explored the link between health and housing and considered ways in which potential threats to health might be addressed. The influence and operation of the housing systems and housing policy in enabling society to meet the basic need for shelter within a decent, affordable home for the maximum number of citizens was considered. The impact of a complex housing system, including the role of key players, was developed, and a beginning made to analyse their ability to interact to achieve healthful housing. Agencies operating within the built environment were considered and a range of issues or problems, themes and debates that arise were discussed. The appreciation of the nature and effectiveness of current national and local policies, and debate of current issues and challenges in managing the built environment, were developed. Finally, the chapter explored the potential to deliver better health and well-being through considering the wider health issues associated with place making, and delivering sustainable communities.

PART 3

Globalization and health and social care considered the contemporary context of health and social care. Globalization was defined and examined to explore how it is having an impact on communities and health and social care services. Flows, barriers, stretched social relations, interpenetration of cultures and the emergence of global infrastructures were discussed. The chapter concluded by examining the impact globalization has had and raising future questions of possible directions for this ongoing process.

Contemporary approaches to management and leadership introduced the concept of management and set out some key stages in its historical development and its expression in the field of health and social care. The chapter examined some of the criticisms that have been made of management theory and practice, and introduced some potential implications for the field of health and social care, which flow from the debates that these critiques have engendered. The notion of discourse, particularly in relation to the concept of managerialism was considered. It was argued that managerialism provides only an attenuated and restricting view of, and guide to, understanding management in the health and social care arena.

Evidence based practice in health and social care examined the knowledge, skills, understanding and the importance of evidence to improve practice. Barriers to implementation were identified and discussed.

Contemporary mental health care examined the history and philosophy of mental health, definitions, and models of care. The influence of debate around defining, models, labelling or diagnosing mental illness has given rise to 'care': a culture of empowerment and person centred care; consent and capacity as criteria driving decisions; learning to live with mental health disturbance rather than trying unsuccessfully to cure it; and bringing all the services together to make access easier and more consistent. The chapter concludes by proposing an 'integrated model of care' for 'positive practice'.

The practice of counselling explored ethics, principles, practice and skills of counselling relationships as an active process of reflective self-exploration.

Substance misuse argued behaviour linked to the use of both illegal and legal drugs is of growing concern across many areas of health and social care provision. This chapter considered the historical development of social policy and legislation linked to substance misuse, from a UK perspective. Biological, psychological and sociological concepts of 'addiction' were discussed, fitting these different perspectives into their historical context and effect on legislation. The range of illegal and legal substances used in contemporary society was discussed in terms of their effects, health risk and patterns of usage both at a cultural and individual level. The chapter concluded by considering substance misuse service provision in the UK along with a brief discussion of the physiological and psychological treatment options available to individuals presenting to such services.

Working with children considered the emergence of children's rights when working with children and young people. It looked at specific understanding of child development to contextualize and understand how and why people in health and social care can work with children and young people to help them express their views, to manage transitions and overcome difficulties. The chapter established a dialectic understanding of children and young people between children's 'rights' (with respect for children as individuals with rights) and 'paternalism' (knowing what is best for children). It reviews current approaches to child development and critically focuses on attachment, resilience, transition, communication and participation as critical and vital elements to working with children.

User involvement: user led approaches in adult care – who is in charge? examined the personalization agenda, drivers for user involvement, policy and legislation, and empowerment. The chapter also addressed the challenges to user involvement such as tensions, staff attitudes, professional agendas, blurred boundaries, service users' voice, benefits, representation and resources. The chapter concluded by considering 'user led organizations' and the role of empowering services, collective and democratic control, and professional judgement.

Young people and youth justice explored the involvement of children and young people in criminality and the ways in which the criminal justice authorities have responded to their activities both in the past and in the present. The chapter was compatible with but not uncritical of the contemporary youth justice system (Hopkins-Burke 2008). By commencing with a reflexive consideration of the involvement of young people in crime and considering some recent statistics, the chapter considered the problem of youthful criminality in an historical and theoretical context with societal attempts to discipline and educate children and young people in the interest of a myriad of groups. The chapter considered the development of a specific juvenile/youth justice system charged with intervention in the lives of young people, from the justice/punishment model to the welfare/treatment model and beyond into the more ambiguous recent territory of 'excluded tutelage' and 'reintegrative tutelage'.

The professionalization of the youth justice workforce discussed the evolution of the modern youth justice system and the elusive nature of professionalization of youth justice. The 'modernization' of this profession by government administrations was discussed before contextualizing youth justice training as justice versus welfare. The tensions of the modernization process with the rise of bureaucracy were contrasted with the feelings and assessment of service users and practitioners. The chapter continued by reflecting on the nature of youth justice and the lack of focus on the historical emergence of this area of health and social care. The development of youth justice training was located within the rise of New Labour's administration and the chapter considered the impact this has had on training and practice within youth justice.

It is hoped that you have enjoyed your journey through *Key Themes in Health and Social Care* and found rich and fertile ground to continue your study, theory and practice in this fascinating field of work. The future presents a range of challenges and potential barriers, which the committed and focused worker and student will make an active contribution to overcome to establish excellence in health and social care.

INDEX

Note: Page numbers followed by 'f' refer to
figures, followed by 'n' refer to notes,
and followed by 't' refer to tables.